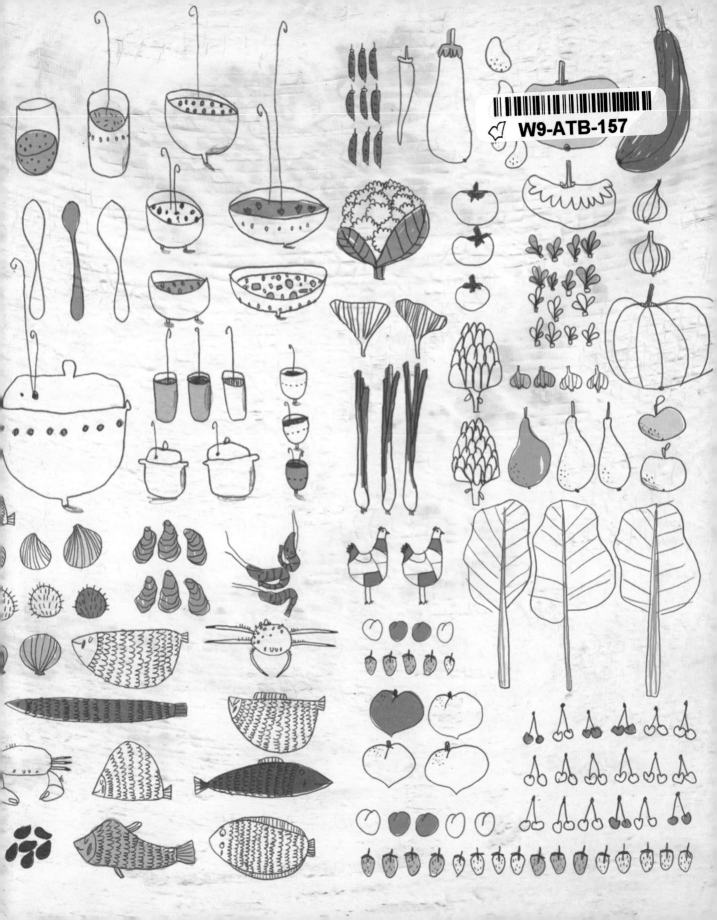

W9-ATB-157

"To Gwénaëlle, who shares my passion for this job, and to our son Arzhel."

First and foremost I must thank all our suppliers: the market gardeners, stockbreeders, fishermen, mushroom pickers, and more, who supply us with all these wonderful healthy products without which we cooks would not amount to much. They are the backbone of this book.

Then I am greatly indebted to **Paule Neyrat** for her prodigious work. She helped me choose the recipes and used her skill in adapting them for anyone to make. Her dual expertise as both cook and nutritionist has been invaluable to me.

I would also like to thank **Christophe Saintagne**, who labored all day, keeping this book going from start to finish, supporting the authors, photographer, designer, and editorial team.

Thanks to:

Françoise Nicol, whose bright and colorful photos are a delight;

Virginie Michelin, for her skillful presentation of the dishes;

Christine Roussey, whose illustrations lend this book its distinctive and imaginative charm;

Pierre Tachon, whose choices as artistic director and designer have brought life and energy to this book.

And of course, thanks to the whole editorial team:

Emmanuel Jirou-Najou, our director of publishing, and **Hortense Jablonski**, our editor.

I owe them all my gratitude for their remarkable work and for the help they have given me in the production of this book, which means such a lot to me.

And I would also like to thank the friends who agreed to come with me on the photo shoots:

At La Bastide de Moustiers: **Jean-François**, **Sandrine** and **Juliette**, **Patrick** and **Isabelle**, **Sébastien** and **Christine**;

At the École de Cuisine Alain Ducasse in Paris: **Béatrice**, **Géraldine**, **Gwénaëlle**, **Gilles**, and **Quentin**.

And last but not least, I would like to thank:

Laetitia Elmaleh, **Romain Corbière**, and all the team at the École de Cuisine Alain Ducasse for making us welcome when photographing the recipes;

Sarah Chailan, **Wilfrid Hocquet**, **Aurélien Stoop**, **Gilles Fraioli**, and all the team at La Bastide de Moustiers for their welcome during the photo shoot around Moustiers. Not forgetting **Gilbert Bonhomme**, the inn's gardener, thanks to whom so many succulent vegetables are served in the restaurant.

The chefs of all the establishments of ALAIN DUCASSE Entreprise across the world, who are the inspiration behind the recipes;

Emmanuelle Perrier, **Alice Vasseur**, **Laetitia Teil**, and **Olivier Guénot**.

And a special mention goes to:

Mustapha Messaoudi, who carves all the mortars that we use in our restaurants and at the École de cuisine Alain Ducasse;

Jean-Louis Nicolaï, market gardener at the market in Aups.

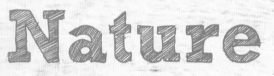

Nature

PHOTOGRAPHY
Françoise Nicol

STYLING
Virginie Michelin

ILLUSTRATIONS
Christine Roussey

ART DIRECTION
Pierre Tachon

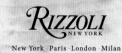

Rizzoli
NEW YORK

New York · Paris · London · Milan

Simple, healthy, and good

Paule Neyrat

Alain Ducasse

Christophe Saintagne

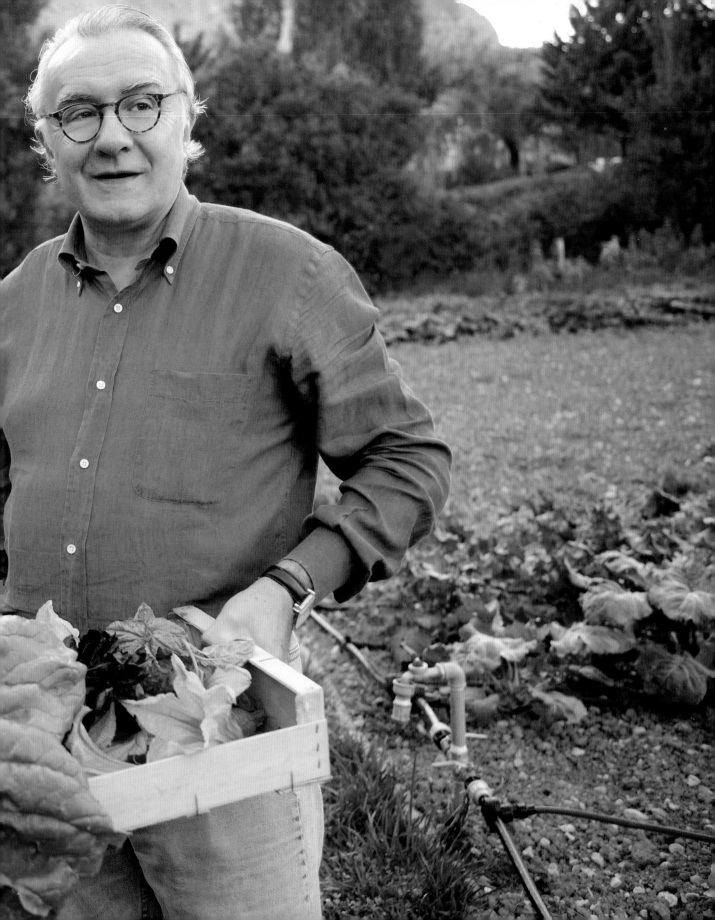

Paule Neyrat— I've always felt that you would never be able to lead the insane life you do, traveling all over the world, if you weren't eating food that was "simple, healthy, and good"!

Alain Ducasse— I was brought up on a farm in the Landes, eating the produce of the farm and garden three times a day. It was something of a paradise on earth and it formed my eating habits and my sense of taste.

PN— That's why we tend to have a pot of Piment d'Espelette on hand when we're cooking your recipes. (If you can't find it, hot paprika makes a good substitute.) But one of your first jobs as a cook was with Michel Guérard, the high priest of light cuisine!

AD— And two years later I was working with Roger Vergé at Mougins, where I fell in love with Provençal cuisine, and where I put down my Mediterranean roots.

AD— I know, you've no need to lecture me! Plenty of fruit and vegetables, raw and cooked, grains, preferably whole grains, a little meat or fish, and all cooked in olive oil. That's the basis of my cuisine and of the recipes in this book.

PN— Without realizing it at the time, you were already observing the famous Mediterranean diet, which became recognized in the '60s and '70s for its usefulness in combating cardiovascular diseases and many cancers.

PN— With a dash of wine, too! And you're forgetting dried fruit, which also features in the book; there's even a dried fruit condiment! It's not hard to make either, and neither are the other recipes, I've made sure of that.

PN— And you'll put on weight too! These recipes call for only one or two spoonfuls of olive oil, or even a splash or just a drop. I've taken great care over this, even though it's not a diet book.

AD— You can't cook well without good ingredients. If you don't treat the ingredient and its flavors with respect, if you drown it in oil for instance, even olive oil, you'll spoil it.

AD— Cooking is a love affair. It's all about falling in love with your ingredients.

PN— And enjoying the process without getting stressed. So I've simplified your recipes quite a bit, and made sure they are well balanced!

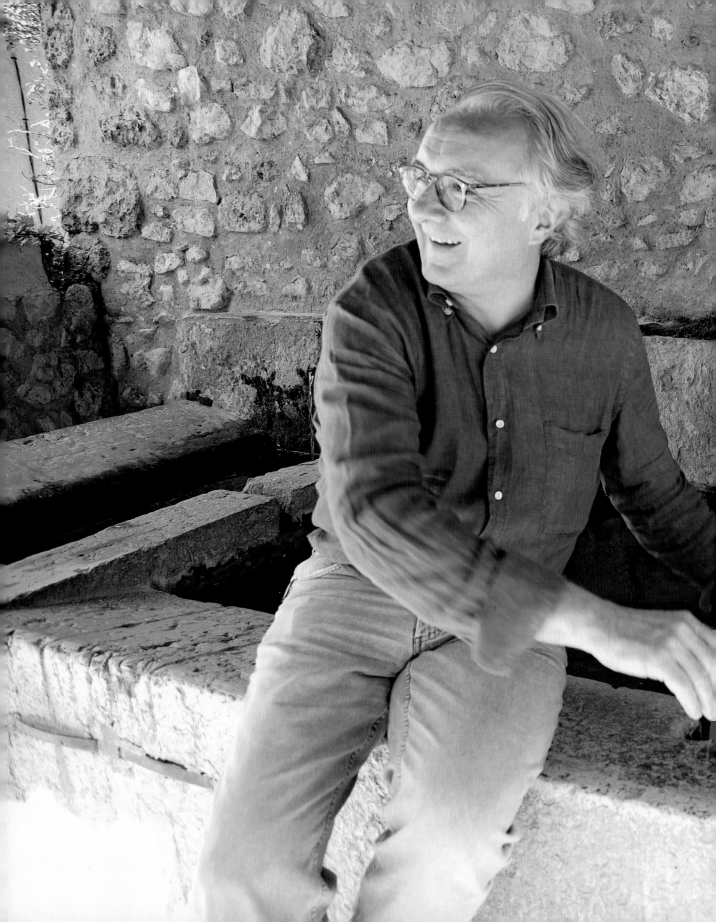

Contents

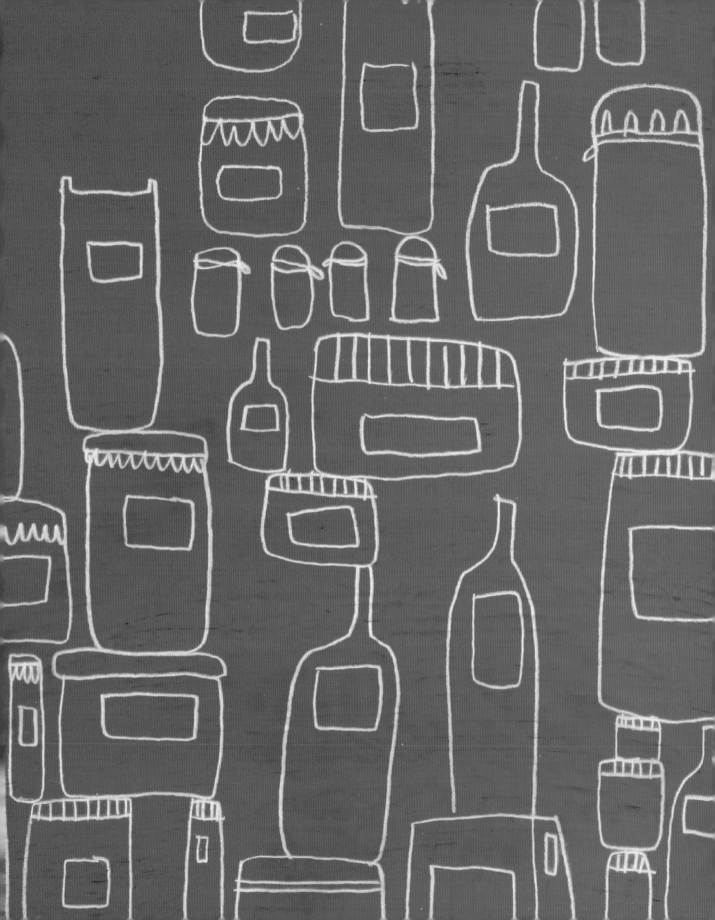

AD— You can of course find almost all these products in large supermarkets or on the Internet. But as I use them so much, I like to always have them at home.

PN— If you make these recipes yourself, they're bound to be healthier and tastier. Not to mention the pleasure of having them always on hand and being able to say: "I made this myself" . . .

Staples

Chicken Stock

AD— Ask your butcher for chicken carcasses. Otherwise, buy chicken giblets. Also, keep any leftover stock from when you make a blanquette (page 315) or pot-au-feu (page 305). PN— Lots of recipes call for chicken stock. You can of course buy various brands in cube or powder form. But the one you're going to make here will be a lot healthier, contain less salt and no additives, and have a more delicate flavor.

…Makes approximately 1½ quarts

…Cut 2¼ pounds of chicken carcasses into large pieces.

…Place them in a cooking pot, cover well with water, and bring to a boil. Skim off all the impurities that form on the surface.

…Meanwhile, peel and quarter 1 onion. Trim and wash 1 small leek, 1 carrot, and half a rib of celery and cut into large chunks.

…When the stock is clear, add the vegetables, 1 bay leaf, 1 sprig of thyme, 3 sprigs of parsley, 10 white peppercorns, and 1 teaspoon of coarse salt.

…Bring back to a boil, then lower the heat and simmer gently for a good 2 hours, skimming the surface from time to time.

…Take out the pieces of chicken and the vegetables with a slotted spoon.

…Strain the chicken stock through a chinois (a fine-mesh conical strainer) or a sieve lined with fine cheesecloth.

…Cool, then refrigerate for several hours to allow the fat to rise to the surface. Then remove the fat.

…Divide the stock into small containers and freeze. You can then thaw them in the microwave as and when you need them.

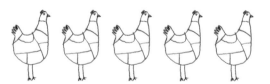

French Shortcrust Pastry–Pâte Brisée

… Makes approximately 1⅓ pounds

… Gather 2½ tablespoons of butter, 3 cups of pastry flour, ¾ cup of potato starch flour, ¾ teaspoon of salt, 2 teaspoons of superfine sugar, 2 eggs, and ½ cup of water or white wine and set aside.

If you are using a food processor

… Put the pastry flour, potato starch flour, salt, sugar, and butter cut into small pieces into the food processor bowl.

… Process for 10 seconds at a medium speed until you have a sandlike consistency.

… Add the eggs and water or white wine and mix. Stop the processor as soon as a dough is formed.

… Remove and shape into a ball.

If you are making it by hand

… Cut the butter into small pieces on a plate and crush with a fork to soften.

… Sift the pastry flour and potato starch flour together, on the worktop. Add the salt and sugar, fold together, and make a well in the center.

… Put in the butter and rub gently into the flour with your fingertips. Then add the eggs and mix, adding the water or white wine little by little until you have a smooth dough.

… Stop working it as soon as a dough is formed, and shape into a ball.

To finish

… Press down on the ball to flatten it slightly. Wrap in plastic wrap and leave to rest in the refrigerator, or freeze for later use. The pastry will keep, tightly wrapped, for three days in the refrigerator or for several months in the freezer.

AD— For a savory tart, use white wine, and for a sweet one, water. PN— Whether you are using a food processor or making it by hand, this French shortcrust pastry doesn't take long to make. It's low in fat and is far better than prepared pastry.

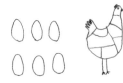

Garlic Confit

AD— When you've used up all the garlic cloves, you can keep the flavored oil for cooking meat or vegetables. The low cooking temperature does not affect its nutritional qualities.

PN— This garlic confit certainly won't leave you with bad breath! So you can use it frequently in vegetable dishes, salads, or gravies. A good way to enjoy the many health benefits of garlic.

… Makes 1 jar

… Separate the cloves from 3 heads of garlic, removing any that are really too small (keep them for a salad or another recipe).

… Remove only the thick outer skin of each garlic clove, then put them in a saucepan.

… Add 2 sprigs of thyme, 2 sprigs of rosemary, 15 black peppercorns, and 1½ teaspoons of coarse salt.

… Barely cover with olive oil.

… Put the pan over very low heat; the oil should tremble gently just under a simmer, and certainly not boil.

… Leave the garlic to cook like this for 45 minutes to an hour.

… Remove the pan from the heat and allow to cool.

… Transfer the garlic cloves and their aromatics into a jar. Cover with the oil you cooked them in.

… Put on the lid and keep tightly closed.

… Take out the cloves with a small spoon as and when you need them, and close the lid tightly. Stored in the refrigerator and well sealed, the garlic confit will keep for several months.

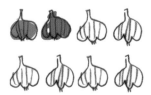

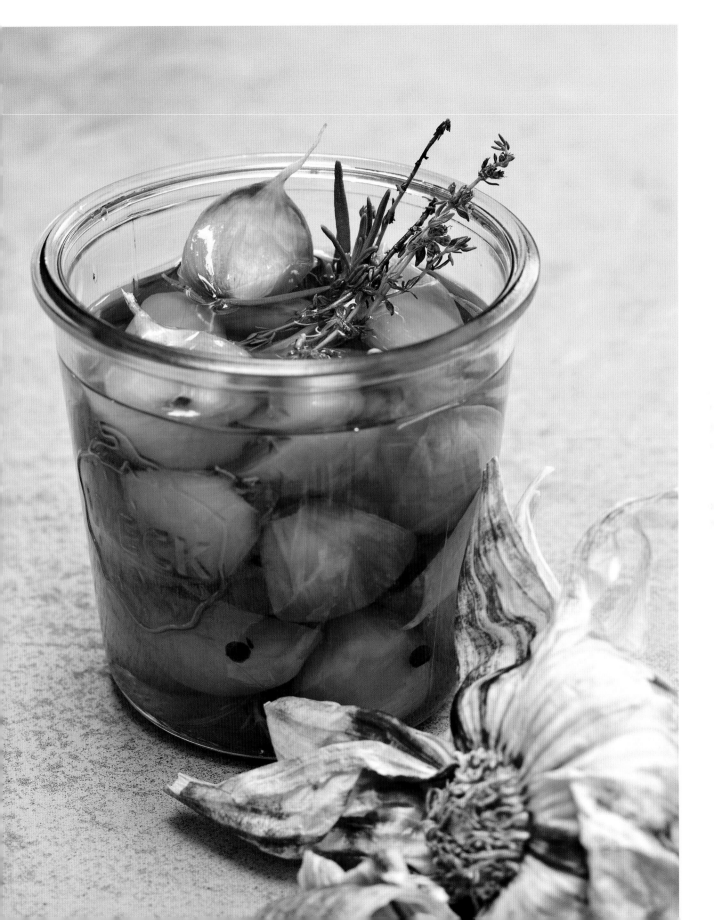

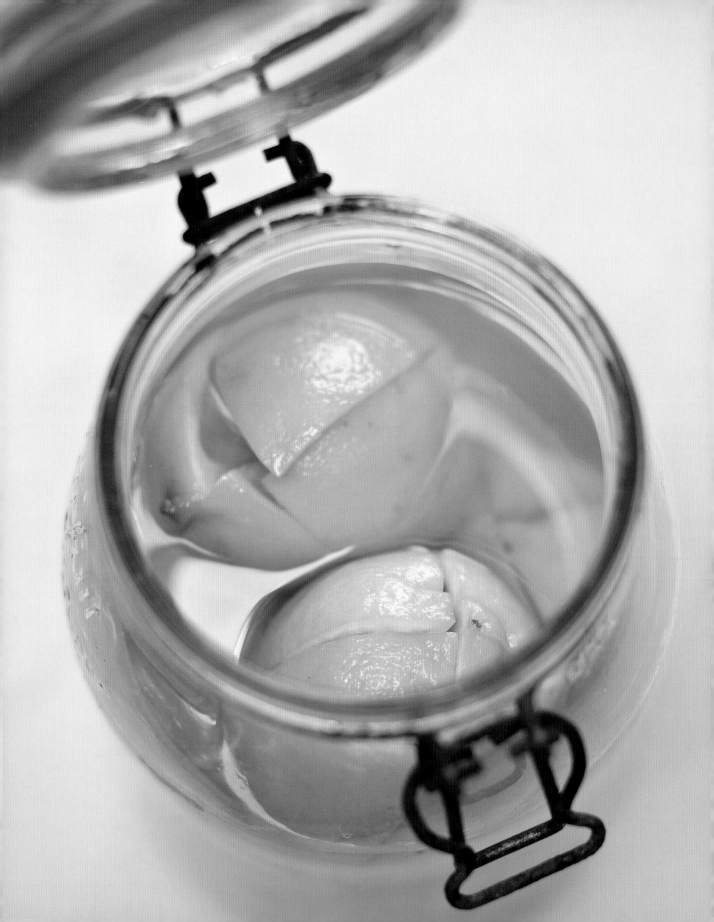

Salt-Preserved Lemons

… Makes 1 large jar

… Make the syrup: heat 2 quarts of water with 4½ cups of superfine sugar in a large saucepan, bring to a boil, then remove from the heat and allow to cool.

… Mix ¾ cup salt with 1 cup superfine sugar.

… Wash 12 yellow unwaxed lemons. Slit into quarters vertically from one end, without separating the pieces, leaving them attached at the other end.

… Gently open out these quarters. Place a generous pinch of the salt and sugar mixture inside each one and close the fruit back up.

… Place the lemons stuffed with salt and sugar in a sterilized jar as you go along, keeping them upright and tightly packed together with the opening at the top (so that the salt doesn't fall to the bottom).

… Pour the rest of the salt and sugar mixture into the jar, then top up with the syrup to cover.

… Put a weight on top of the lemons to prevent them from floating up and seal the jar airtight.

… Store in the refrigerator away from light for at least two months. The preserved lemons will keep for several months in the refrigerator.

AD— You can find salted lemons on the market, but they tend to be far too expensive and not necessarily that good, certainly not as good as these! PN— You can use the peel of salted lemons for a tagine or to spice up other slow-cooked dishes, adding a touch of sunshine, and the lemon pulp to dress salads without piling on the calories.

Tomato Confit

AD— When you use these preserved tomatoes, drain the oil from them thoroughly. You can use this fragrant oil later in your cooking or for dressings.

PN— These preserved tomatoes are particularly rich in antioxidants. Use them liberally in salads, pasta, rice, or vegetables, to add piquancy to the flavor.

… Makes approximately 1 pound

… Blanch 2¼ pounds of ripe vine or plum tomatoes. Quarter them and remove the seeds. Peel 3 garlic cloves.

… Preheat the oven to 215°F.

… Put the tomato quarters in a large bowl. Sprinkle with ¼ cup of olive oil and a little salt. Mix gently with your hands until the tomatoes are well coated and seasoned.

… Cut 1 garlic clove in half and rub the baking sheet with it, sprinkle the leaves from 4 sprigs of thyme (5 sprigs required in total for recipe) over it, then spread out the tomato quarters so that they don't touch one another. Pour all the juice remaining in the bowl over the tomatoes.

… Put the sheet in the oven and keep the door slightly open, wedging it with a spoon, to let in a light breath of air.

… Cook for 2 to 3 hours, checking from time to time. Turn over any tomatoes that are dry on the top and too moist underneath and gradually take out those that are cooked.

… Allow to cool. Put in a plastic container or jar and cover with olive oil. Add 2 thinly sliced garlic cloves and a sprig of thyme to flavor your oil.

… Store in the refrigerator. The tomato confit will keep, chilled, for up to two weeks.

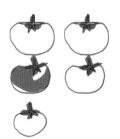

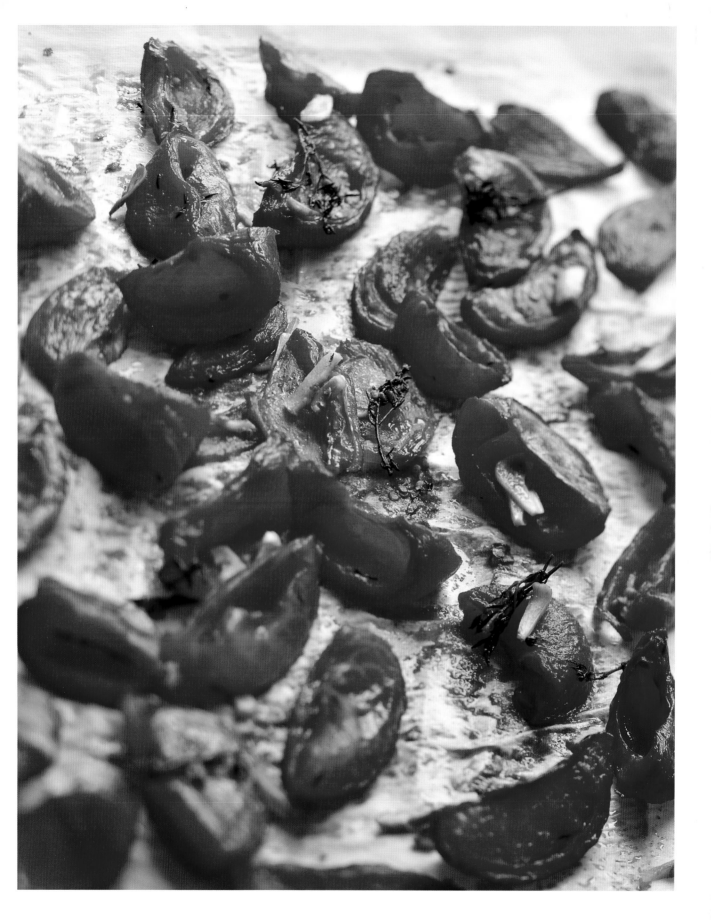

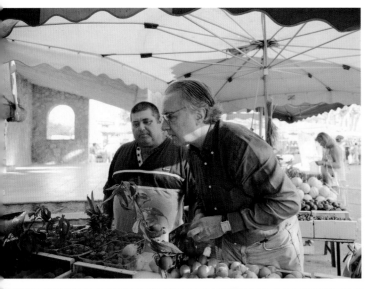
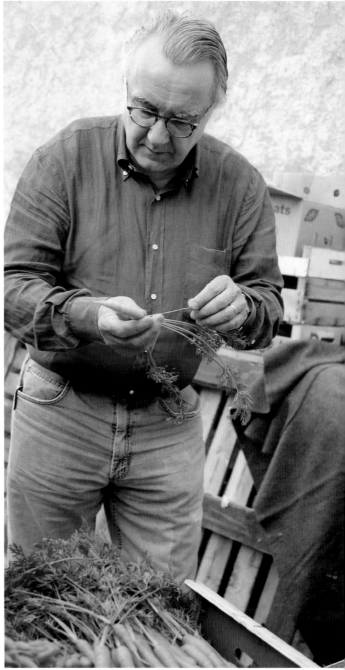
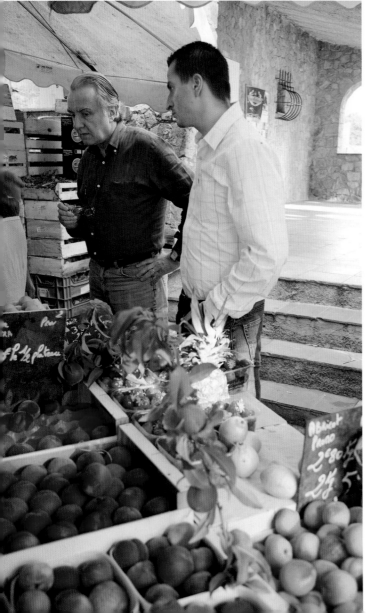

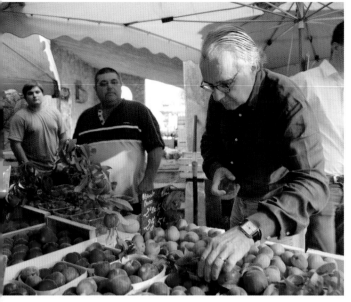
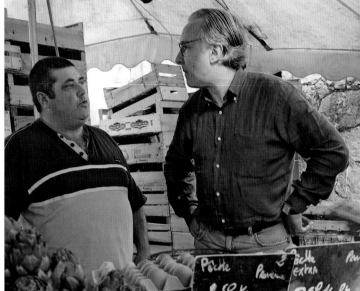
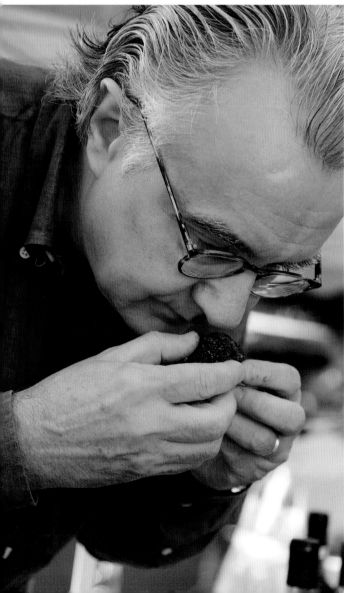
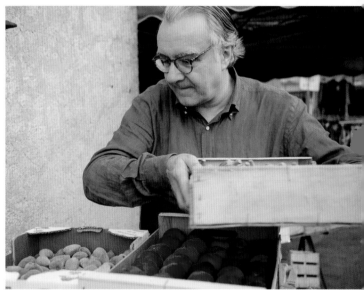
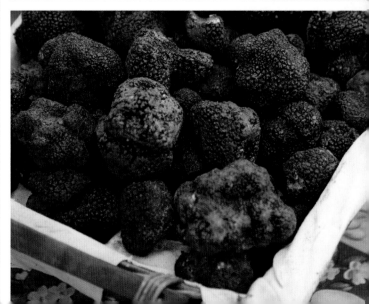

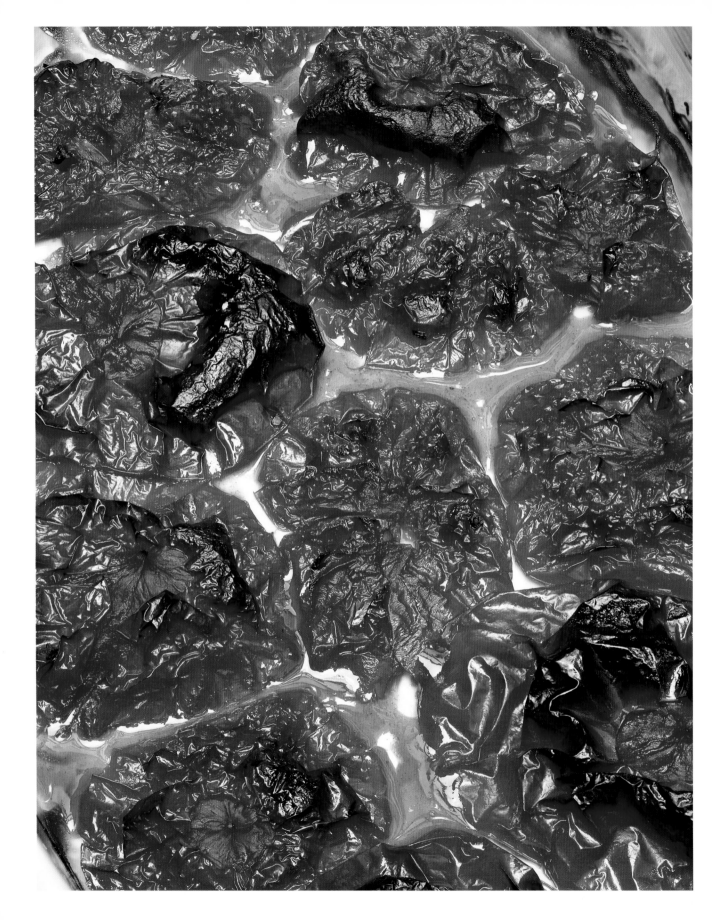

Chopped Cooked Tomatoes

… Makes approximately 1 pound

… Preheat your oven to 325°F.

… Wash 8 large ripe tomatoes, cut out any hard base around the stems, and cut in half widthwise.

… Squeeze their juice into a bowl and set aside.

… Sprinkle a pinch of salt and 2 pinches of superfine sugar on a baking sheet, then arrange the tomatoes in rows, skin side up, close together but not overlapping.

… Cover with parchment paper, held down with 2 spoons so that it doesn't move, and put in the oven for 1 hour.

… Take the sheet out of the oven, take off the parchment paper, then take off the tomato skins. Strain the reserved tomato juice and pour it over the tomatoes.

… Return the sheet to the oven and continue to cook (uncovered) for approximately 1 hour, until the edges of the sheet begin to caramelize.

… Continue to cook for an additional 5 minutes, scraping the juices two or three times and returning the sheet to the oven each time.

… Transfer the tomatoes to a plastic container and keep in the refrigerator or freeze. The tomatoes will keep one week in the refrigerator or for several months if frozen.

… If you are going to use them right away, add 2 tablespoons of olive oil to add flavor and a glossy sheen.

AD— These chopped cooked tomatoes come in very handy, not only for the recipes in this book but for any pasta, risotto, or vegetable dish. Make large quantities in the summer when tomatoes are cheap, then freeze them.

PN— As well as being delicious when nice and ripe and in season, the tomato is well known for its health benefits, as it contains lots of antioxidants: carotenoids, vitamin C, vitamin E, polyphenols, and lycopene. Lycopene becomes even more active when the tomatoes are cooked, making this preparation particularly valuable.

My Ketchup

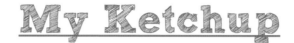

AD— *If you prefer a hot spicy ketchup, remove only one of the chiles.*
PN— *Do we need to tell you that this ketchup is far healthier than commercial versions? So it's a whole lot better for children, who are crazy about it. In winter you can make it with canned chopped tomatoes.*

… Makes approximately 7 ounces

… Blanch and seed 3 ripe tomatoes, carefully removing their juice and chopping them.

… Peel and thinly slice 1 inch of ginger and half a stem of lemongrass.

… Put 3 tablespoons of superfine sugar in a saucepan and heat until it turns a light amber caramel. Then add the tomatoes and stir well.

… Cook for 2 to 3 minutes.

… Then add the ginger, lemongrass, 1 teaspoon of Chinese five-spice powder, 2 tablespoons of sherry vinegar, 2 teaspoons of honey, and 2 whole hot chiles (such as bird's eye chile). Allow to simmer for 15 minutes, stirring frequently.

… Take out the chiles, then blend the mixture until nice and smooth.

… Then strain your ketchup in a fine conical strainer and store, refrigerated, in a plastic bottle (or carefully clean and reuse an old ketchup bottle). The ketchup will keep for one week in the refrigerator.

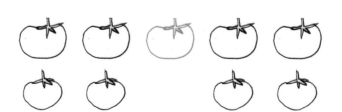

With Jean-Louis at the Aups market.

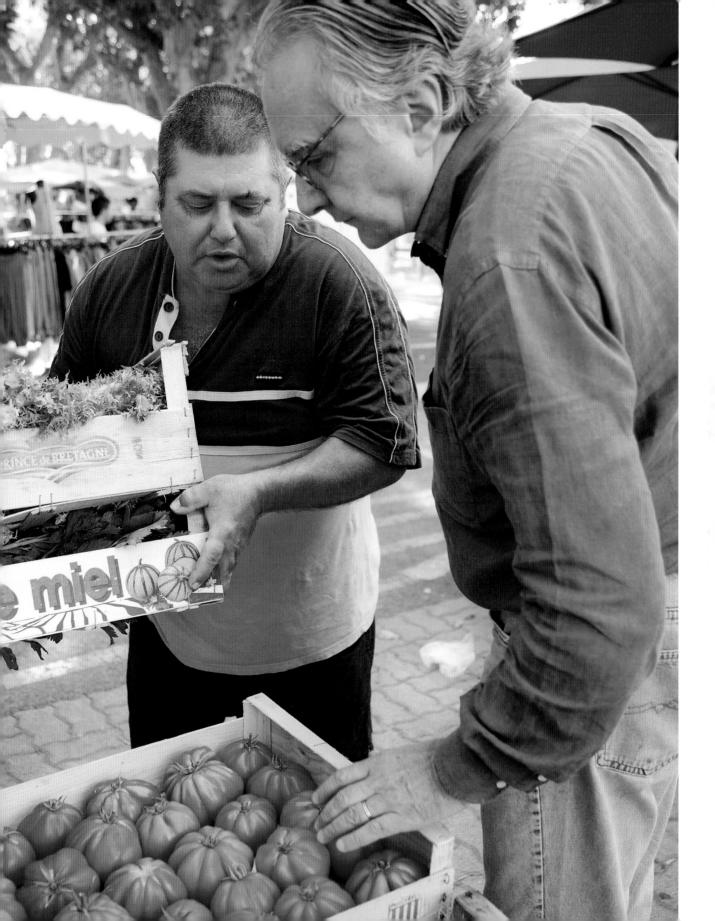

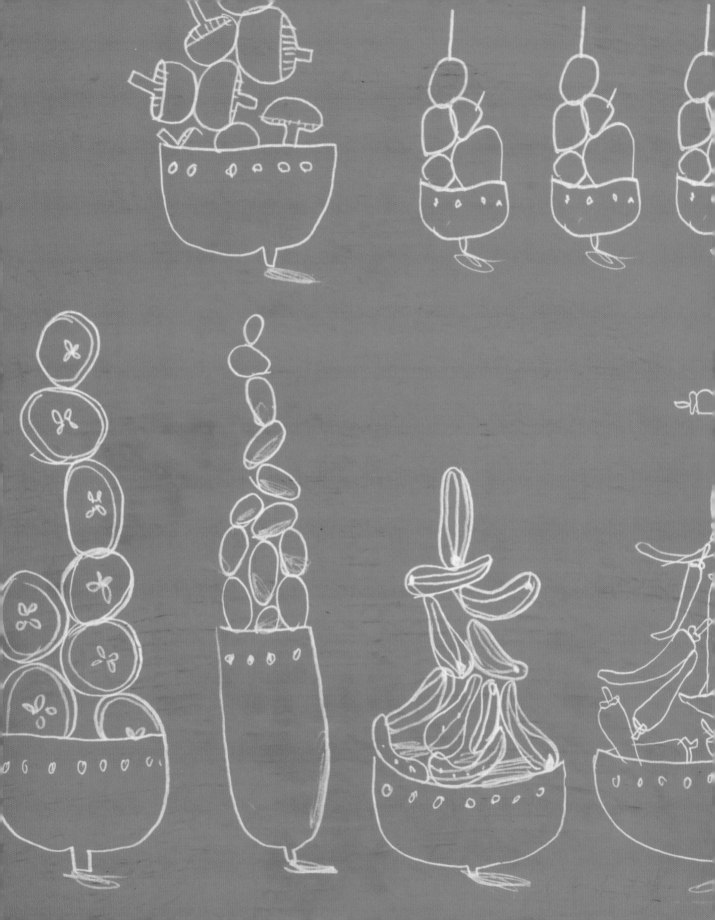

PN— Use as an accompaniment and to spice up simply steamed or poached vegetables, grilled meat, or fish. All these condiments are "light" and packed full of beneficial nutritional elements.

AD— Or use them as a topping for crostini when friends pop round for an aperitif, or on larger slices of toast for a simple supper. They're all quick to make and there's a wide variety to inspire you.

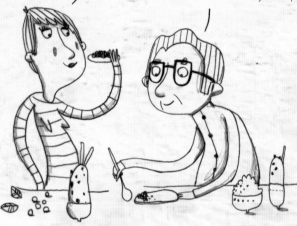

Condiments

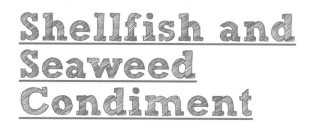

Shellfish and Seaweed Condiment

AD— Don't add any salt to this condiment; the seaweed and shellfish will take care of that.
PN— This condiment provides plenty of iodine, minerals, and trace elements of all different kinds! Whelks are packed with them, as are oysters and seaweed.

… Serves 4

… Wash and brush 1 medium Yukon gold potato and boil in salted water without peeling.

… Peel and mince 1 shallot, put it in a saucepan, add ¼ cup of red wine vinegar, put over low heat, and cook until completely reduced.

… Meanwhile, remove the shells of 10 ounces of cooked whelks (or small clams) and open 4 oysters over a bowl to catch their water. Rinse ¼ cup of seaweed to get rid of the salt. Then thinly slice the whelks, oysters, and seaweed.

… Peel the potato and put it in a mortar with 1 egg yolk.

… Crush, gradually adding 3 tablespoons of olive oil and the oyster water. When you have a nice smooth paste, add the oysters, whelks, seaweed, and the shallot in vinegar.

… Stir well. Add freshly ground black pepper and 2 teaspoons of sesame seeds, mix, and store in the refrigerator.

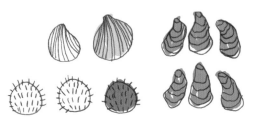

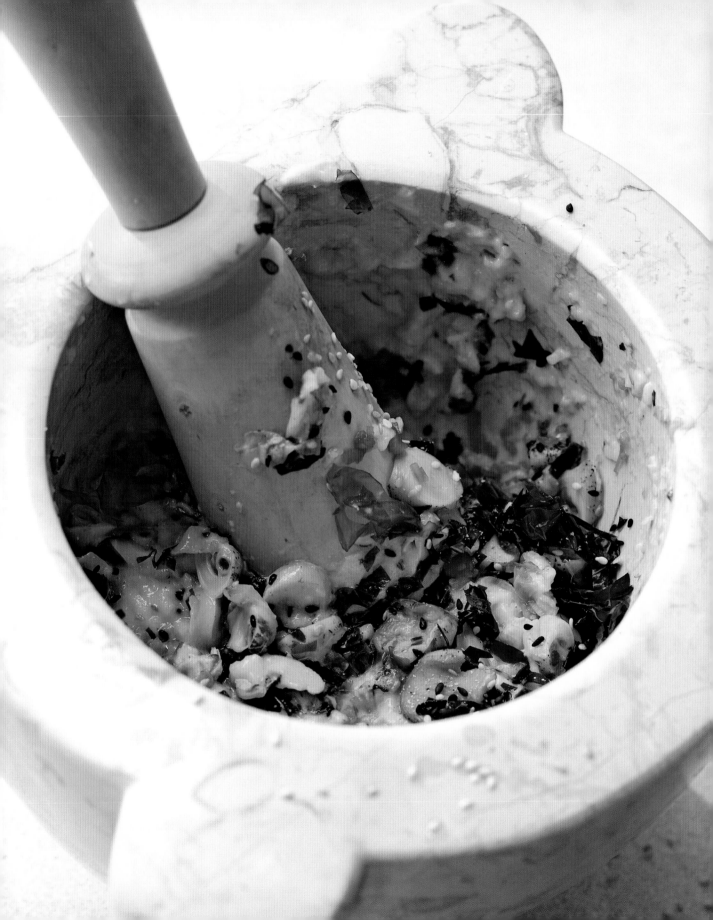

Guacamole

*AD— Choose ripe avocados.
To remove the pit, stick a fork
into it and twist.
PN— This is an excellent source of
oleic acid, a fatty acid that helps
lower cholesterol and is good for
the heart. Olive oil is bursting with
it, and avocados contain quite a
lot too. With the antioxidants from
the tomato and onions, and the
vitamin C from the lemon, this
guacamole is a genuine health food,
and it takes just a few minutes
to prepare.*

———

*Piment d'Espelette is a seasoning
from the Basque region of Spain;
hot paprika may be substituted if
Piment d'Esplette cannot be found.*

… Serves 4

… Blanch and seed 1 small tomato and finely dice the flesh.

… Peel 3 pearl onions and dice similarly.

… Halve 2 avocados and remove the pits.

… Remove all the flesh with a small spoon and crush with a fork.

… Mix it with the tomato and onions, 1 teaspoon of Piment d'Espelette or
hot paprika, and the juice of 1 lime.

… Then pour in 2 tablespoons of olive oil, stirring vigorously. Add salt and
freshly ground black pepper.

… Store in the refrigerator.

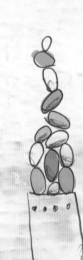

Asparagus-Tabasco Condiment

… Serves 6

… Peel and wash 15 small green asparagus spears. Cut the tips into 1½-inch lengths and set aside.

… Thinly slice the stalks. Heat 1 tablespoon of olive oil in a sauté pan and add the sliced asparagus, salt lightly, and sauté over medium heat for 3 minutes without browning.

… Add ¾ cup of chicken stock (page 10) or water, and cook for an additional 5 minutes.

… Blend and add 3 tablespoons of olive oil until you have a nice smooth puree. Empty into a bowl.

… Thinly slice the asparagus tips, finely chop 3 tarragon leaves, and add these.

… Season with 1 tablespoon of sherry vinegar, 1 teaspoon of Tabasco, salt, and freshly ground black pepper.

… Refrigerate until serving.

AD— I like this condiment to be quite hot, but if you prefer it less so, start with a few drops of Tabasco and adjust to your own taste.

PN— If your asparagus spears are thin, there's no point in peeling them. Just remove the white base. That way you will get even more fiber and vitamins.

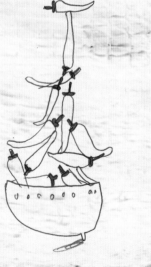

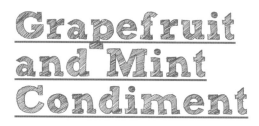

Grapefruit and Mint Condiment

AD— The grapefruit and pomelo are related fruits. The true pomelo is extremely bitter. For this condiment, I prefer pink grapefruits. The redder the flesh, the sweeter the juice.

PN— This condiment gives you a real boost because of its richness in vitamin C, which is plentiful in the grapefruit! The pinker the flesh, the richer the carotenoid content, which combines its antioxidant action with that of the vitamin C. An excellent cocktail for the skin and the arteries.

Mignonette pepper is a traditional French blend of white peppercorns, black peppercorns, coriander seeds, and herbs. It can be found in specialty shops and online, or coarsely ground white or black pepper may be substituted.

… Serves 4

… Preheat the oven to 200°F.

… Peel and remove the inner membrane of 5 pink grapefruits, then separate the segments over a bowl to catch the juice.

… Squeeze the remaining parts of each fruit in one hand to collect all the juice. Set aside in the refrigerator.

… Sprinkle a baking sheet with 3 pinches of superfine sugar and 1 pinch of salt, then add the grapefruit segments.

… Put the sheet in the oven and cook for 45 minutes.

… Shred 10 mint leaves.

… Remove the tray from the oven, add the grapefruit juice, mint, a good pinch of mignonette pepper, and 1 tablespoon of olive oil.

… Scrape with the back of a fork to thoroughly mix in all the caramelized parts.

… Taste and correct the seasoning.

… Store this grapefruit condiment in the refrigerator.

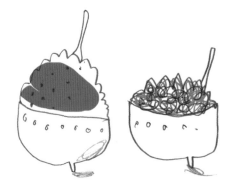

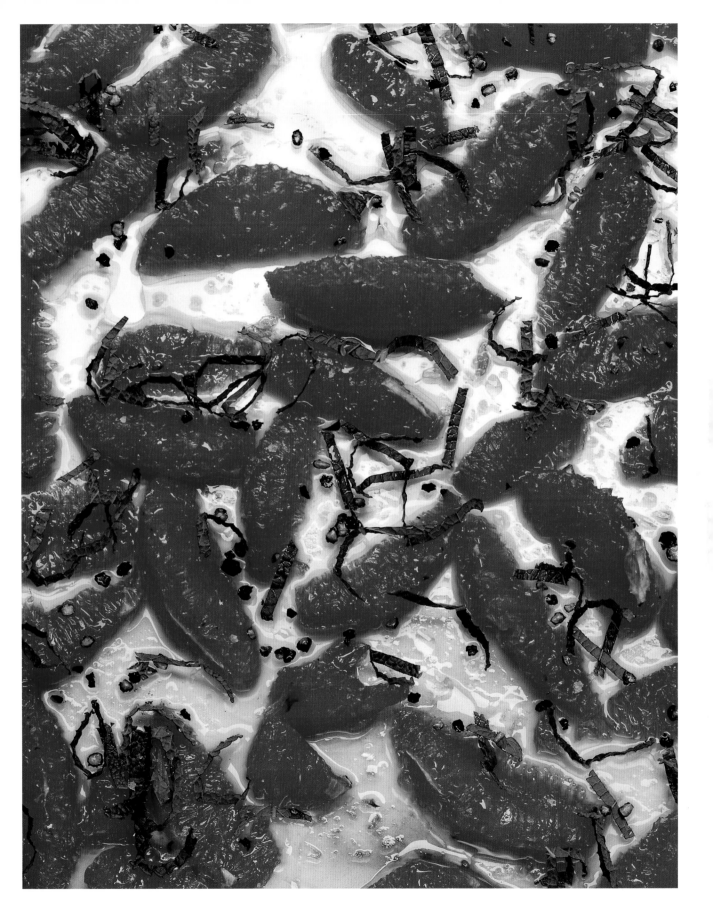

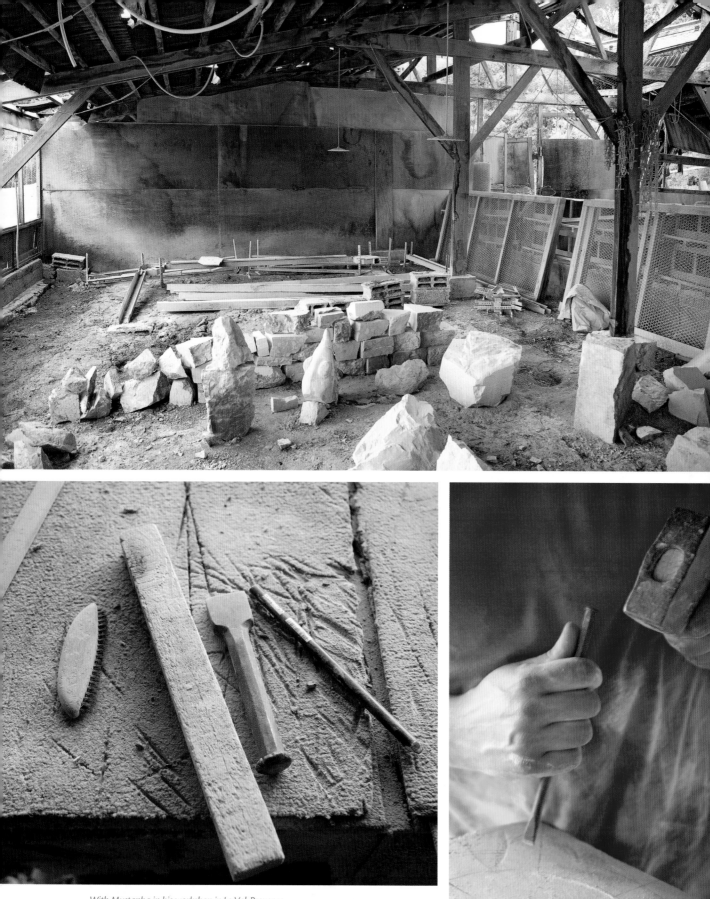

With Mustapha in his workshop in Le Val, Provence.

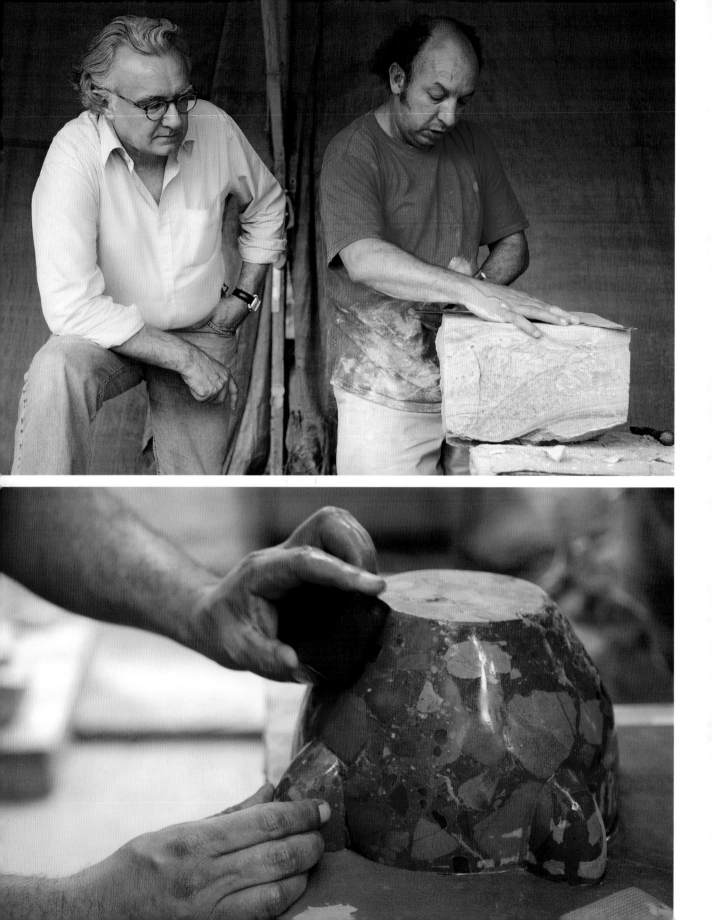

Creamy Garlic Condiment

AD— When fresh garlic is out of season, discard the sprout from inside the garlic cloves and immerse the cloves in salted boiling water for 30 seconds before blending.
PN— Garlic is amazingly rich nutritionally and is good for you in even small quantities. Eating garlic every day (1 or more cloves) helps lower cholesterol and blood pressure. It also has antimicrobial, anti-allergy, and antioxidant properties.

… Serves 4

… Peel 5 cloves of fresh garlic, chop them, and put in a blender.

… Add the whites of 3 eggs, the juice of 1 lemon, and 2 tablespoons of fromage blanc (fresh white cheese).

… Blend slowly, gradually adding 2 to 3 tablespoons of olive oil until you have a smooth cream.

… Add a little salt.

… Transfer to a bowl. Pour a thin film of olive oil over the surface to prevent oxidation. Cover the bowl with plastic wrap and refrigerate.

… Serve nice and cold.

Hummus

… Serves 4

The day before

… Soak 1 cup of dried chickpeas.

On the day

… Peel 1 onion and 1 carrot and put them in a saucepan with 1 bay leaf. Drain the chickpeas, add them to the pan, and cover well with water. Bring to a boil and cook for 1 hour 30 minutes and add salt only at the end of cooking.

… Peel 1 clove of garlic and cut it into 2 or 3 pieces.

… With a slotted spoon, drain the chickpeas and blend with the garlic and 1 or 2 ladles of the cooking water to obtain a nice smooth cream.

… Add the juice of half a lemon, 1 teaspoon of ground cumin, 1 teaspoon of ras al-hanout, 2 pinches of paprika, and 1 teaspoon of tahini (sesame paste) and blend a little more to incorporate well.

… Taste the hummus and check the seasoning.

… Store in the refrigerator.

AD— For an even more refined hummus, drain the chickpeas into a large bowl of water and ice cubes. This will help you remove the outer skins easily. And if you're short of time, you can always use canned chickpeas.

PN— Chickpeas are the most useful of the pulses, not only because they are high in carbohydrates, protein, and minerals, but also because they contain antioxidants, carotenoids, and vitamin E.

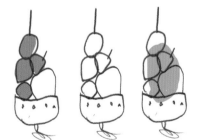

Light Pesto

AD— *If you have some garlic confit (page 12), use this: take 6 cloves of garlic confit and 1 fresh clove of garlic. The word* pesto *derives from the Italian* pestare, *"to crush or grind," because of its traditional method of preparation in a mortar before the existence of food processors.*

PN— *Basil is extremely rich in antioxidant carotenoids and minerals, and garlic is a true medicine. Antimicrobial, anti-allergy, and antioxidant, garlic strengthens the immune system. So use this light pesto without restraint!*

… Serves 4

… Peel 4 garlic cloves and cut them in half. Remove any small sprouts in the center.

… Immerse 3 of them in boiling water for 2 minutes, then drain in a colander and refresh under the tap.

… Remove the leaves from 2 bunches of basil. Grate ¾ ounce of fresh Parmesan.

… If you have a mortar, crush the cooked garlic cloves, the raw garlic clove, the Parmesan, ¼ cup of pine nuts, and the basil until the mixture is quite thick and pasty, then gradually pour in 6 tablespoons of water and 6 tablespoons of olive oil, stirring as you go.

… Otherwise, blend them all together in a blender.

… Adjust the seasoning by adding salt and freshly ground black pepper and keep in the fridge, as this light pesto should be served cold.

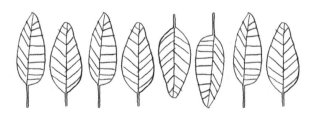

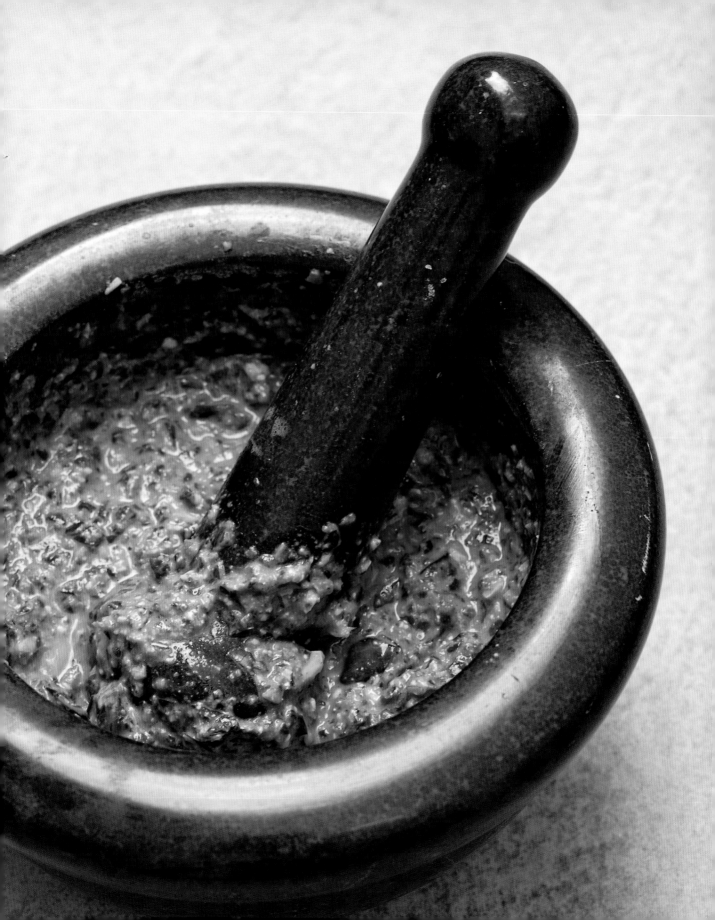

Baba Ghanoush

AD— Baba ghanoush (or baba ganoush) is the Arabic name for an eggplant dip. I've adapted it to my own taste by adding lots of herbs and goat's curd, which sweetens it. You can substitute a spoonful of fromage blanc for the goat's curd.

PN— Fresh herbs are particularly rich in minerals and vitamins. They make up for the lack of these properties in the eggplant, which is not much of a star in that respect.

Fresh curd can be found at specialty cheese shops or sourced online. Fromage blanc or cottage cheese may be substituted.

… Serves 4

… Preheat your oven to 425°F.

… Wash 2 medium eggplants, wipe dry, and prick here and there with a fork, then place them on a baking sheet.

… Bake in the oven for 1 hour, or until they are well browned and toasted.

… Take them out and allow to cool so as not to burn your fingers. Cut them in half lengthwise and remove the flesh with a small spoon and put it in a blender or a mortar.

… Also collect a little of the toasted skin: approximately 10 percent of the weight of the flesh (for example, for 3 ounces flesh, ⅓ ounce skin), and add it to the flesh.

… Crush the mixture in the mortar, or blend roughly to produce a nice compote rather than a liquefied puree. Transfer to a large bowl.

… Remove the stems, wash, and chop the leaves of 2 sprigs of marjoram, 2 sprigs of mint, 2 sprigs of cilantro, and 2 sprigs of flat-leaf parsley. Peel and crush 1 garlic clove.

… Stir into the eggplant mixture with a spoon. Add 1 tablespoon of fresh goat's curd and 2 tablespoons of olive oil. Season with salt and freshly ground black pepper and stir again.

… Keep the baba ghanoush in the fridge, as it should be served nice and cold.

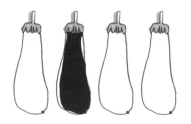

Anchoïade

… Serves 4

… Wash and peel a quarter of 1 fennel bulb, slice thinly with a mandoline, then chop these shavings finely with a knife.

… Peel and crush 2 cloves of garlic with a garlic press.

… Rinse 16 salted anchovy fillets under running water, pat dry, then chop roughly.

… Crush 1 rounded tablespoon of pitted black olives.

… In a bowl, mix the fennel with the garlic, anchovies, crushed olives, and 3 tablespoons of olive paste. Pour in ¼ cup of olive oil, then a splash of wine vinegar, stirring well with a small whisk.

… Taste your anchovy paste and adjust the seasoning with freshly ground black pepper; the flavor should be fairly salty.

… Then put in the fridge, as this anchoïade should be served nice and cold.

AD— I prefer the anchovies from Collioure, which are still salt-cured in the traditional way. They really are the best. Collioure holds the "site remarquable du gout" ("site of culinary excellence") award and its anchovies are protected by a PGI (Protected Geographical Indication) designation. They're guaranteed to have been fished in the Mediterranean.

PN— Omega-3s from the anchovies, oleic acid from the olive oil and olives—all this is good news for your arteries!

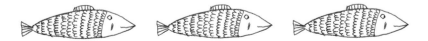

Tapenade

AD— I always prefer the black olives from Nice. Granted they're small and harder to pit, but they have an incomparable flavor. Tapenade is traditionally made in a mortar, so if you've got one, take the time to make it this way!

PN— Olive oil is the mainstay of the famous Mediterranean diet. It's rich in oleic acid, which helps lower bad cholesterol, as do olives, of course. But it also has a beneficial effect on intestinal transit and the gallbladder.

… Makes approximately 7 ounces

… Pit 5 ounces of black olives from Nice with a small knife.

… Peel half a garlic clove and if there is a central germ sprout, remove it.

… Rinse 1 salted anchovy fillet well under the tap and remove the bones.

… Roughly chop 5 basil leaves.

… In the bowl of the blender, combine the olives, garlic, anchovy, basil, and 1 tablespoon of capers.

… As you blend, gradually add 7 tablespoons of olive oil until you have a smooth but still slightly chunky paste.

… Store the tapenade in the refrigerator.

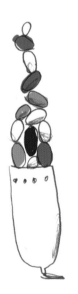

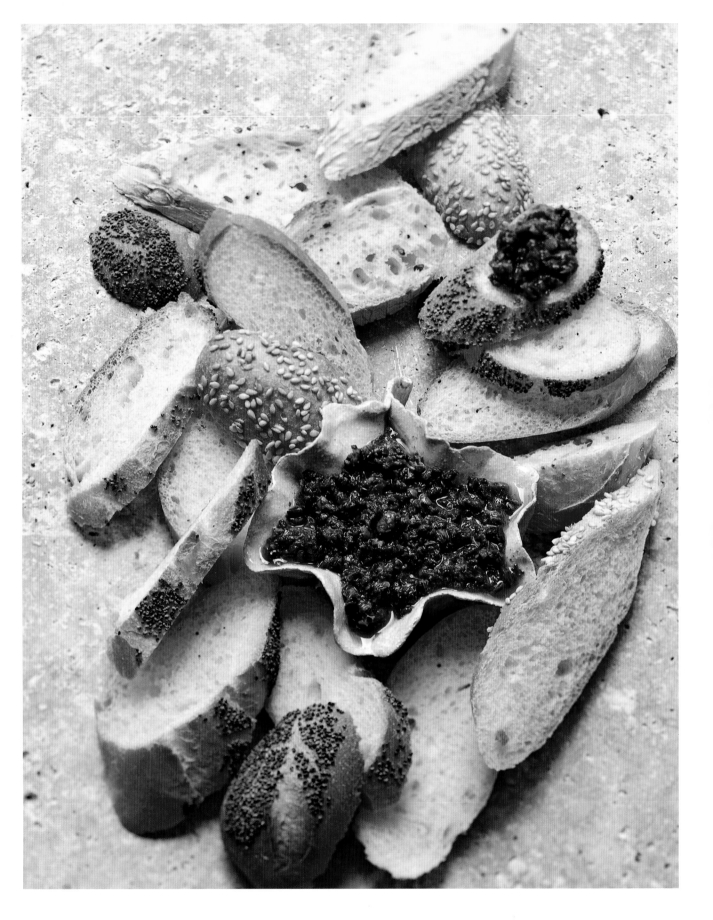

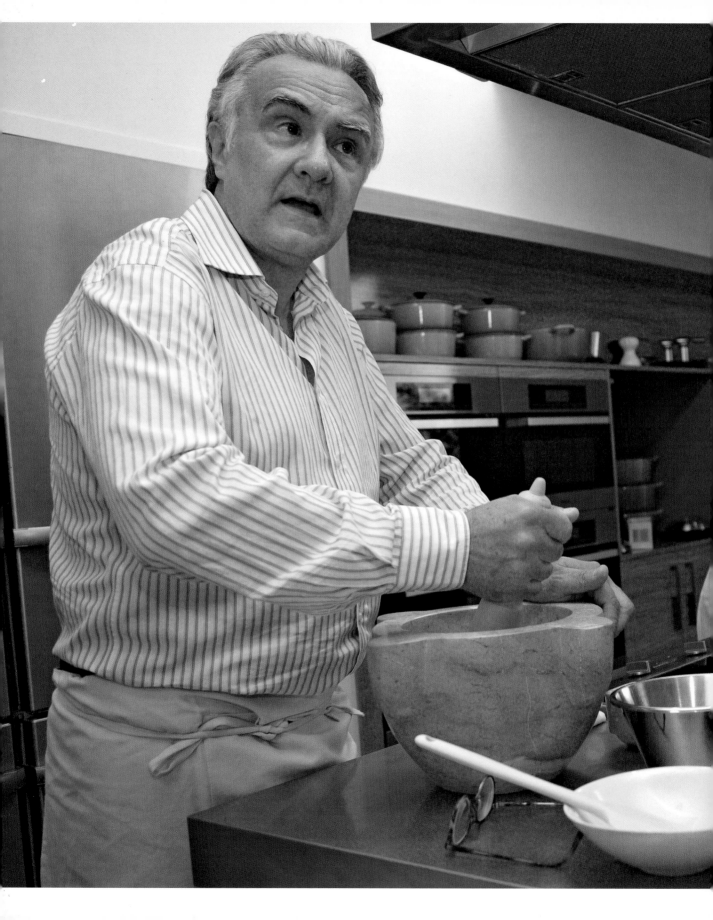

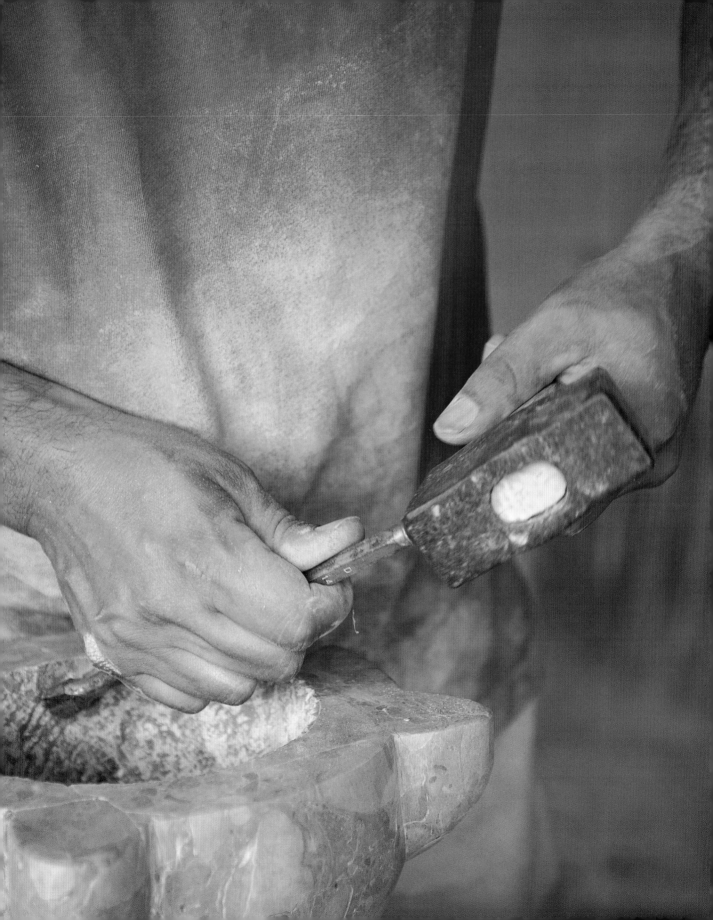

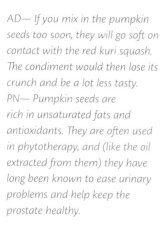
Pumpkin Seed Condiment

AD— If you mix in the pumpkin seeds too soon, they will go soft on contact with the red kuri squash. The condiment would then lose its crunch and be a lot less tasty.

PN— Pumpkin seeds are rich in unsaturated fats and antioxidants. They are often used in phytotherapy, and (like the oil extracted from them) they have long been known to ease urinary problems and help keep the prostate healthy.

… Makes approximately 10 ounces

… Peel 1 red kuri or hokkaido squash and cut into small cubes. Peel 2 garlic cloves.

… Steam them together (in a steamer, couscous pot, or a sieve placed over a saucepan of boiling water) until the squash is nice and soft.

… Then mash with a fork and add, mixing well as you go, 1 teaspoon of prepared mustard, 1 teaspoon of olive oil, and 3 tablespoons of grated Parmesan. Put in a bowl and set aside.

… In a hot skillet very lightly brushed with oil, slightly toast 6 tablespoons of hulled pumpkin seeds and season with salt and freshly ground black pepper.

… Transfer them to a paper towel, then crush them in a mortar or a blender.

… Rinse, dry, and chop the leaves from 3 sprigs of parsley. Set them to one side.

… Only add the pumpkin seeds and chopped parsley to the bowl of garlicky squash just before serving.

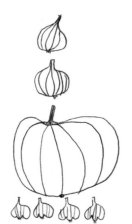

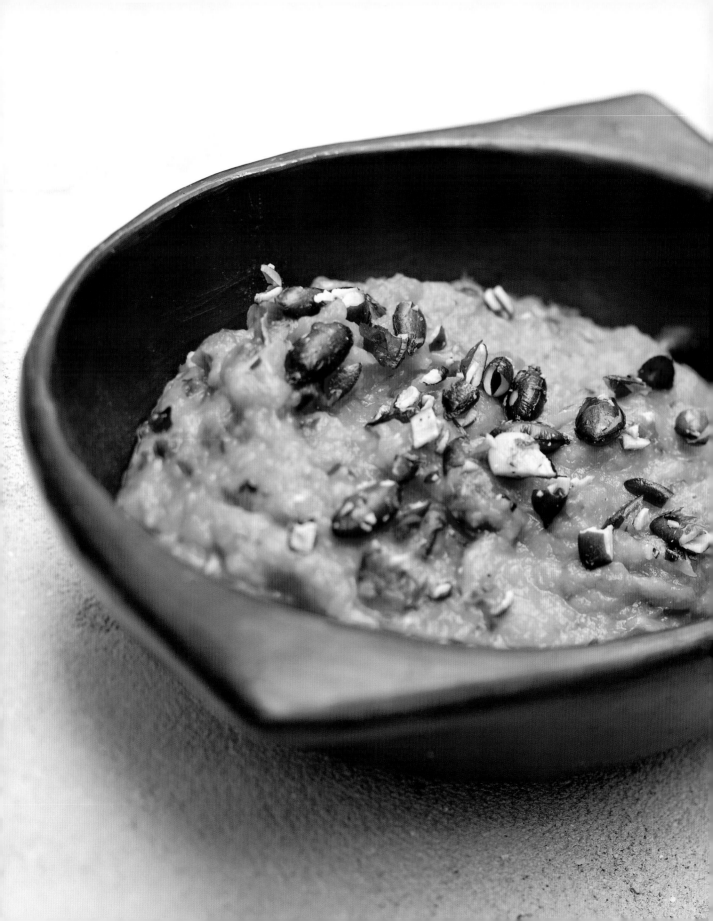

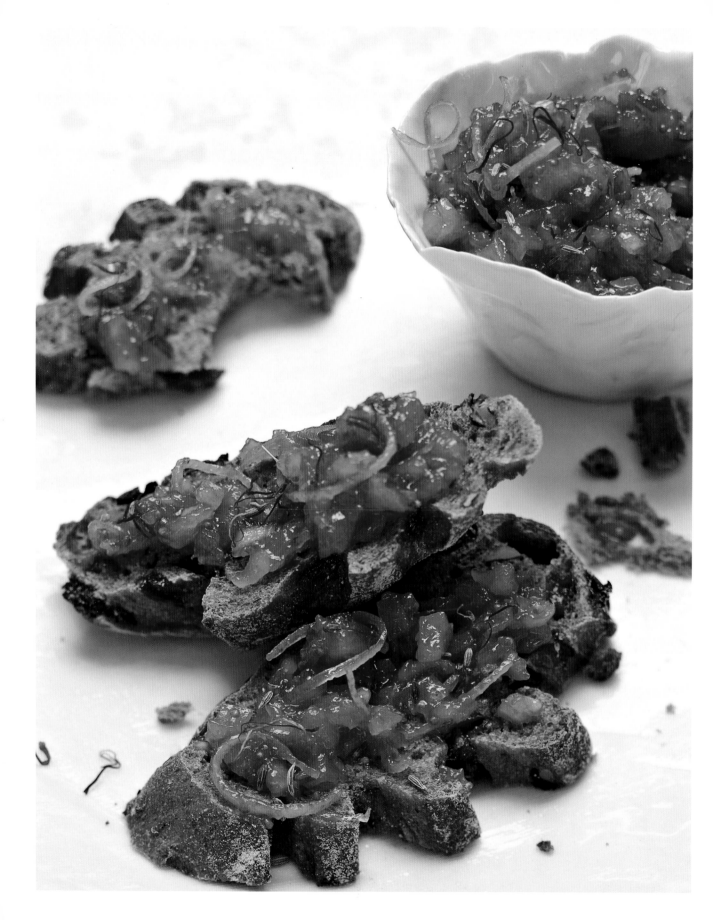

Dried Fruit Condiment

... Serves 4

... Chop 8 dried apricots, 8 dates, and 4 dried figs into tiny dice (brunoise).

... With a vegetable peeler, cut off the zest of 1 unwaxed orange (2 oranges required in total for recipe). Immerse the zest in boiling water for 2 minutes, drain in a sieve, and cool immediately under the tap. Cut into the finest possible slivers (julienne) and set aside.

... Squeeze the juice of the orange into a small saucepan and bring to a boil. Then add the dried fruit brunoise and stir. Take the saucepan off the heat and allow the mixture to swell for approximately 5 minutes.

... Pour 1 tablespoon of honey into a small sauté pan and heat until it takes on the appearance of a pale caramel.

... Squeeze the juice of a second orange and pour it onto the honey. Stir well and bring to a boil. Add the contents of the pan of dried fruit and simmer for 5 to 6 minutes.

... In the meantime, lightly crush 1 teaspoon of cumin seeds and set aside on a saucer.

... Add this at the end of cooking, along with 6 saffron threads, 5 tablespoons of white balsamic vinegar, and the julienne of orange zest. Mix and then transfer to a bowl. Cover with plastic wrap and set aside.

... This dried fruit condiment can be served warm or at room temperature.

AD— If you're making this condiment in advance, keep it in the fridge and pop it in the microwave for 10 seconds before serving.

PN— This condiment is packed with mineral salts. It's also rich in fiber and entirely fat free.

Gribiche Sauce

AD— Taste this sauce before you season with salt and pepper. There is no point in making it too salty. PN— The herbs are an excellent source of vitamins and minerals of all kinds, and the yogurt provides calcium and protein. This sauce goes particularly well with grilled meat or steamed vegetables.

…Hard boil 2 eggs (10 minutes). Cool them and remove the shells.

…Rinse, pat dry, and chop the leaves from a small bunch of flat-leaf parsley, a small bunch of tarragon, and a small bunch of chervil.

…Chop 1 tablespoon of capers and cut 5 gherkins into very thin rounds.

…Strain 1 cup fat-free yogurt through a very fine sieve into a large bowl.

…Mix in ½ tablespoon of prepared mustard, 3 tablespoons of wine vinegar, the chopped herbs, the chopped capers, the slices of gherkin, and ¼ cup of olive oil, stirring well.

…Place a cheese grater over the bowl and grate the hard-boiled eggs into the mixture. Stir in gently. Season to taste and store in the refrigerator.

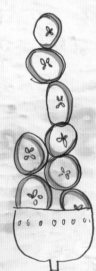

Cucumber and Apple Condiment

… Serves 4

… Peel 1 cucumber weighing about 10 ounces and cut into small cubes.

… Place them in a sieve, sprinkle generously with salt, and leave for 15 to 20 minutes.

… Peel and core 2 Granny Smith apples and cut into small cubes.

… Blanch and seed 2 tomatoes and cut into small dice.

… Rinse and pat dry a small bunch of cilantro and 10 chives. Cut the leaves from the cilantro, and chop both these herbs.

… Squeeze the juice of 2 lemons into a ramekin and mix into it 1 teaspoon of garam masala and 1 teaspoon of Piment d'Espelette or hot paprika.

… Combine all these ingredients in a large bowl with ½ cup of plain yogurt and mix gently.

… Check the salt seasoning and keep refrigerated before serving.

AD— Garam masala is a spice mixture (coriander, cumin, ginger, cinnamon, black pepper, nutmeg, oregano, cardamom, chiles, cloves, and bay leaf) originating in North India. It's fairly hot; garam means "hot" in Hindi. If you don't have any, substitute 2 pinches of curry powder.

PN— Cucumber is always easier to digest when it is sliced and sprinkled with salt before eating. But if you are able to digest it without problems, you can skip this step.

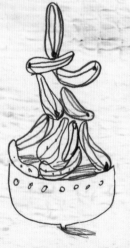

Tzatziki

AD— To dice the brunoise, lay each half cucumber flat on your cutting board. With a knife, cut lengthwise into small strips, then cut again widthwise.

PN— When salted, cucumber is easy to digest. This vegetable is not particularly rich in vitamins and minerals, but the mint and parsley contain plenty, and the yogurt provides calcium.

… Serves 4

… Rinse 1 cucumber weighing approximately 10 ounces. Do not peel it, but cut it in half lengthwise and remove all the seeds with a small spoon.

… Then cut it into small dice (brunoise). Salt generously and leave to marinate for 15 minutes. Rinse in cold water and drain on a dish towel.

… Rinse a small bunch of mint and 2 to 3 sprigs of flat-leaf parsley. Take off the leaves and chop them.

… Squeeze the juice of half a lemon.

… In a large bowl, combine the diced cucumber, ½ cup Greek-style yogurt, the chopped mint and parsley, 1 pinch of Piment d'Espelette or hot paprika, and the lemon juice.

… Add salt and mix well. Taste and correct the seasoning.

… Refrigerate for at least 1 hour, as this tzatziki should be served very cold.

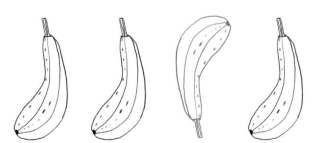

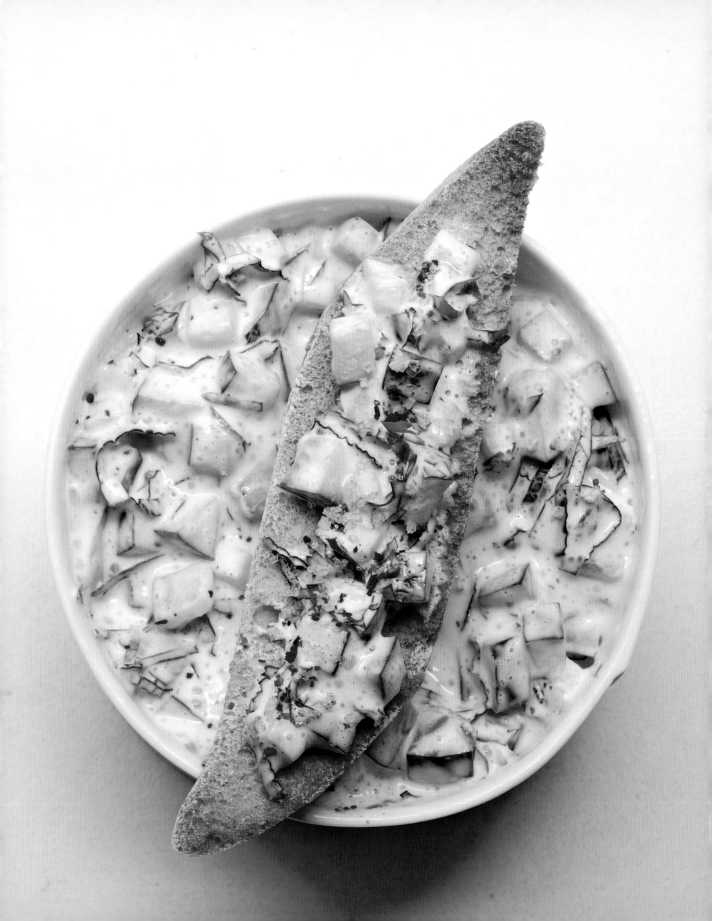

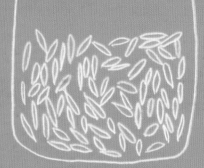
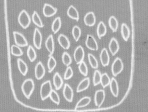
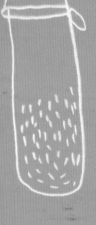
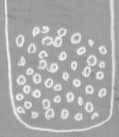
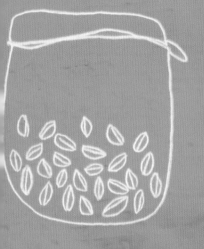
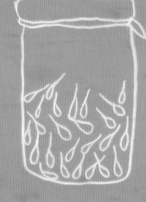
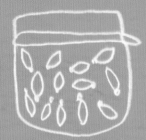
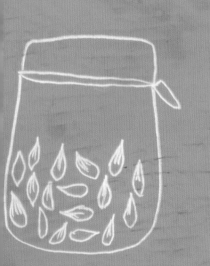
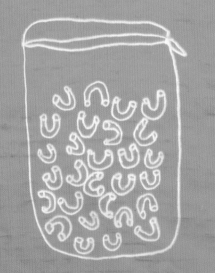
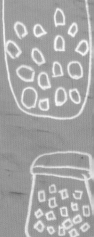
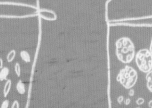
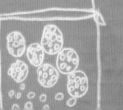
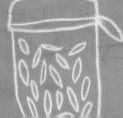
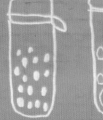
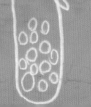
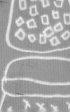

AD— Why are there so many recipes for tartines (open sandwiches), tarts, pizzas, crêpes, pasta, rice, and other grains such as fonio and quinoa? Well, to start with, because they're so good to eat!

PN— And not just that, grains are necessary for a balanced diet and therefore for good health. Half of our daily calories should come from carbohydrates, and grains of all kinds are the foods that contain the most. They also contain a whole array of vital nutrients, especially in their whole grain form.

Grains, Breads, and Pasta

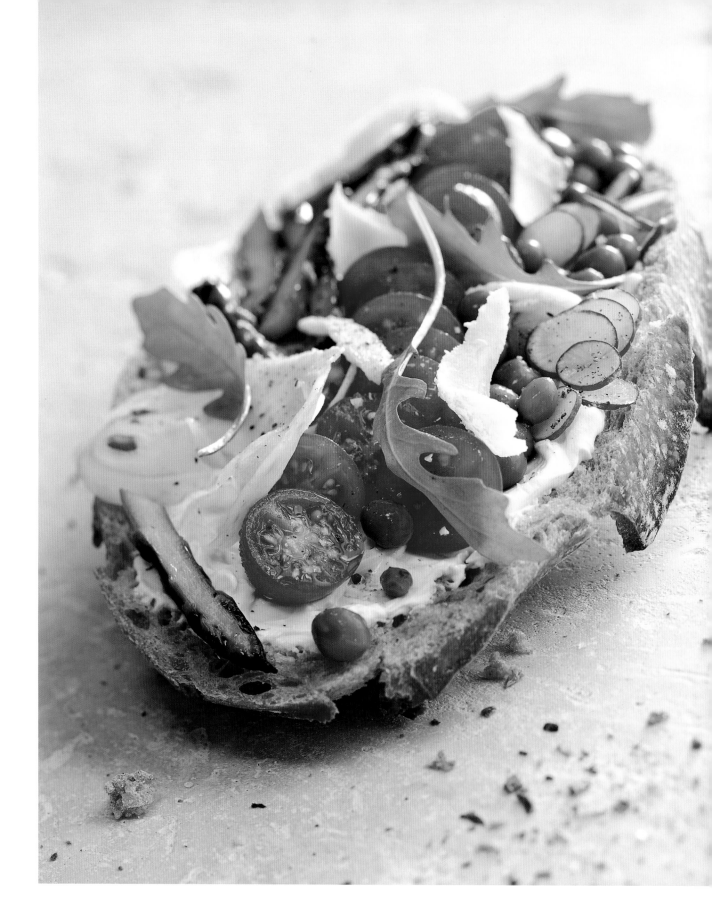

Spring Tartines

… Makes 4 tartines

… Bring a saucepan of salted water to a boil and get a bowl ready with water and ice cubes.

… Cut the tips of 16 small green asparagus spears into 2- to 2½-inch lengths, rinse, and immerse in the boiling water along with a good handful of peas.

… Drain and immediately plunge them into the ice water to keep their color. Leave for 2 minutes, then drain with a slotted spoon and lay on a dry dish towel.

… Peel and wash about 10 radishes and slice into thin rounds (about ⅛ inch) with a mandoline.

… Rinse a quarter of a fennel bulb and slice into thin slivers of the same size.

… Wash and dry about 20 cherry tomatoes and halve them.

… Remove the stalks, wash, and dry a handful of arugula.

… Toast 4 slices of whole-wheat or multigrain bread on one side only.

… Spread approximately 5 ounces of cream cheese, preferably Saint-Moret, over the slices of bread.

… Line the halved cherry tomatoes along the center of each slice.

… Then layer the slivers of fennel, radish slices, and peas on top.

… Slice the asparagus tips lengthwise and scatter them over.

… Then shave 1½ ounces of Parmesan with a vegetable peeler and add these.

… Finish with the arugula leaves.

… Add a generous twist of freshly ground black pepper. Keep cool (not for too long!) until it's time to eat.

AD— You might feel that these tartines are rather long in the preparation, but it shouldn't take you more than 15 to 20 minutes. You can prepare the other vegetables while the peas and asparagus are cooking.
PN— These tartines are a fine example of a healthy balance: bread and vegetables (carbohydrates, fiber, and vitamins), plus cheese (protein and calcium). Wrap them in plastic wrap and they're perfect for a lunchbox.

Herb Tartines

AD— There's no vinegar in the seasoning, as this would overwhelm the delicate flavor of the herbs. If you want a little acidity, add a few drops of lemon juice at the last minute. A young olive oil with an "herby" flavor is good here too.

PN— This is a well-balanced tartine: fiber and carbohydrates from the whole-wheat bread, vitamins and minerals in the herbs, calcium from the cheese, animal and vegetable protein from the cheese and bread.

… Makes 4 tartines

… Remove the stalks, wash, and dry 2 handfuls of arugula.

… Pick off the smallest leaves from half a bunch of basil, set them aside, and finely chop.

… Wash, separate the leaves from the stalks of a small bunch of chervil and a sprig of tarragon, and chop roughly.

… Grate 2 ounces of pecorino or other hard sheep's cheese.

… Combine all the herbs and the cheese in a large bowl and toss.

… Season with a splash of olive oil (1 or 2 tablespoons, no more). Set aside.

… Peel 1 garlic clove, soak it in olive oil, and rub it on 4 slices of whole-wheat or multigrain bread.

… Heat a nonstick skillet and lightly brown the slices of bread on both sides.

… Spread the herb mixture on top. Add freshly ground black pepper and serve.

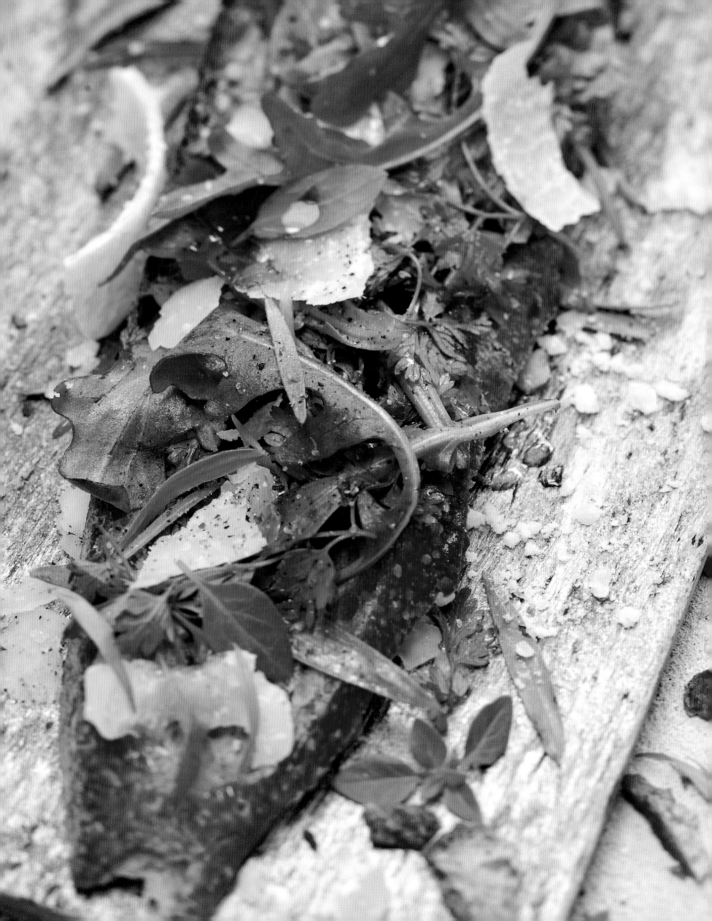

Purple Artichoke and Asparagus Tapenade Tartines

AD— If you can't get hold of purple artichokes, use green bulb artichokes and boil them in salted water. If you can't get caper berries, use capers instead.

PN— The caper berry is the fruit of the caper bush, the (smaller) caper is the bud. Frozen artichoke bottoms have the same nutritional value as fresh. They can save you time, but their flavor is less refined than that of fresh purple artichokes.

… Makes 4 tartines

… Break the stem off 4 large purple artichokes and remove the tough leaves. Cut the top off with a large sharp knife. Then cut around each artichoke with a small knife until you come to the tender leaves. Place them in water with the juice of 1 lemon as you go.

… Steam the artichokes for approximately 20 minutes.

… While the artichokes are cooking, peel and wash 4 asparagus spears. Cut off the hard bottom section and slice the asparagus into fine shavings with a mandoline.

… Remove the choke with a small spoon, then cut each artichoke bottom into 4 or 5 thin slices.

… Lightly brush 4 slices of French-style country bread or multigrain bread with olive oil on one side only, then toast on the same side until golden.

… Spread 4 tablespoons of tapenade (page 40) onto the slices of bread. Scatter the artichoke bottoms and slivers of asparagus on top, without pressing them down.

… Cut 8 caper berries marinated in vinegar in half and add them.

… Sprinkle with a few crystals of sea salt and a few drops of olive oil and a generous twist of freshly ground black pepper.

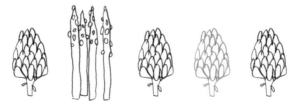

Jabugo Ham and Tomato Tartines with Capers and Olives

… Makes 4 tartines

… Blanch 3 ripe tomatoes of different colors, quarter them, and remove all the seeds. Cut the flesh into small pieces and put them in a large bowl.

… Cut 12 pitted black (preferably Taggiasche) olives into rounds and mix with the tomatoes.

… Then add 1 tablespoon of small capers.

… Add 1 to 2 tablespoons of olive oil, salt very lightly, and add pepper.

… Wash, dry, and separate the leaves from 3 or 4 sprigs of flat-leaf parsley, and 3 or 4 sprigs of basil. Rinse and dry 3 or 4 chives.

… Set aside several nice parsley leaves and a few basil leaves for decoration. Then chop the rest of the herbs, add to the tomatoes, and toss together.

… Toast 4 good-sized slices of whole-wheat or multigrain bread and cover with the aromatic tomatoes.

… Then spread 4 ounces of flakes of Jabugo ham on top.

… Garnish your tartines with the reserved herb leaves.

AD—Taggiasche olives are the Rolls-Royce of the olive world, but you can substitute other black olives; likewise, other herbs. Jabugo is a superb Spanish ham produced in the village of Jabugo according to an old tradition unique to this village, from wild Iberian pigs fed on bellota (acorns). You can use a different kind of cured ham, but it must be in very fine flakes.

PN— Don't skimp on the herbs; they're full of vitamins! But go easy on the salt, as the olives, capers, and ham should provide enough.

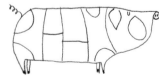
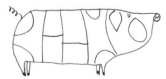

Sheep's Curd, Fig, and Honey Tartines

AD— *If you can't get Basque products, substitute goat's (or even cow's) curd and use a different kind of tangy pressed cheese. What matters here is the combination of curd, figs, honey, and cheese.*
PN— *And this combination, with the good carbohydrates from the bread, is great from a nutritional point of view!*

Fromage blanc or cottage cheese may be used if fresh curd cannot be found. Ossau-Iraty is a classic sheep's milk cheese from the French Pyrénées; Parmesan works similarly well with the figs if Ossau-Iraty cannot be found.

… Makes 4 tartines

… Toast 4 slices of multigrain bread in the toaster.

… Drop a tablespoon of sheep's curd (4 tablespoons required in total) on each one without spreading it. Sprinkle a pinch of mignonette pepper (see page 30) over.

… Strip the leaves off a small sprig of thyme and a small sprig of rosemary and distribute them over each tartine.

… Cut 8 fresh figs into 3 slices each and arrange on each tartine.

… On each one drizzle a teaspoon of *miel de montagne* (mountain honey) (4 teaspoons required in total) and a splash of olive oil.

… Then cut ¾ ounces of Ossau-Iraty cheese into slivers with a vegetable peeler and distribute over each tartine.

… Serve immediately.

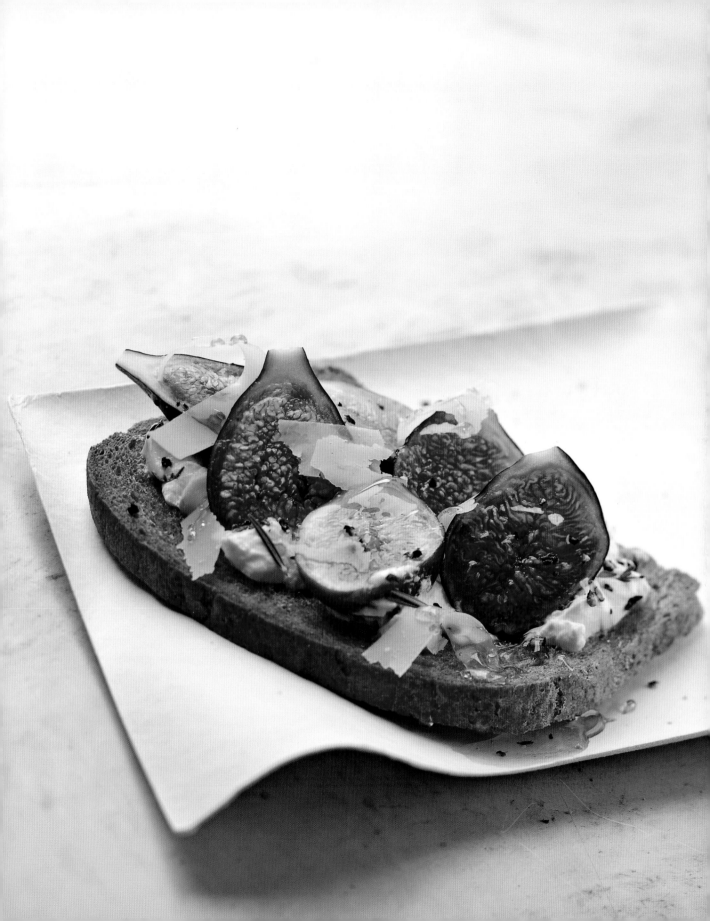

Ham and Ricotta Tartines

AD— If you have some pesto (page 36) on hand, you can use this instead of the basil and olive oil in the ricotta. Get your delicatessen to slice the ham extremely thinly. And opt for Parma ham if you can find it.

PN— It's best to remove the stalks from the arugula as they're not easy to digest if you have a delicate colon. With protein in the ham and ricotta, calcium in the two cheeses, and slow carbohydrates in the bread, these tartines make a perfect quick lunch.

… Makes 4 tartines

… Put ½ cup of ricotta and 2 tablespoons of grated Parmesan in a bowl.

… Chop the leaves from 4 sprigs of basil. Add to the bowl and mix well. Add freshly ground black pepper. Keep cool.

… Wash, dry, and remove the stalks from a handful of arugula. Place in another bowl.

… Cut 4 very fine slices of cured ham into shavings and mix gently with the arugula.

… Lightly toast 4 large slices of whole-wheat or multigrain bread and spread them with the basil-flavored ricotta.

… Sprinkle the ham and arugula mixture on top. Add a twist of freshly ground black pepper and serve.

Fava Bean Tartines

… Makes 4 tartines

… Shell 1 pound of small fresh fava beans and remove their skins. Take off the outer skin by pressing each bean between your thumb and index finger.

… Trim, wash, and dry 8 radishes and slice thinly with a mandoline.

… Trim and wash 3 scallions and cut them at an angle into very small pieces.

… Chop 5 mint leaves.

… Toast 4 slices of country or multigrain bread.

… Lightly salt 3½ ounces of goat's curd and spread it on the slices of toast.

… Sprinkle the chopped mint, fava beans, and pieces of scallion on top.

… Drizzle lightly with olive oil, then season with sea salt and freshly ground black pepper.

… Sprinkle the slices of radish on top as a garnish.

… Serve these tartines cold.

AD— This small variety of fava bean is harvested before the beans are fully ripe. They have a pale green pod with small beans, and are sold in French markets in the springtime.

PN— If you can't get hold of goat's curd, use an unstrained fresh white cow's milk cheese. It doesn't taste the same but has the same nutritional value.

———
Fromage blanc may be used if fresh curd cannot be found.

Vegetarian Sandwiches

AD— *You can vary this recipe by using small rolls or a crusty baguette split open, and vary the herbs according to what's available in the market.*

PN— *With fiber and carbohydrates from the whole-wheat bread and vegetables, plant protein, and also a little animal protein, from the ricotta and Parmesan, this is a very well balanced sandwich. Combine with a yogurt and some fruit, and you have a perfect office lunch.*

... Makes 4 sandwiches

... Cut 8 large slices lengthwise from a whole-wheat loaf, and rub them with 1 garlic clove cut in half.

... Wash 1 eggplant and 2 zucchini and cut into slices about ¼ inch thick. Brush them lightly with oil, salt them, and grill or broil for 1 minute on each side. Drain on paper towels.

... Chop the leaves of 4 sprigs of basil and mix them in a bowl with ¼ cup of ricotta, 1 tablespoon of grated Parmesan, and a small splash of olive oil.

... Wash a handful of arugula and dry well, then remove the stalks.

... Slice 2 tomatoes into rounds, then arrange over the 4 tartines with the slices of grilled eggplant and zucchini.

... With a peeler, shave 1½ ounces of Parmesan and spread on top.

... Spread the other 4 slices of bread with basil-flavored ricotta and arrange the arugula leaves on top.

... Give a generous twist of freshly ground black pepper and lay the ricotta tartines on top of the slices covered with vegetables. Press lightly to hold them together.

... Wrap in plastic wrap until you are ready to eat.

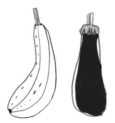

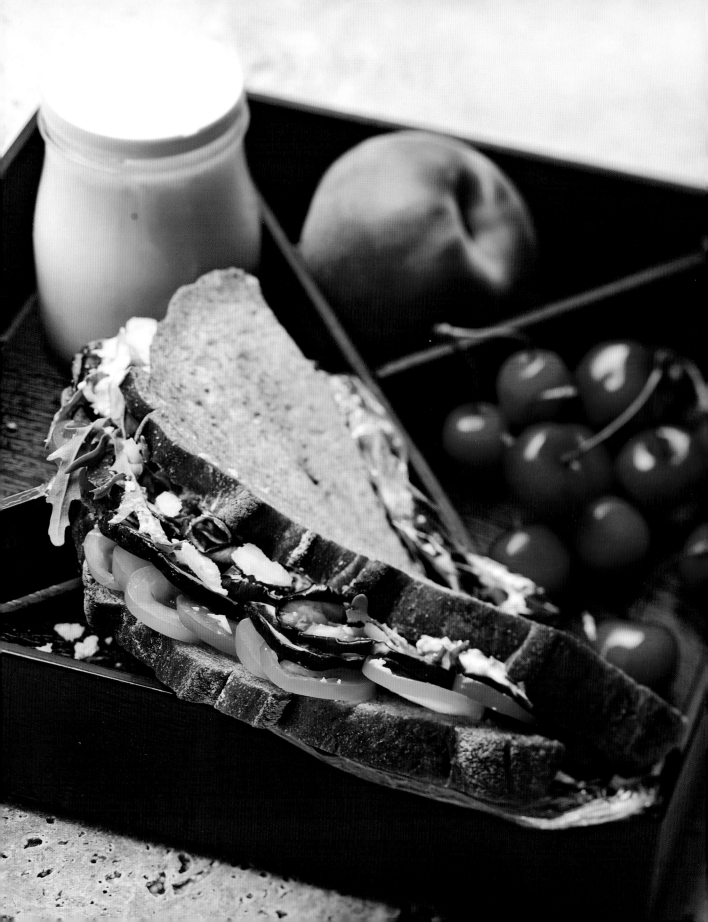

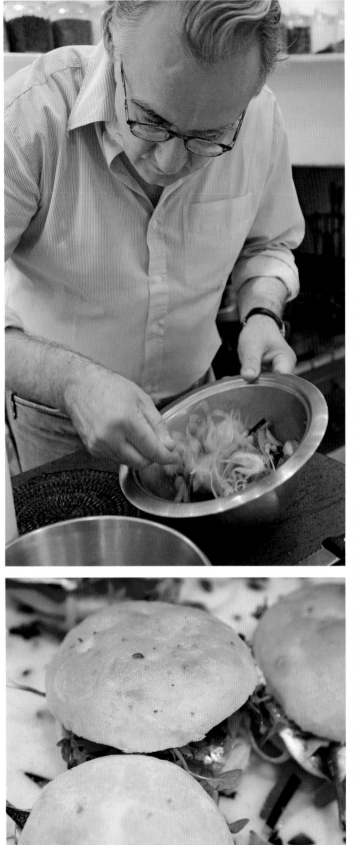
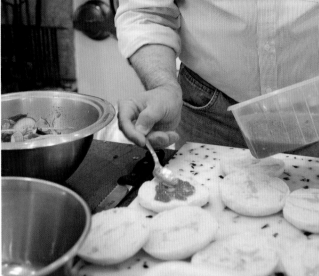
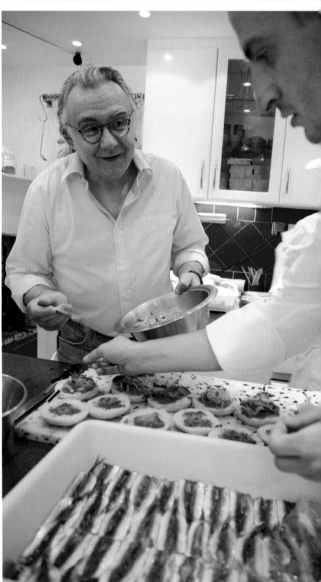

With Wilfrid in the kitchen at La Bastide de Moustiers.

Pan-Bagnat
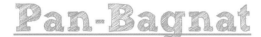

… Serves 4

Prepare the bread

… Cut 4 flat round whole-wheat rolls about 6 inches in diameter in half through the middle. Peel and halve 1 garlic clove and rub each half roll with it.

… Wash 6 tomatoes and cut in half; squeeze gently to collect the juice in a bowl. Sprinkle the half rolls with it, then drizzle a little olive oil and a little wine vinegar on top. Sprinkle with a little sea salt and some freshly ground black pepper. Set aside.

Prepare the quail eggs

… Cook 8 quail eggs in boiling water for 5 minutes. Allow to cool, then shell and cut them in half. Set them aside.

Prepare the salad and tomatoes

… Wash and spin 12 leaves of romaine lettuce. Cut the half-tomatoes into slices ¼ inch thick and cut 12 segments of tomato confit (page 16) in half. Set all this aside.

Prepare the vegetables

… Clean 8 radishes, 1 zucchini, 2 scallions, 1 small celery heart, 1 silverskin or large pearl onion, half a yellow pepper, and 1 small fennel bulb.

… Slice the radishes and the zucchini very finely. Cut the scallions and celery at an angle into 1/16-inch slices. Slice the onion into very thin rounds. Cut the pepper into strips ¾ inch by 1/16 inch. Cut the fennel bulb in half, then cut each half into 1/16-inch slices. Strip the leaves off a small bunch of basil.

… Combine all these vegetables and the basil in a large bowl. Season with a little olive oil and a little wine vinegar, salt, and freshly ground black pepper. Then add 12 pitted Niçoise olives and mix well.

To finish your pan-bagnats

… Drain 3½ ounces of tuna in oil. Drain 8 fillets of anchovies in oil.

… Arrange the tomato rounds, tomato confit, and romaine on 4 half rolls. Spread the vegetable mixture on top. Add the whole anchovies, tuna, and quail eggs. Add freshly ground black pepper.

… Close up the rolls and press gently. Let them rest for 10 minutes before serving.

AD— Pan-bagnat (literally "bathed bread") originated around the classic salade Niçoise. In the past, an hour before serving the salad they would add crumbled stale bread. It produced a delicious bread soaked in oil and tomato juice. This led to the idea of putting this salad inside bread.

PN— And it's a perfect example of the Mediterranean diet, which protects you from just about everything. Bread (carbohydrates), vegetables (fiber, vitamins, antioxidants), a little fish (protein), and olive oil. Whereas the classic ham sandwich . . .

Poppy Seed Tarts with Tomato and Tuna

AD— Use a good sharp knife to slice the tuna! This pastry dough keeps very well in the refrigerator, rolled out and covered in plastic wrap. Use it for other tarts or for a pizza.

PN— This pastry is particularly rich in healthy fiber from the whole-wheat flour and oats. With the omega-3s in the tuna and anchovies and the antioxidants from the tomatoes, this tart is a genuine "functional food"!

… Serves 4

Make the pastry

… Put 1 cup of whole-wheat flour and 1 pinch of salt in a bowl. Make a well and add 3½ tablespoons of butter cut into small pieces. Rub well with your fingertips until the mixture has the consistency of coarse breadcrumbs. Add ¼ cup rolled oats, 1 tablespoon of poppy seeds, and, gradually, 5 tablespoons of water. Knead to form a dough.

… Shape into a ball and leave to rest for 30 minutes at room temperature.

Prepare the topping

… In the meantime, cut 8 ounces of fresh white tuna fillet into thin slices (flakes). Season with Piment d'Espelette or hot paprika.

… Rinse and dry a handful of arugula. Also rinse 12 salted anchovy fillets under the tap.

Bake the pastry

… Preheat the oven to 350°F.

… Roll out the pastry into a circle ¹⁄₁₆ inch thick. Cut into quarters and arrange on a baking sheet, placing a small coffee cup on top of each to create a hollow in the center.

… Bake for 10 to 12 minutes, until the pastry is golden.

To finish your tarts

… Take out the baking sheet, but don't turn off the oven.

… Spread ½ cup of chopped cooked tomatoes (page 21) over the bottom of each tart, alternating with anchovies, tuna flakes, and 12 segments of tomato confit (page 16).

… Return the tarts to the oven for 3 minutes, until just warmed through.

… Meanwhile, season the arugula with a splash of olive oil and the juice of a quarter of a lemon.

… Remove the tarts from the oven, add the arugula, and serve immediately.

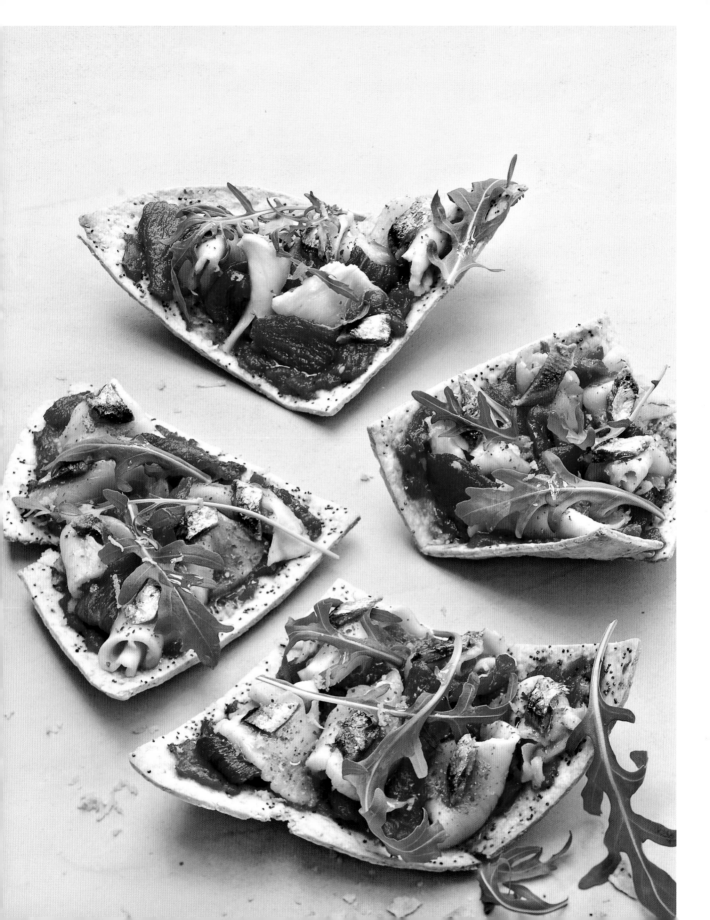

Vegetable Pie

AD— Check when the pie is done by inserting a skewer or knife into it. It should come out dry. If you make your pâte brisée in advance, begin by placing it in the pie dish and put it in the fridge while you prepare the vegetables.

PN— A pie bursting with antioxidants, gentle fiber, vitamins, minerals, and not much fat: How much better could it be?

… Serves 4

… Make 14 ounces of pâte brisée (page 11) if you don't have some stored away.

… Wash 1 pound of Swiss chard. Plunge the leaves into salted boiling water for 2 minutes. Drain and squeeze to extract as much water as possible. Chop them and set aside.

… Wash 1 fennel bulb and 2 zucchini. Thinly slice the fennel. Cut the zucchini in half lengthwise and remove the seeds before thinly slicing these, too. Peel 1 red onion and slice thinly. Peel and crush 1 garlic clove.

… Heat a skillet with 2 tablespoons of olive oil and sweat the fennel, zucchini, onion, and garlic with the leaves of 2 sprigs of thyme for 10 minutes. Then add the Swiss chard and ½ cup of shelled peas, ½ cup of shelled fava beans, and salt and cook gently for 5 minutes.

… While this is cooking, rinse, dry, and chop the leaves of a small bunch of parsley and a small bunch of chervil. Wash and finely chop a small bunch of chives. Crush 2 tablespoons of pitted black olives.

… In a bowl, mix 3 tablespoons of crème fraîche with 2 egg yolks (3 yolks required in total for recipe).

… After 15 minutes of cooking, take the skillet off the heat and gradually incorporate all these ingredients, stirring well. Also add 2 tablespoons of grated Parmesan. Mix well. Taste and adjust the seasoning, adding salt if needed.

… Preheat the oven to 350°F.

… Cut the ball of pastry in half and roll out each half. Lay one of the rolled-out pieces in a 9-inch round baking pan. Pile the contents of the skillet on top in a dome shape, then cover with the other piece of pastry and press the edges together.

… Mix the last egg yolk with a little water and brush the whole surface of the pie. Sprinkle the top with 3 pinches of sesame seeds. Pierce a hole in the center of the pie to allow the steam to escape.

… Put in the oven for 30 minutes. Then allow to rest for 15 minutes. Serve it in its baking pan.

My Take on Pissaladières

... Serves 8

Make your dough

... Put 2 cups all-purpose flour in a bowl. Make a well in the middle and add all together 3 pinches of salt, 1 teaspoon of baker's yeast, 5 tablespoons of olive oil, and ⅓ to ½ cup of cold water.

... Stir with your fingers, then knead until you have an even, smooth, and elastic dough.

... Form into a ball and leave to rise in the bowl covered with a dish towel at room temperature for 30 minutes.

Prepare the onions and fennel

... In the meantime, trim, wash, and thinly slice 5 good-sized onions and 2 fennel bulbs.

... Heat a little olive oil in a flameproof casserole dish and sweat the onions and fennel for 10 minutes without coloring. Add 4 crushed garlic cloves, 1 sprig of thyme (3 sprigs required in total for recipe) and 1 bay leaf, season with salt, and cook gently for about 15 minutes, stirring occasionally.

Make your pissaladières

... Preheat your oven to 350°F.

... Cut the ball of dough in half and roll out each half to a thickness of ⅛ inch. Place each in a 9-inch pie dish forming a rim of ½ inch.

... Remove the garlic cloves, thyme, and bay leaf from the onion and fennel mixture, and spread it evenly over each tart. Pick the leaves off the remaining 2 sprigs of thyme and sprinkle them over the surface of each pissaladière.

... Bake in the oven for 15 to 20 minutes.

... Take the pissaladière out and increase the oven temperature to 400°F.

... Spread 3½ ounces of fresh anchovy fillets and 30 black olives (Taggiasche, preferably; see page 59) on top and return to the oven for 5 minutes.

... When you take them out, sprinkle with a few grains of sea salt and freshly ground black pepper.

... These pissaladières can be eaten hot or at room temperature.

AD— The Italians invented pizza, and the people of Nice the pissaladière! And now I've added fennel. You can save time by using prepared bread dough from your baker and frozen onions.

PN— Adding fennel is a good idea because its nutritional reputation is well known and its benefits (minerals, carotenoids, and so on) combine with those of the onion to make this a genuine natural health food.

Baker's yeast is fresh yeast. It contains no artificial additives and can be kept in the refrigerator for up to four weeks. If using dry yeast instead, replace with approximately one-third the amount of fresh yeast. Here, use about ⅓ teaspoon.

Zucchini and Sainte-Maure Pizza

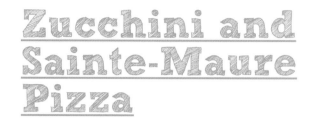

AD— Sainte-Maure de Touraine is a superb goat cheese, which is now protected by the AOP label. It is rolled in fine charcoal ash before aging.

PN— Zucchini are not particularly well endowed with vitamins and minerals. But combined with basil, which has lots, and tomato confit, the result is very good for you. Especially with cheese, to add some calcium.

If Sainte-Moure de Touraine cannot be found, any fresh goat cheese— preferably coated in ash and slightly aged—may be used.

… Serves 4 to 6

Make the pizza dough

… Dissolve 1 teaspoon of baker's yeast or a quarter of a packet of dried yeast (see page 71) in a little warm water. Put 1 cup of fine pastry flour, 2 pinches of salt, 1 teaspoon of olive oil, and 2 tablespoons of cold water in the bowl of a standing mixer.

… Mix at a slow speed until you have an even dough. Shape into a ball. Cover with a damp cloth and leave to rise at room temperature for at least 30 minutes.

Prepare the zucchini

… In the meantime, wash 4 green and yellow zucchini, cut two of them into thin rounds (about 1/16 inch) and the other two into small cubes (1/4 inch), removing the seeds. Trim and thinly slice 1 white onion. Rinse, dry, and pick the leaves from a bunch of basil, then chop them.

… In a skillet with a little olive oil, gently sauté the zucchini cubes with 1 crushed garlic clove and the leaves of 1 sprig of thyme with the lid on for 10 minutes, then crush with a fork. Salt lightly, add the chopped basil, and mix well.

Make your pizza

… Roll out the dough into a rectangle 1/8 inch thick. Place it on a baking sheet lined with parchment and put in the oven for just 3 minutes.

… In the meantime, cut half a Sainte-Maure de Touraine cheese into rounds.

… Take the baking pan out and spread the zucchini mixture on top nice and evenly. Arrange alternate rounds of raw zucchini, rounds of Saint-Maure, sliced onion, 20 segments of tomato confit (page 16), and 20 pitted black olives (preferably Taggiasche) decoratively on top.

… Put the pizza in the oven and bake for 10 to 15 minutes.

… When you take it out, add a twist of freshly ground black pepper.

… Serve immediately.

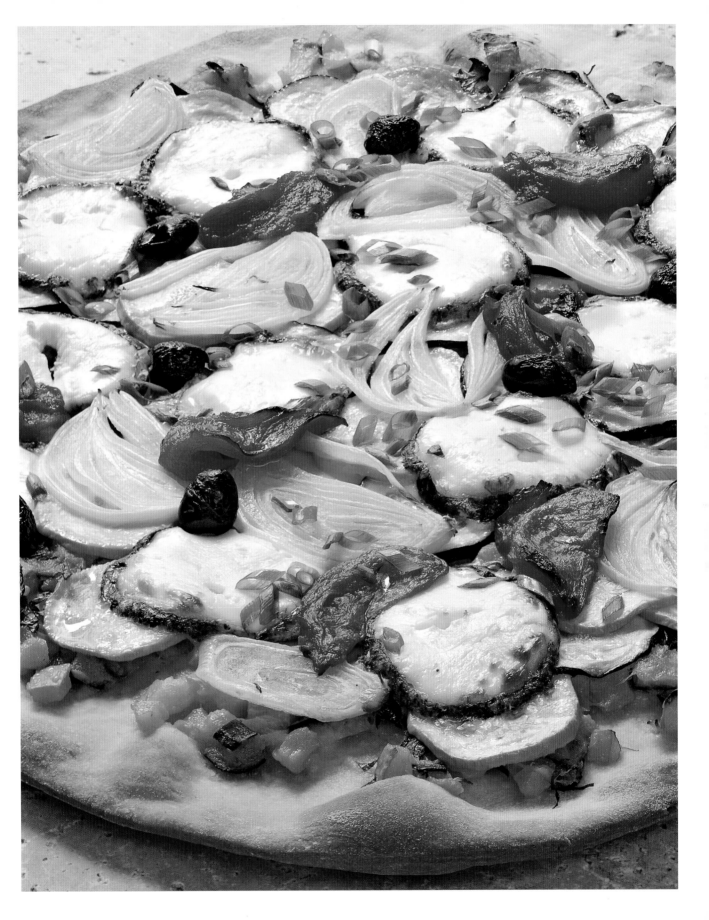

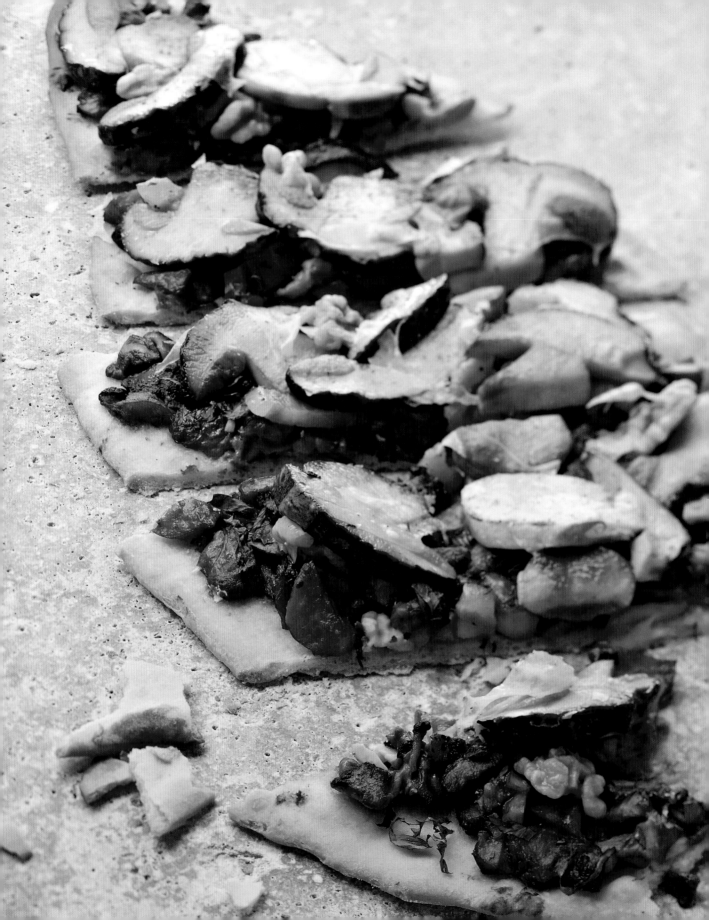

Pizza with Porcini Mushrooms

… Serves 4

Make the pizza dough

… Using 1 teaspoon of baker's yeast (see page 71), 1 cup of fine pastry flour, 2 pinches of salt, 1 teaspoon of olive oil, and ⅓ cup of cold water, make the same pizza dough as for the zucchini pizza (page 72).

Prepare the porcinis

… In the meantime, clean 1¾ pounds of fresh medium porcini. Cut four of them into ¼-inch-thick slices and dice the rest. Dice 3½ ounces of smoked bacon. Trim 5 scallions, cut the white parts into rounds, remove the tough part of the greens, and chop the rest into small pieces.

Cook the diced porcinis

… Heat 1½ tablespoons of duck fat (4½ tablespoons required in total for recipe) in a flameproof casserole dish. Brown the bacon lightly, then sweat the chopped scallion greens for 2 minutes. Add the diced porcinis, season with salt, and cook gently for 20 minutes, adding a little water if necessary until the porcinis are nice and soft.

Cook the sliced porcinis

… Meanwhile, heat a skillet with the remaining 3 tablespoons of duck fat. Cook the sliced porcinis until lightly golden on each side. Add salt. Lay them on paper towels.

Prepare and bake your pizza

… Heat your oven to 400°F. Peel 2 garlic cloves, chop the leaves of 5 sprigs of flat-leaf parsley, and add to the cooked diced porcinis.

… Roll out the dough lengthwise to ⅛ inch thick. Place on a baking sheet lined with parchment. Spread the cooked diced porcinis on top. Then decorate with the sliced porcinis, 8 walnut halves, and the scallion whites. Bake in the oven for about 20 minutes.

… Take the pizza out of the oven. Shave 1 ounce of Parmesan into flakes and sprinkle over the pizza. Return to the oven for 1 to 2 minutes, until melted. Add freshly ground black pepper and serve.

AD— This pizza dough freezes very well rolled out on a sheet of parchment paper. You can then use it straight from the freezer without any need to thaw.
PN— A healthy pizza! B vitamins, minerals, and fiber in the porcinis, plus healthy fatty acids from the duck fat. If this is not available, use olive oil rather than butter.

Buckwheat Crêpes with Andouille Sausage and Leeks

AD— If you add the stiff egg whites at the end, the batter will be lighter and the crêpes will also be thicker.

PN— Use a nonstick skillet in good condition for these crêpes; otherwise you will have to oil it too much to keep them from sticking. With a salad and a nice dessert, this makes a perfect Sunday-evening dinner.

… Makes 4 large crêpes

Make the batter

… Put ½ cup of buckwheat flour and ⅓ cup of pastry flour in a bowl. Mix together and make a well in the center.

… Separate the whites and yolks of 2 large eggs and drop the yolks in the well. Mix in, gradually adding 1½ cups of lowfat milk.

… Cut 3 tablespoons of lightly salted butter into pieces and melt in a small pan until lightly golden. Pour into the batter, beating well as you do so.

… Beat the egg whites until stiff, then fold them gently into the batter, stirring constantly in the same direction so that they don't collapse.

… Cover the bowl with a clean dish towel and leave the batter to rest for 1 hour.

Cook the leeks

… Wash 2 small leeks, cut off the base, remove the green part, take off the outer leaf, and cut them at an angle into slices about ⅛ inch thick.

… Heat a splash of olive oil in a nonstick sauté pan, add the leeks, season with salt, and sweat for 2 minutes, keeping them crunchy. Remove from the pan with a slotted spoon and lay them on a plate.

Cook the crêpes

… Take the skin off 12 thin slices Andouille de Guéméné or other coarse-grained smoked pork sausage and shred them.

… Return the nonstick sauté pan to the heat. When it's hot, scatter a spoonful of leeks and 3 slices of andouille, and cook for just 20 seconds.

… Then pour a small ladle of batter and spread it over the whole surface of the pan. Cook until the edges of the crêpe begin to color, then flip or turn it with a spatula and cook the other side for approximately 1 minute.

… Lay the crêpe on a plate and keep warm.

… Cook the other three crêpes in the same way.

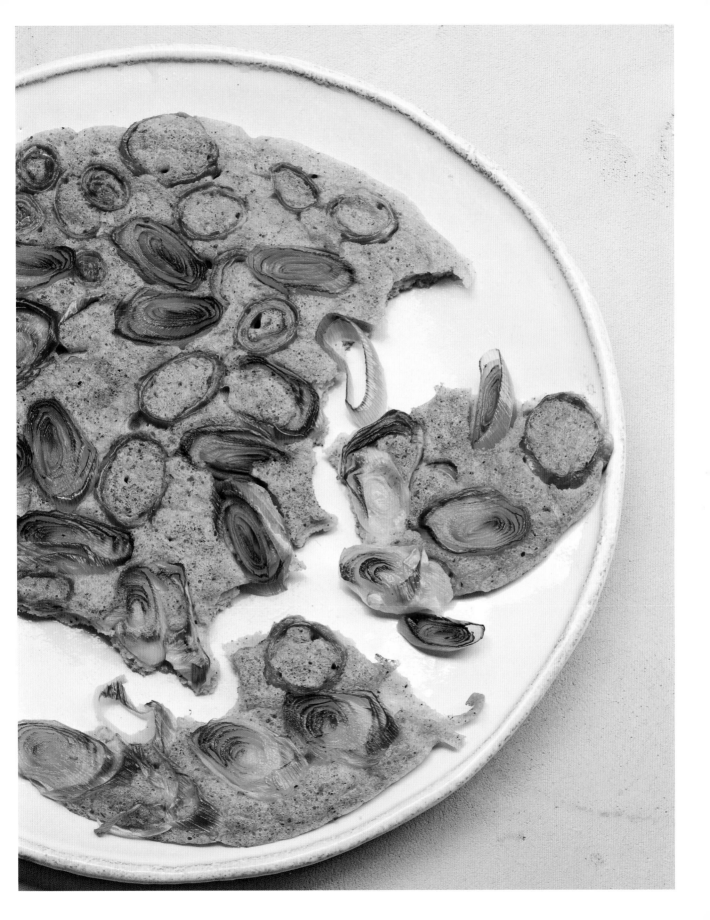

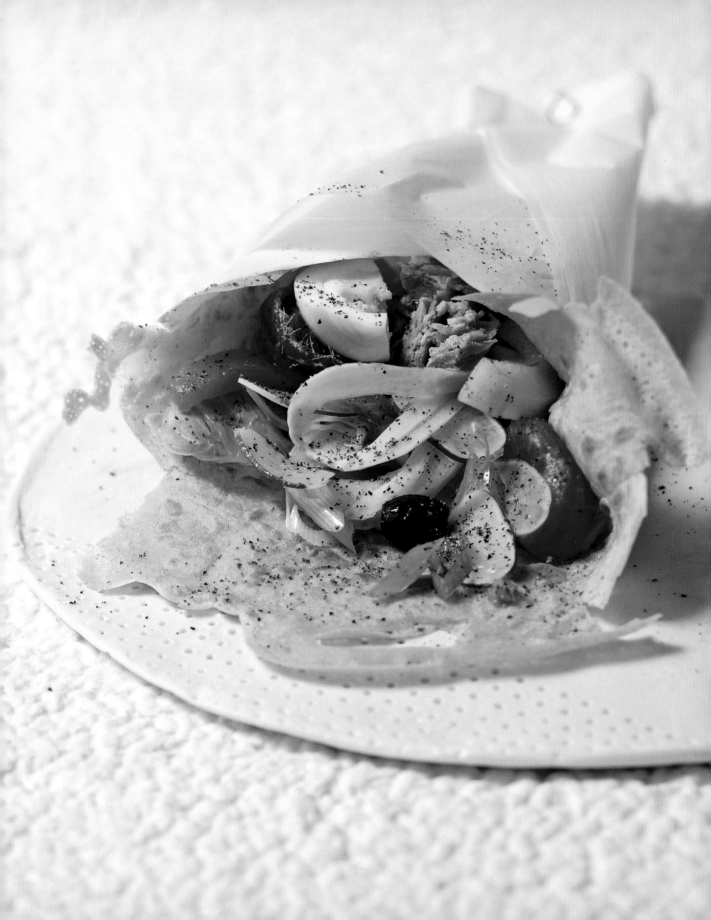

Socca with Niçoise-Style Vegetables

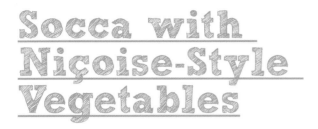

… Serves 4

<u>Make the socca batter</u>

… Put 1½ cups of chickpea flour, 2 pinches of fine salt, and 5 tablespoons of olive oil in a bowl. Stir, then gradually add 2 cups of cold water, beating vigorously. Leave the batter to rest in the refrigerator.

<u>Prepare the eggs and vegetables</u>

… Hard boil 2 eggs (10 minutes). Cool and shell them.

… Wash and trim half a fennel bulb, 6 radishes, half a cucumber, 2 tomatoes, 4 scallions, and the heart of 1 head of romaine lettuce.

… Cut the fennel and radishes into thin slices with a mandoline. Cut the cucumber, tomatoes, and scallions into small slivers. Cut the romaine leaves in half lengthwise.

… Pick the leaves from a small bunch of basil and chop them roughly with a knife.

… Drain the oil from half a jarred roasted red pepper and cut this into small slivers too. Cut 8 segments of tomato confit (page 16) and 4 anchovy fillets in oil in half. Roughly crumble 3½ ounces of tuna belly fillets in oil. Cut the hard-boiled eggs into rounds.

… Rub a large bowl with 1 garlic clove and combine all the above together in it.

… Season with 2 tablespoons of tapenade (page 40), 1 to 2 tablespoons of olive oil, salt, and freshly ground black pepper.

<u>Cook the socca</u>

… Heat a nonstick sauté pan with a splash of oil. Pour in a small ladle of batter and cook for 2 minutes. Make thin crisp crêpes in this way until you have used up all the batter.

<u>To finish your soccas</u>

… Arrange the vegetables on each crêpe then roll them up.

… Secure with a small wooden skewer and arrange on the serving dish or wrap in a paper cone. Optionally, serve your soccas with pesto (page 36).

AD— You can also cook the socca in the oven at 450°F: Oil a socca dish (10-inch diameter), cover with a thin layer of batter, and put in the oven for about 15 minutes, until golden.

PN— With carbohydrates from the socca, plenty of fiber, minerals, and vitamins from all the vegetables, and protein from the eggs and tuna, this is a well-rounded dish.

Crunchy Panisses with Fresh Goat Cheese and Pumpkin Seed Condiment

AD— It's perfectly possible to make these panisses the day before and fry them at the last minute. When you're making them, you must stir frequently to prevent them from sticking to the bottom of the pan. PN— Fresh soft goat cheese is as rich in calcium as cheese made from cow's milk. And chickpea flour contains as much slow-release carbohydrate and protein as wheat, without any gluten.

… Serves 4

Make the panisses

… Heat 2 cups of water with 1¾ tablespoons of butter and a splash of olive oil.

… Put 2¾ cups of chickpea flour in a large bowl and gradually pour in 2 cups of cold water, beating until you have a uniform mixture.

… Strain through a fine conical strainer, pour into the boiling water containing the butter and oil, and simmer over low heat for 20 minutes, beating very frequently.

… Oil a loaf pan, pour in the batter, and pat down to remove the air. Cover with plastic wrap and allow to cool, then refrigerate for 6 hours.

Prepare the condiment

… Place 8 ounces of strained fresh soft goat cheese (with its whey) in a bowl.

… Chop the leaves from 1 sprig of basil and 1 sprig of cilantro, crush 2 cloves of garlic confit (page 12) with a fork and add them to the cheese along with a splash of olive oil. Keep cool.

… Heat a skillet and lightly toast a small handful of pumpkin seeds. Set aside on a paper towel.

Cook the panisses

… Take the panisse from the pan, cut into sticks, and pat dry if damp.

… Heat a skillet with 2 or 3 spoonfuls of olive oil and fry the panisses, turning them until golden and crisp. Drain on paper towels and sprinkle with salt and freshly ground black pepper.

To finish your dish

… While the panisses are cooking, add the toasted pumpkin seeds to the fresh cheese. Adjust the seasoning to taste. Pour the condiment into a small bowl. Arrange the panisses on a dish and serve.

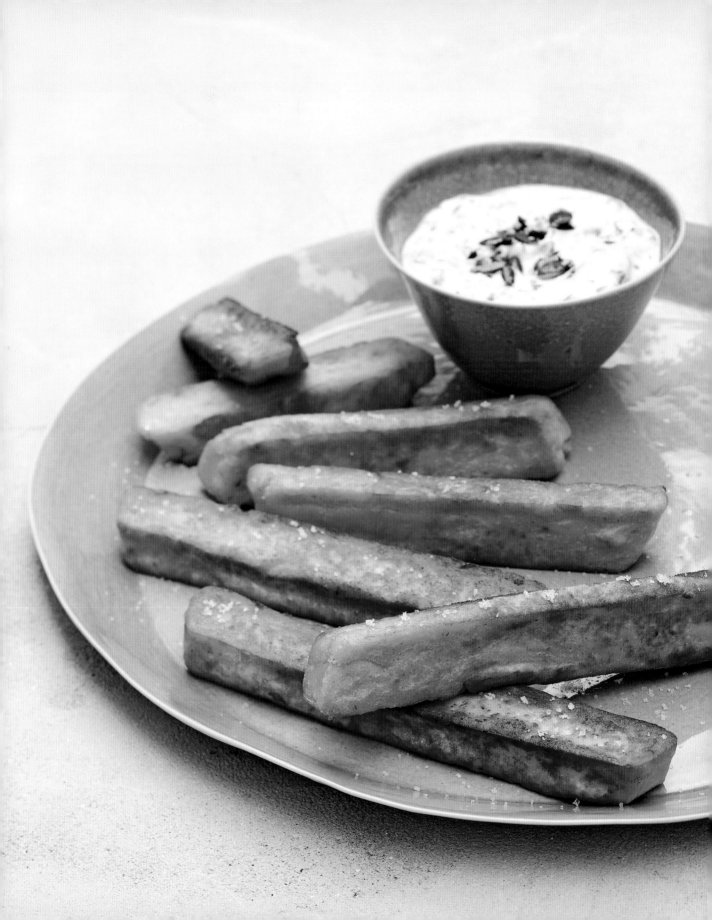

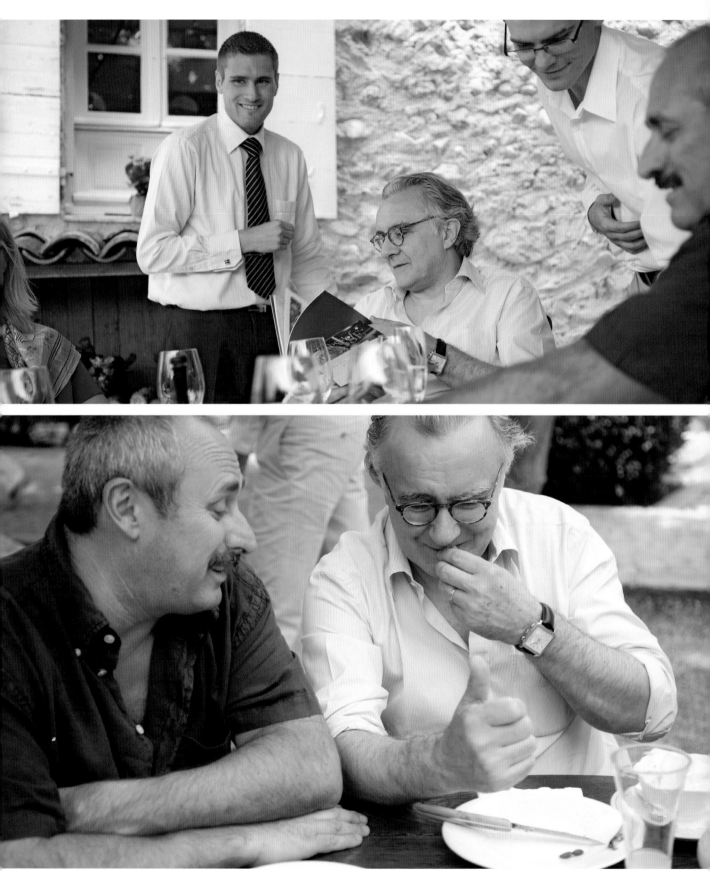

Lunch with friends on the terrace at La Bastide de Moustiers.

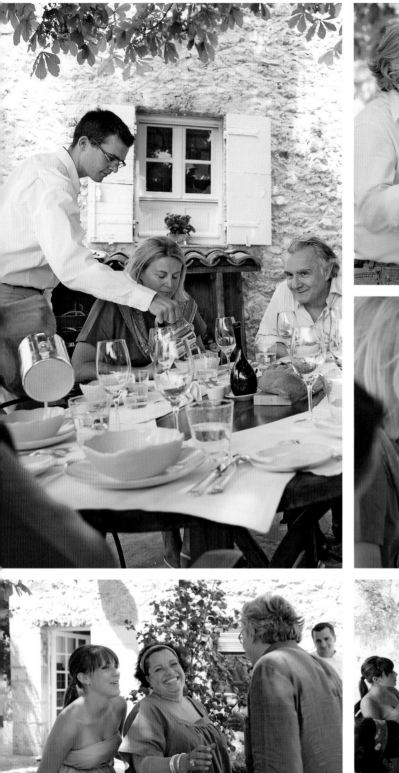

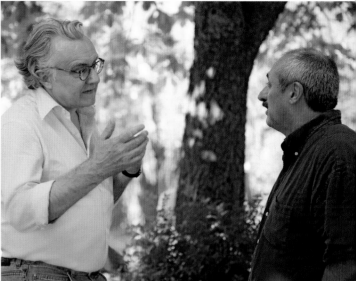

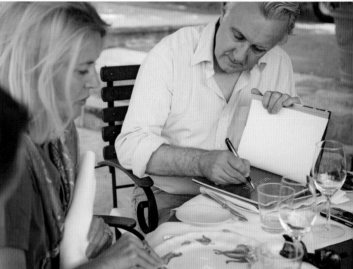

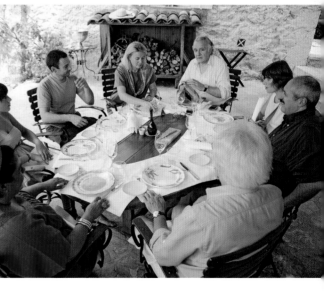

"Nature is all about cooking with feeling, cooking from the heart for the people you love, about sharing and feeling good together."

Individual Casseroles of Whole-Wheat Pasta, Broccoli, and Daube

AD— If you don't have individual small casseroles or ovenproof glass dishes, finish cooking the pasta in a large casserole dish, sealing the lid in the same way. The rosemary is in the sealing pastry dough simply for the pleasure of its aroma as it cooks!

PN— A remarkably rounded dish: meat (protein), pasta (carbohydrates), vegetables (fiber, vitamins), and cheese (calcium). The fiber in whole-wheat pasta combines well with that in the broccoli.

… Serves 4

Prepare the broccoli

… Remove and wash the florets of 2 large heads of broccoli (keep the stalks for a soup) and boil in salted water for just 3 minutes. Remove with a slotted spoon and immerse immediately in ice water. Then drain and set them aside. Don't throw away the broccoli cooking water; you will need 2 cups of it for cooking the pasta.

Prepare the pasta

… Heat a splash of olive oil in a skillet, add 8 ounces of whole-wheat pasta, and stir well. Then add 1 cup of the broccoli cooking water, stir, and cook until absorbed. Add an additional 1 cup of this water. Cook the pasta until al dente (try it).

Prepare the mini casseroles

… While the pasta is cooking, heat 1 pound of daube with its gravy (page 312) and set the oven to 350°F.

… Also prepare the sealing pastry: Mix 2½ cups flour with ½ cup of cold water and the leaves of 5 sprigs of rosemary. Work the pastry until it's smooth. Shape into a ball.

… In 4 small casseroles or ovenproof glass containers, distribute the meat from the daube. Then drain the pasta and place it on top. Arrange the broccoli, 12 segments of tomato confit (page 16), and ¾ cup of grated Parmesan on top of that.

… Add 5 tablespoons of sherry vinegar to the gravy of the daube, stir, and pour over the dishes.

… Cut the sealing pastry into 4 pieces, shape into long sausages, and flatten each one into a ⅛-inch-wide strip. Use these to seal the lids of the casseroles (or glass dishes). Brush the pastry with 1 beaten egg (mixed with a little water) and put in the oven for 10 minutes.

… When you take them out of the oven, shake each casserole (or glass dish) to soak all the ingredients with the gravy. Serve immediately.

Pappardelle with Pesto

… Serves 4

… Boil 8 ounces of pappardelle in salted water (for the time stated on the package).

… While they are cooking, heat a nonstick skillet and lightly toast 2 to 3 tablespoons of pine nuts. Cool them on a paper towel.

… With a vegetable peeler, cut 1½ ounces of Parmesan into fine shavings, and set aside.

… When the pasta is cooked, drain and transfer to a sauté pan.

… Add 2 ounces of light pesto (page 36) and, over low heat, mix well to coat the pappardelle. Check the seasoning.

… Pick the leaves off 1 sprig of basil.

… Transfer the pasta to a warm dish or serve directly from the skillet.

… Add the Parmesan shavings and basil leaves. Serve immediately.

AD— The noun pappardelle comes from the Italian verb pappare, which means "to wolf down"! If you can get hold of good-quality fresh pappardelle, don't hesitate. It will cook in just 2 to 3 minutes. PN— Not only do pine nuts add a nice crunch, they also contain very good unsaturated fatty acids. So, along with those in the pesto and its vitamins, and the carbohydrates from the pasta, these pappardelle are excellent from a nutritional point of view.

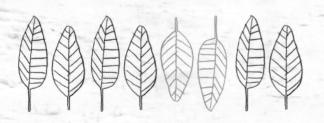

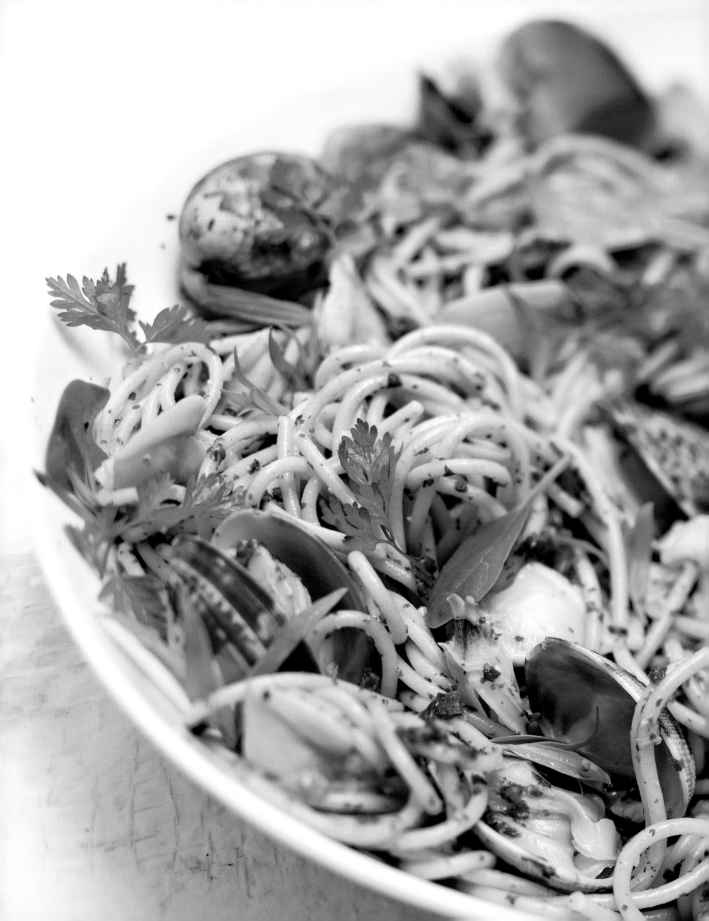

Whole-Wheat Spaghetti with Clams in an Herby Marinière Sauce

… Serves 4

Prepare your ingredients

… Rinse 32 clams in several changes of water to get rid of any sand.

… Peel and mince 1 shallot. Wash and pick the leaves from a small bunch of parsley, a small bunch of chervil, a sprig of tarragon (don't throw away the stems), and a handful of baby spinach. Put some aside to use at the end and roughly chop the rest. Peel and finely dice 2 garlic cloves.

Cook the spaghetti

… Put 8 ounces whole-wheat spaghetti in a large pan of salted boiling water and cook for the time stated on the package.

Open the clams

… While the spaghetti is cooking, heat a splash of olive oil in a sauté pan and brown the shallot. Add half of the garlic and the herb stems, mix well, and cook for just 30 seconds. Then add the clams and pour ⅓ cup of white wine over, stir, and cook with the lid on for 1 to 2 minutes, until they open.

… Drain. Strain the liquid through a fine strainer. Remove the shells.

Prepare the herby marinière sauce

… Wipe out your sauté pan and heat with a splash of olive oil. Put in the rest of the chopped garlic, chopped herbs, and spinach and cook lightly for 1 minute, stirring regularly.

… Transfer to a blender and puree, gradually adding the juice from the clams until the sauce is smooth and the consistency of soup.

To finish your dish

… Drain the spaghetti, return it to its saucepan, then add the herby sauce and clams. Mix delicately to coat the pasta with sauce, then add a splash of olive oil, the herbs, and the reserved baby spinach leaves. Serve hot.

AD— To make sure the liquid from the clams is fully strained, place a piece of paper towel in the colander or line your conical strainer with a paper coffee filter.

PN— Clams are a source of minerals. They must be extremely fresh. Scrupulously reject any that have opened, even if the fishmonger tells you that it is normal. The whole-wheat spaghetti is a welcome source of fiber.

Casarecce with Head Cheese and Onions in Vinegar

AD— An attractive mix of flavors and colors. Prepare the onions in vinegar the day before if you don't have a lot of time. And make a large quantity while you are at it, as they keep very well in their vinegar.

PN— Head cheese is low in lipids (fats) and cholesterol, but high in protein and it contains quite a lot of B group vitamins. As for the onions, they supply lots of antioxidants.

―――――

Casarecce resemble short pieces of partially rolled pappardelle. Any long, hollow-shaped pasta that works well with a chunky sauce, such as penne or rigatoni, can be used.

… Serves 4

Prepare the onions in vinegar

… Peel 2 red onions and cut each into 8 wedges.

… Put 1 cup of red wine vinegar and 1 teaspoon of superfine sugar in a pan and bring to a boil. Add 10 black peppercorns and the peel of 1 orange. Turn the heat down to the minimum and allow to infuse for 5 minutes.

… Then add the onion wedges and simmer gently for approximately 20 minutes.

… Set them aside in a bowl and allow to cool.

Prepare the pasta

… Put 8 ounces of casarecce in salted boiling water and cook for 8 to 10 minutes (according to the directions on the package).

… While this is cooking, cut 7 ounces of head cheese into long narrow strips (about 2 by ⅛ inch).

… Peel and wash 4 scallions, keeping 4 inches of green. Cut the green stalks into thin slices and cut the whites into thin wedges.

… Sweat the bulbs in a flameproof casserole dish with a splash of olive oil for 2 minutes, then add 1 tablespoon of capers and the strips of head cheese, mixing well as you add them. Cook gently for 1 to 2 minutes, until the head cheese melts.

… Then add the red onion wedges and stir in gently.

… Drain the pasta, add it into the casserole dish, and stir.

… Add the chopped onion stalks. Drizzle with a little olive oil and 4 full tablespoons of the onion vinegar. Stir well to coat the pasta.

… Transfer to a hot dish or serve straight from the casserole dish.

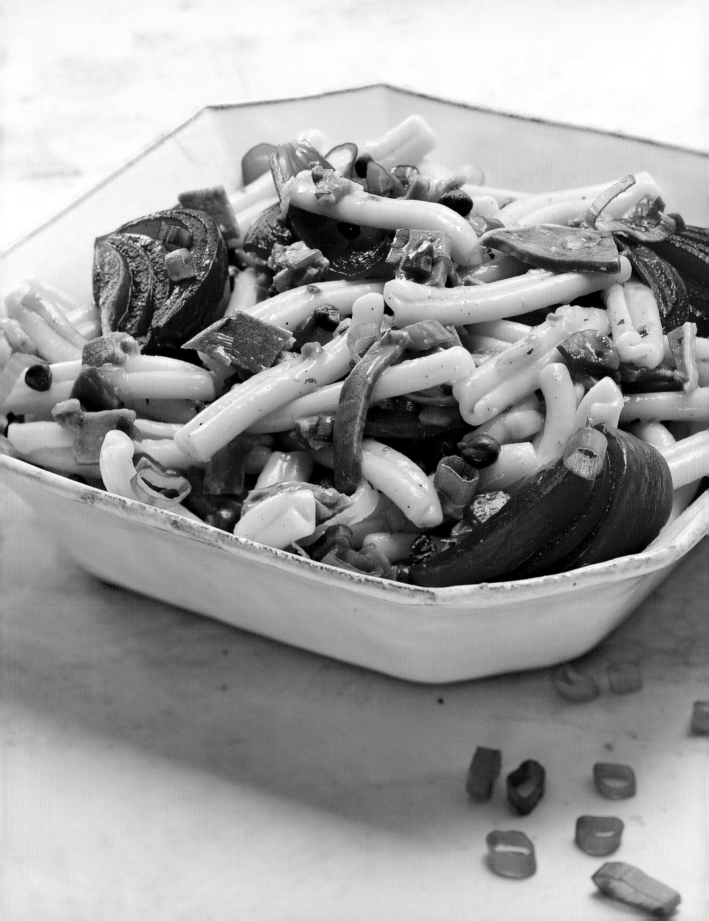

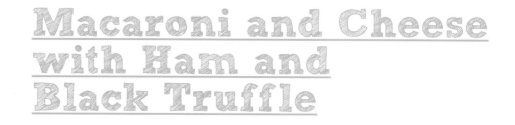

Macaroni and Cheese with Ham and Black Truffle

AD— A sophisticated take on childhood macaroni cheese and ham without breaking the bank (a small can of truffle shavings is not expensive). Make sure the serving dish is nice and hot.

PN— Most of the alcohol from the cognac and port evaporates on cooking, so you can also serve this macaroni to children. A good opportunity to educate their taste buds with a dish that is also well balanced, with carbohydrates, vegetable and animal protein, and calcium.

… Serves 4 to 6

… Cut 3½ ounces of mild ham and 2 ounces of Gruyère or Emmental cheese into small dice.

… Peel, wash, and thinly slice 2 scallions.

… Cook 8 ounces of macaroni in salted boiling water (according to the time stated on the package).

… While this is cooking, drain the contents of 1 small can of black truffle trimmings, taking care to preserve the liquid.

… Cut 3½ tablespoons of butter into small pieces and melt in a small pan. Add the truffle trimmings and cook for just 1 minute.

… Add 1 teaspoon of cognac and 1 teaspoon of ruby port, stir, and reduce slightly, then add the reserved truffle liquid and the sliced scallions.

… Drain the macaroni and transfer to a hot serving dish.

… Add the truffle butter and half of the diced ham and Gruyère, and mix well.

… Sprinkle the rest of the ham and cheese on top and serve immediately.

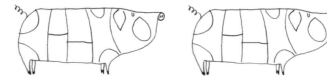

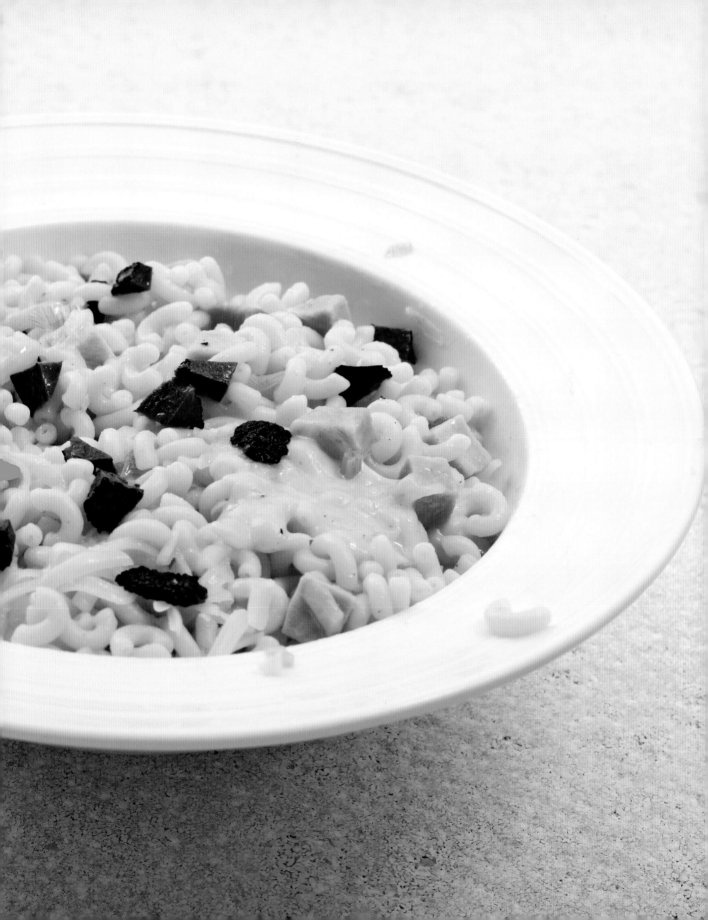

Orecchiette with Garden Peas

AD— This recipe can easily be made with other types of pasta than orecchiette. You can also vary the aromatic herbs, using rosemary or savory, for example.
PN— When peas are out of season, use frozen ones. They have the same nutritional value as fresh peas. Add them to the casserole dish a little sooner, as they take slightly longer to cook than fresh peas.

… Serves 4

… Cut 3½ ounces of pancetta into very small lardons. Peel 1 white onion and cut into 8 wedges. Heat 3 cups of chicken stock (page 10).

… Heat a flameproof casserole dish with a drop of olive oil and melt the lardons for 2 minutes. Add the onion wedges and cook over low heat for 3 minutes without allowing to color.

… Add 8 ounces of orecchiette to the casserole dish and stir several times to coat with fat. Then pour in 1 or 2 ladles of chicken stock to come halfway up the pasta. Pick the leaves from 2 sprigs of thyme, add them, and stir well.

… Cook gently until the orecchiette have absorbed the liquid. Add stock little by little as it is absorbed by the pasta, stirring well each time.

… It takes 15 or 20 minutes for the pasta to cook. After 10 minutes, add 12 ounces of shelled garden peas and mix well.

… When the pasta is cooked (taste to check and adjust the time accordingly), pour in 5 tablespoons of meat or roast chicken juices and stir.

… Adjust the seasoning, add a splash of olive oil, and stir again to coat the pasta.

… Serve in the casserole dish or arrange on plates and finish with a generous twist of freshly ground black pepper.

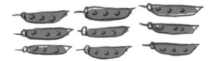

Touring La Bastide de Moustiers with Sarah, the director.

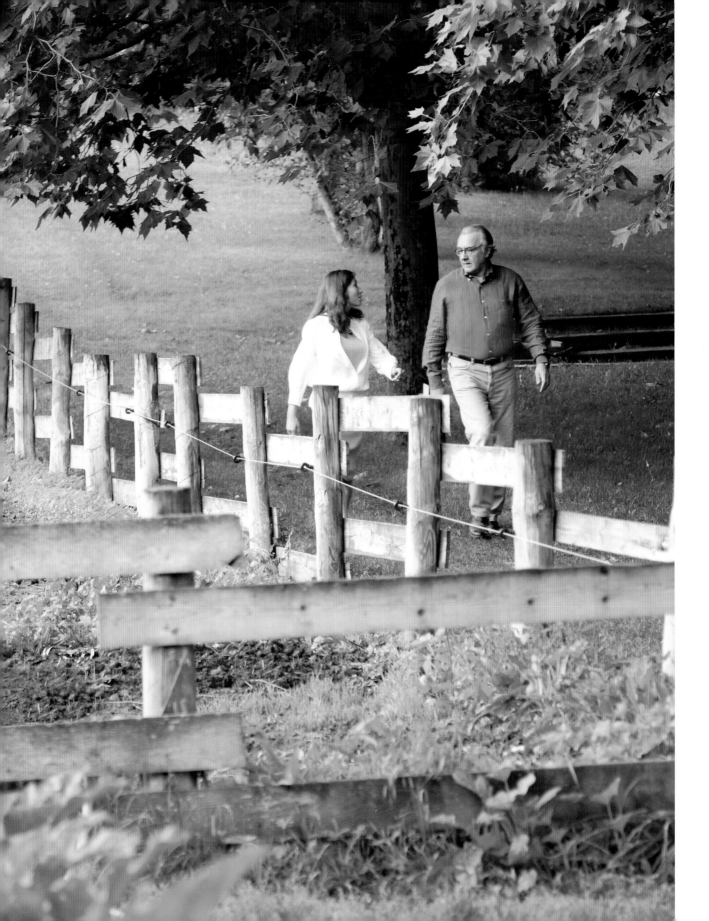

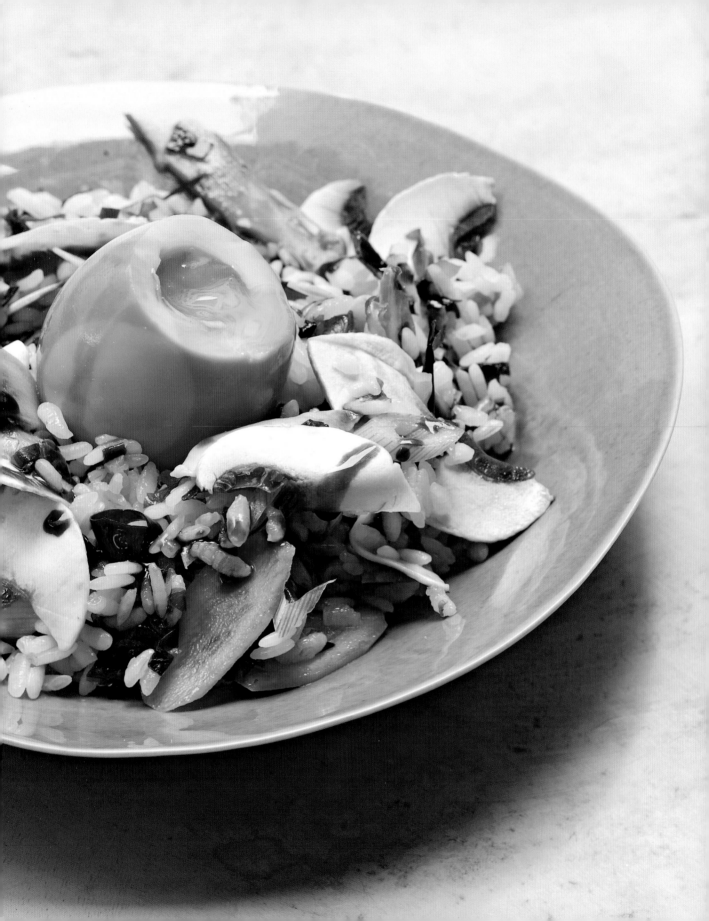

Steamed Rice with Marinated Soft-Boiled Eggs

... Serves 4

Prepare the marinated eggs

... Immerse 4 eggs in boiling water for 6 minutes. Allow to cool, then shell.

... Peel and chop 2 garlic cloves and 2 inches of ginger. Place in a bowl along with 3 tablespoons of wasabi (keep aside one small teaspoonful). Add 1 cup of soy sauce, 5 tablespoons of aromatic vinegar, and 5 tablespoons of water, stirring well to dissolve the wasabi. Immerse the eggs in this marinade and set aside for 2 hours at room temperature.

Prepare the rice

... Rinse 10 ounces of sushi rice in a sieve, then pour into a large bowl, cover with water, and leave to soak until the rice grains are nice and white.

... Boil water in the pot of a couscoussier or steamer. Drain the rice and spread it evenly in the steamer basket. Cover and cook for 15 to 20 minutes, then turn off the heat and leave the rice to swell in the basket for about 10 minutes.

Prepare the seaweed and sliced vegetables

... While the rice is cooking, soak 1 tablespoon of seaweed in fresh water to eliminate the salt and then slice. Clean 2 large mushrooms, and peel and wash 1 carrot with its top and 4 green asparagus spears. Cut the asparagus tips into 3- to 4-inch lengths. Cut all these vegetables into thin slices with a mandoline and set aside.

Make the sauce

... Take a large ladleful of the egg marinade and strain it through a tea strainer. In a bowl or sauce boat, mix with the reserved teaspoon of wasabi and ¼ cup of olive oil.

To finish your dish

... When the rice is cooked, transfer it to a bowl, then lift and turn it over several times with a spatula, while adding 5 tablespoons of white wine vinegar, the seaweed, and sliced vegetables. Arrange on a serving dish.

... Drain the eggs of their marinade and place them on top of the rice. Serve the sauce separately.

AD— There's no need to add salt to the rice. It gets enough seasoning from the seaweed and the sauce. PN— An excellent cocktail of animal and vegetable protein (eggs and rice), slow carbohydrates (rice), fiber, and vitamins from the vegetables. A fine nutritional balance! You do need a salad or starter, though, to up your quota of vegetables.

Pumpkin Rice

AD— To preserve the juices
and flavors, avoid stirring
the pumpkin in the early stages
of cooking. Remove the garlic
skin before serving.

PN— Pumpkin is wonderfully
rich in antioxidant carotenoids,
which are good for the skin, heart,
and all the cells of the body.
It also provides fiber and quite
a lot of vitamins.

... Serves 4

... Preheat the oven to 350°F.

... Peel 1 large slice of pumpkin and cut the flesh into ½-inch cubes. Similarly cut 1 slice of bacon ¼ inch thick.

... Place them in an ovenproof dish with 4 tablespoons of olive oil and 4 garlic cloves unpeeled and crushed, add salt, mix well, and put in the oven for 25 minutes.

... Take out the dish, add 8 ounces of Spanish short-grain rice, sprinkling it evenly, and return to the oven for 2 minutes. Then add one and a half times the rice's volume in cold water and return it to the oven for 20 minutes, checking the cooking of the rice regularly. If it is drying too quickly, add a little more water.

... While the rice is cooking, heat a nonstick skillet and gently toast 2 tablespoons of hulled pumpkin seeds. Cool on a kitchen towel, crush, and mix with 2 tablespoons of grated Parmesan.

... When the rice is cooked, take out the dish and sprinkle the seed and Parmesan mixture over the surface, add freshly ground black pepper, and return to the oven on the top rack to brown. Serve nice and hot in the cooking pot.

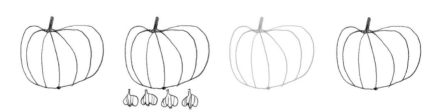

Plain Risotto

… Serves 4

… Peel and finely dice 1 white onion. Heat 2 cups of chicken stock (page 10).

… Heat 2 tablespoons of olive oil and 1 tablespoon of butter (2 tablespoons in total required for recipe) in a sauté pan. Add the onion and sweat for 3 minutes without letting it color. Add a little salt.

… Add 6 ounces of Arborio or Carnaroli rice and cook for 2 minutes over very low heat, stirring until it becomes translucent and all the grains are coated.

… Add ⅓ cup of dry white wine and wait until it is completely absorbed.

… Then pour in hot chicken stock to cover and stir.

… When the rice has absorbed this stock, pour in a little more and continue to cook, stirring until it is absorbed.

… Repeat the process until the rice is fully cooked, 18 to 20 minutes. Check the seasoning.

… Off the heat, add the last 1 tablespoon of butter and stir it in until melted.

… Then do the same with ½ cup of grated Parmesan. Serve immediately.

AD— Short-grain rice is indispensable for risotto! But these two, Arborio and Carnaroli (which come from Piedmont in Italy), are really the cook's favorites. They produce an incomparably creamy texture. Vialone Nano is also excellent, but harder to come by.

PN— Rice is one of the few grains that has no gluten. It takes only half an hour to prepare this succulent starchy dish, to which you can add all kinds of vegetables and/or shellfish to create a complete meal.

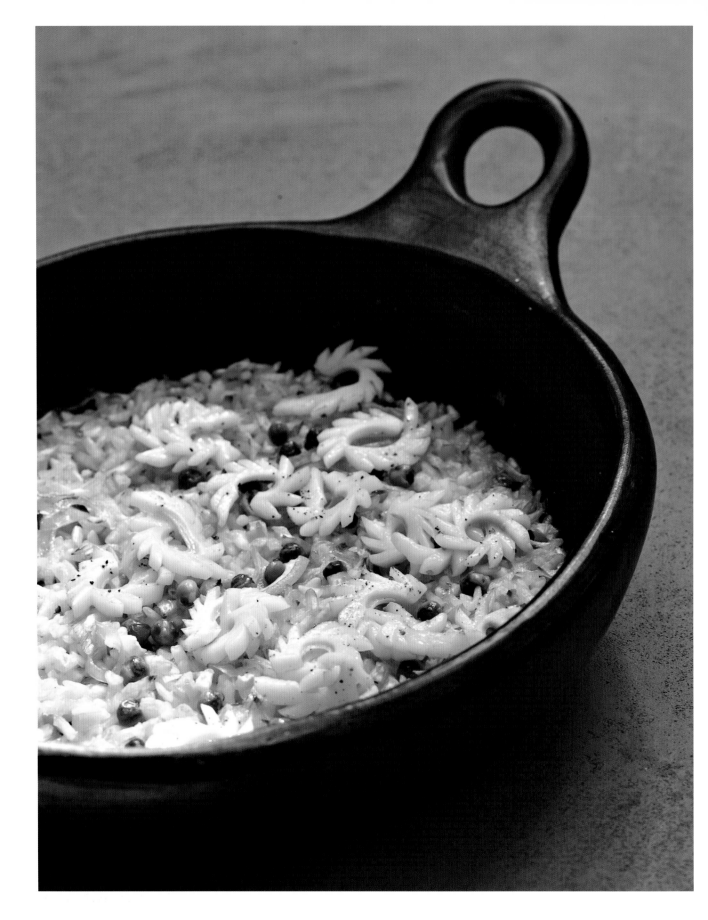

Spanish Rice with Squid and Lemon

… Serves 4

Prepare the squid

… Separate the body and head of 1 squid weighing approximately 12 ounces. Then separate the tentacles and clean out the inside of the body. Rub off the small membranes with coarse salt, then rinse with plenty of water.

… Thinly slice the tentacles.

… With a very sharp knife, cut the skin of the body in a lattice pattern, then cut it into medium-size slivers. Set all the squid aside in a cool place.

Prepare the rice

… Preheat the oven to 350°F.

… Peel and dice 1 white onion. Rinse half a bulb of fennel and dice very finely (brunoise).

… Cut half an unwaxed lemon into wedges.

… Heat an ovenproof dish with ¼ cup of olive oil and sweat the diced vegetables and squid tentacles for approximately 2 minutes, stirring.

… Add 12 ounces of short-grain Spanish or Italian rice and a pinch of salt and cook for 2 minutes over low heat, stirring. Then add the lemon wedges and ¾ cup of shelled fresh peas, then add approximately 2 cups of cold water.

… Spread the rice evenly over the surface and put in the oven for 20 minutes. Check the progress of the rice regularly and if it's becoming too dry, add a little water. When it's cooked, the rice should be soft in the center of the dish and crunchy around the edge.

… Then heat a skillet with a drop of olive oil and sauté the slivers of squid for just 10 seconds. Arrange them over the rice, and add 4 basil leaves and a twist of freshly ground black pepper.

… Serve nice and hot in the cooking dish.

AD— Round-grain Italian (riso della Zelata) or Spanish (arroz bomba) rice has the ability to absorb a lot of liquid and swell up considerably while remaining quite firm. It is important not to rinse it before cooking.

PN— Rice and squid provide a good measure of protein, so there's no need for additional meat or fish. Serve with a vegetable starter, a cheese or other dairy product, and a piece of fruit, and you will have a well balanced meal.

Steamed Rice and Spring Vegetables

AD— This is an essentially Mediterranean dish, and all the flavors are concentrated when you steam it like this. Be careful with the salt, as you will need less if you're using chicken stock and more if you're using water.

PN— Yes, very much a Mediterranean dish, and with all the basic ingredients of the Mediterranean diet that is so good for your health: grains, vegetables, and olive oil.

… Serves 4

… Scrape and wash 16 small green asparagus spears, cut the tips into 2½-inch lengths, and slice all the tender part of the bases into rounds. Remove the outer leaves and wash 1 small leek and cut into rounds. Cut 16 runner beans into 1-inch lengths.

… Trim 4 young violet "poivrade" artichokes, cut into halves or quarters, remove the chokes, and sprinkle with lemon juice.

… Peel and wash 4 small spring onions and cut into rounds (don't throw away the stalks). Prepare 1½ cups of shelled fresh peas and 1½ cups of shelled fava beans.

… Preheat the oven to 350°F.

… Heat 2 cups of chicken stock (page 10) or water in a pan.

… Heat a flameproof casserole dish with 2 tablespoons of olive oil. Add all the vegetables together, season with salt, and cook on the stovetop for 2 minutes, stirring gently.

… Add 7 ounces of basmati rice and stir until it is translucent. Pour in the chicken stock (or water), stir briefly, taste, and correct the seasoning.

… Cover the casserole dish with a lid and put in the oven for 17 minutes.

… Then take it out and leave to rest for 10 minutes.

… Rinse a quarter of a salt-preserved lemon (page 15) and slice thinly. Cut off the tips of the onion stalks you set aside and chop the rest. Rinse and thoroughly dry a handful of arugula.

… Gently stir the rice and vegetables, and add the preserved lemon, onion stalks, and arugula along with a splash of olive oil. Serve immediately in the casserole dish or on individual plates.

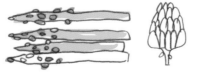

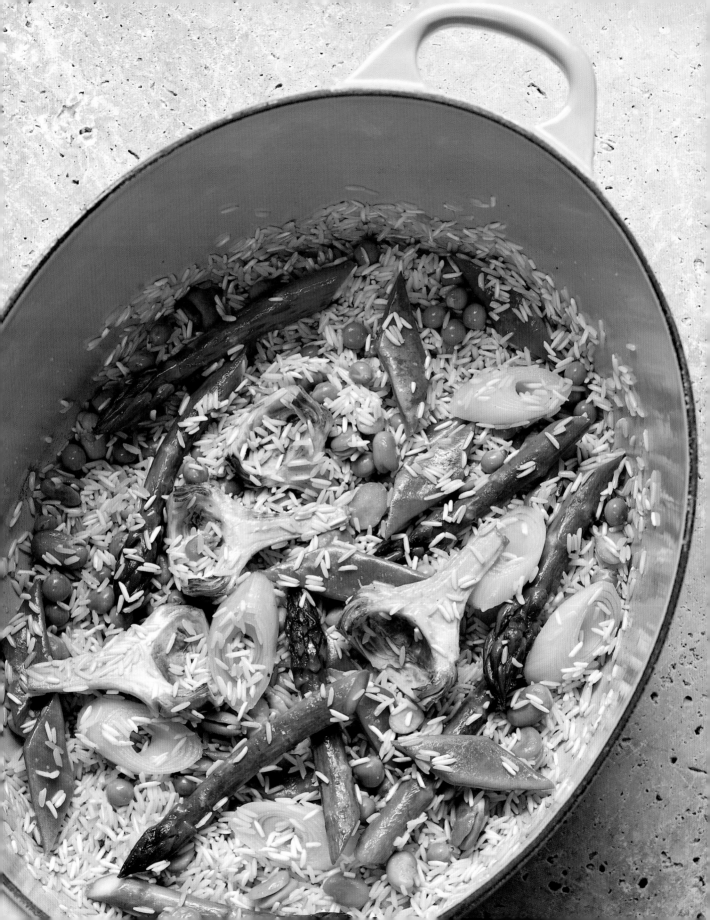

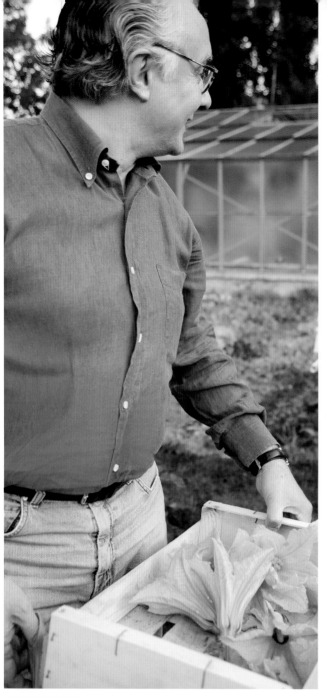
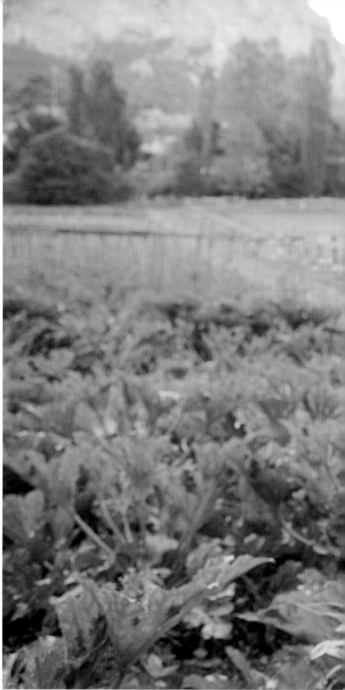
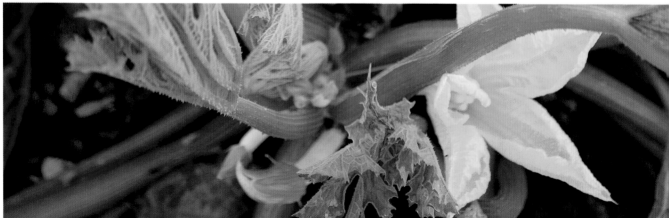

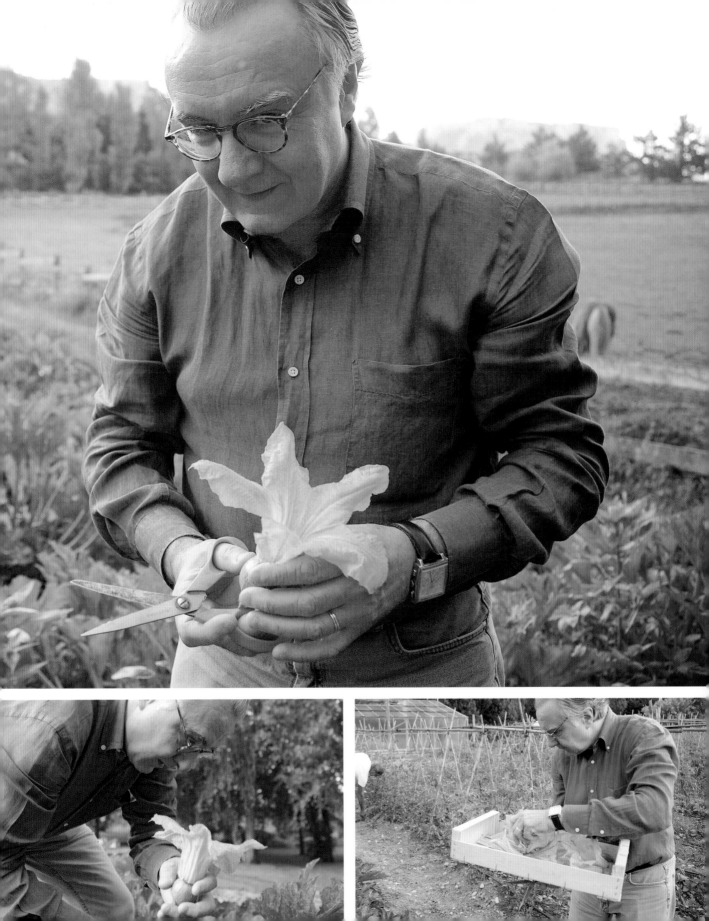

Casserole of Quinori, Crunchy Vegetables, and Herb Pesto

AD— Quinori is a mix of red quinoa, long-grain brown rice, chickpeas, white quinoa, and sesame seeds.

PN— A superb cocktail of vitamins, minerals, fiber, slow carbohydrates, and vegetable protein, without a trace of gluten. This dish is highly nutritious, so there's no need for meat or fish on the menu, but a little cheese (to complete the protein) and a piece of fruit would be welcome.

———

If quinori cannot be found, quinoa may be used instead, but reduce the quinoa's cooking time in the oven from 15 minutes to 12. Both argan oil and oat milk may be found at health food stores or online.

… Serves 4

Prepare the vegetables

… Peel and wash 2 young carrots with tops, 4 spring onions, 5 green asparagus spears, 12 radishes, and 1 small tender fennel bulb. Cut the asparagus tips into lengths of about 3 inches. Slice all the vegetables into the finest possible slices with a mandoline or a vegetable peeler and keep cool.

Cook the quinori

… Preheat the oven to 325°F. Peel and chop 1 white onion. Rinse 1 cup of quinori.

… Heat a flameproof casserole dish with 2 tablespoons of olive oil and sweat the onion for 2 minutes, stirring. Add the quinori and stir. Then add twice its volume in water (2 cups) and stir again. Bring to a boil, then cover and put in the oven for 15 minutes. Then add ¼ cup of chopped cooked tomatoes (page 21) to the quinori and return the casserole dish to the oven for an additional 5 minutes.

Prepare the herb pesto

… While the quinori is cooking, wash and pick the leaves of 2 sprigs of chervil, 2 sprigs of cilantro, 3 sprigs of parsley, and 3 sprigs of basil. Peel and mince 1 garlic clove.

… Put in a blender with 2 tablespoons of pine nuts, 2 tablespoons of argan oil, and 6 tablespoons of oat milk.

… Blend until the mixture is nice and smooth. Add salt and freshly ground black pepper and pour the pesto into a sauce boat.

To finish your dish

… Combine the sliced vegetables in a large bowl and season with 2 teaspoons of olive oil, a pinch of salt, and 3 twists of freshly ground black pepper.

… Take the casserole dish out of the oven and add the vegetables to the top. Cover immediately and transfer the casserole dish to the table along with the sauce boat containing the herb pesto.

… Lift the lid so that everyone can enjoy all the aromas. Then delicately stir the vegetables into the grain and serve. Diners can then help themselves to the herb pesto.

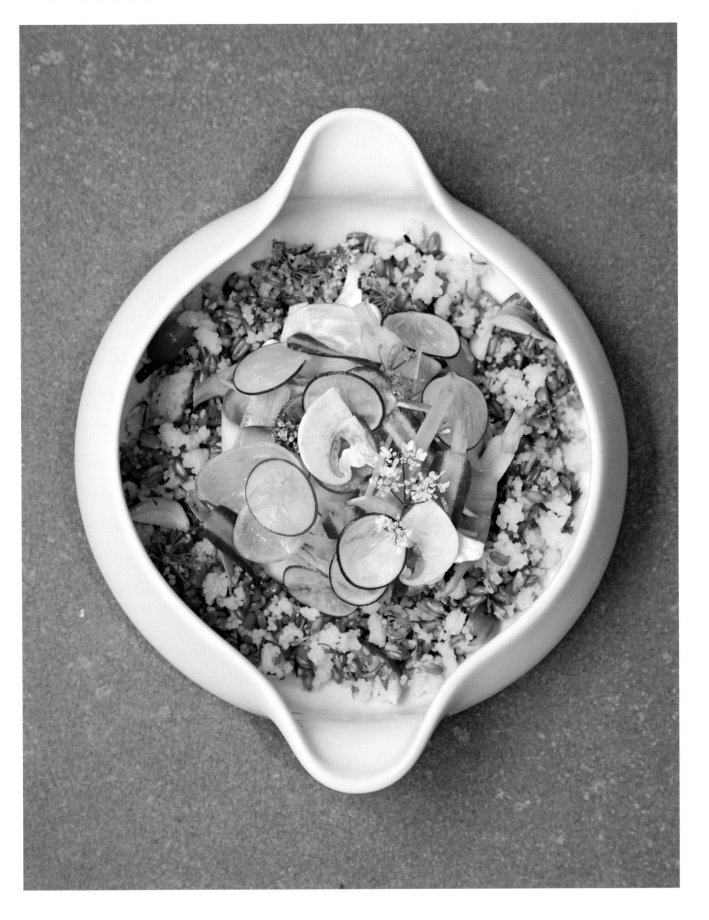

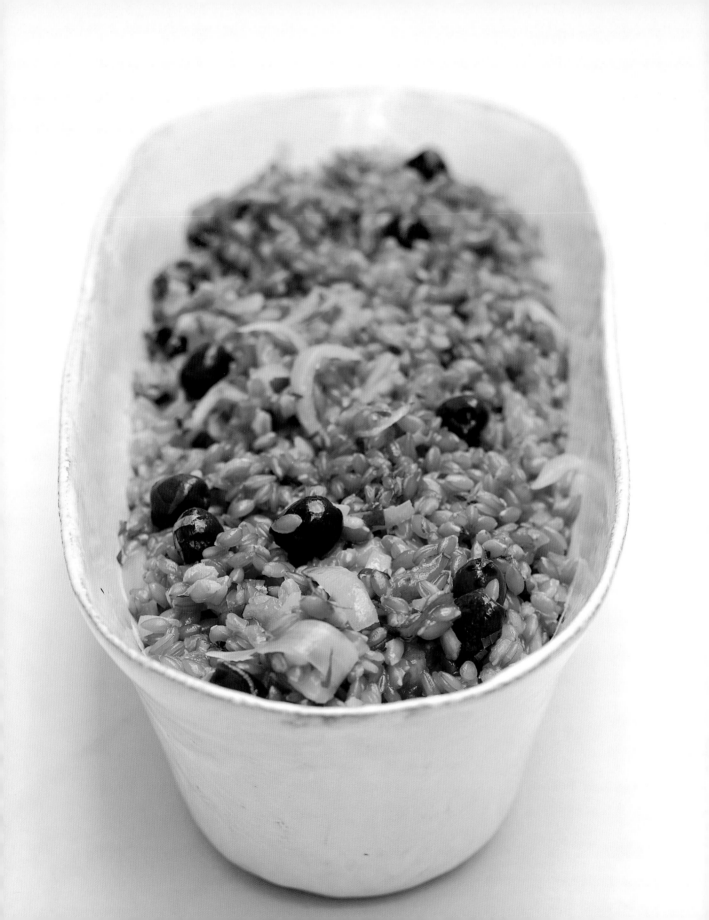

Einkorn and Pepper Casserole

… Serves 4

<u>The day before</u>

… Put 12 ounces of einkorn to soak in a bowl and keep in a cold place for 12 hours.

<u>On the day</u>

… Peel 1 small yellow pepper, 1 small red pepper, 1 small green pepper, and 1 white onion and cut into long thin strips (approximately 1½ by ⅛ inch).

… Peel and mince 1 garlic clove.

… Heat 1 quart of chicken stock (page 10) in a saucepan.

… Heat a flameproof casserole dish with 2 tablespoons of olive oil and sweat the onion and peppers with a pinch of salt for 4 minutes. Stir frequently.

… Add the einkorn, garlic, and a sprig of basil (2 sprigs required in total for recipe). Stir and cook for 1 minute, then add ½ cup of white wine. Allow to reduce almost entirely, then pour in chicken stock to cover. Simmer, adding more chicken stock in stages as it is absorbed.

… Taste and stop cooking when the einkorn is how you like it, slightly firm or softer. Adjust the seasoning.

… While the einkorn is cooking, pick the leaves from the reserved sprig of basil and chop finely.

… When the einkorn is cooked, remove the casserole dish from the heat, grate ¾ ounce of Parmesan directly into it, and stir gently, adding 2 tablespoons of olive oil and 2 tablespoons of pitted black olives. The dish should be sufficiently moist and "creamy."

… Add the chopped basil and serve straight from the casserole dish.

AD— Serve this dish as a starter or as an accompaniment to a grilled filet of beef or a fish such as tuna or swordfish.
PN— Like all grains, einkorn contains a lot of carbohydrates but it's much richer than others in protein, fiber, minerals of all kinds, and B vitamins.

———

Einkorn was one of the earliest cultivated forms of wheat. It can often be found at health food or organic stores or sourced online. Spelt may be substituted in place of the einkorn, but the cooking time should be increased by about 5 minutes.

Baby Vegetables Stuffed with Millet

AD— Use your imagination
with the stuffing, adding olives,
anchovies, cilantro, and so on to
the millet. Other vegetables such as
artichokes or peppers work well
with a stuffing of this kind.
PN— A meatless stuffing based on
grains! This is very well balanced
nutritionally and will satisfy
any vegetarian urges. You can
increase the numbers or stuff
larger vegetables.

… Serves 4

… Wash and dry 8 round zucchini weighing 2 ounces, 8 mini eggplants weighing 1½ ounces, 8 vine tomatoes weighing 2 ounces, and 8 spring onions with stalks weighing ½ ounce.

… Cut the top off each vegetable and set aside. Also set aside the stalks of the onions.

… With a small spoon, remove the flesh from all the vegetables and put in a bowl.

… Heat a saucepan of salted water and, when it boils, immerse the emptied zucchini, eggplants, and onions and their tops for 5 minutes. Drain.

… Clean 10 ounces of mushrooms and chop roughly. Also roughly chop the flesh of the vegetables. Slice the onion stalks.

… Put this mixture in a sauté pan heated with a splash of olive oil, add salt, and sweat for 6 minutes. Then add 1¼ cups of millet, stir well, and cook for an additional minute. Gradually add 1½ cups of chicken stock (2½ cups required in total for recipe) (page 10) in stages as it is absorbed by the millet. Cook for a total of about 15 minutes.

… While it is cooking, snip the leaves from a small bunch of basil. Peel and chop 1 garlic clove. Roughly chop 8 segments of tomato confit (page 16) and add these ingredients to the sauté pan.

… Stir, adjust the seasoning with salt and freshly ground black pepper, and take the sauté pan off the heat.

… Preheat the oven to 225°F.

… With a small spoon, stuff each vegetable with this mixture. Place them in a baking dish and replace their tops.

… Add a splash of olive oil and the reserved 1 cup of chicken stock to the dish and put in the oven for 1 hour. Serve in the dish.

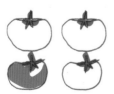

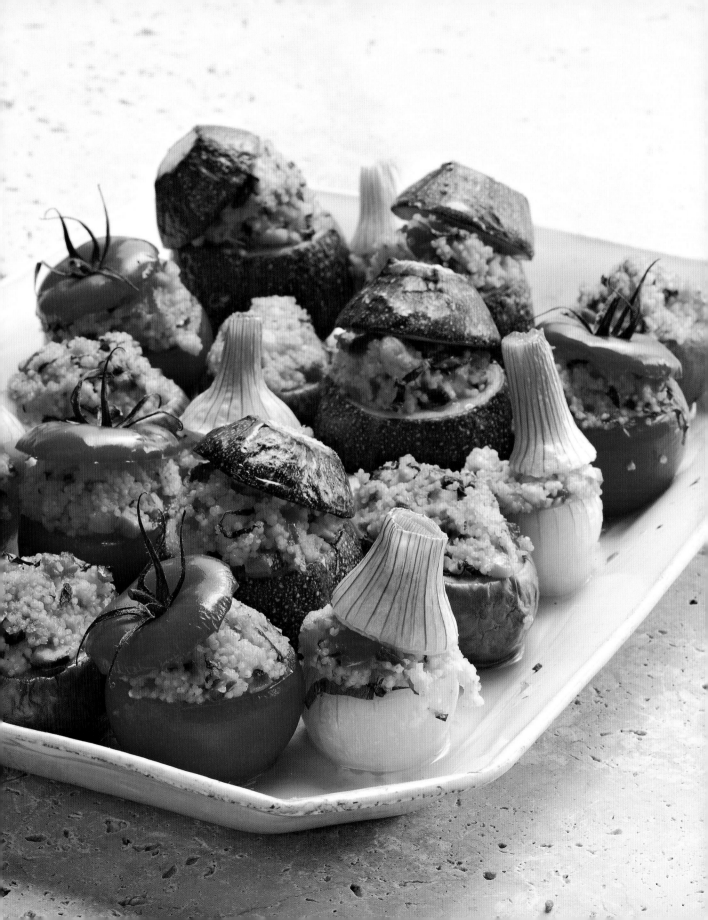

Deviled Oysters with Quinoa

AD— You can of course open the oysters in the traditional way, but then you must strain their water in a conical strainer lined with a paper cone to remove any small pieces of shell.

PN— It may look like a grain, but quinoa is not a true cereal; it's the fruit of an annual herbaceous plant. But it has all the qualities of a grain and more besides, because it is a lot richer in protein.

… Serves 4

… Blanch and seed 2 tomatoes and cut into small pieces.

… Peel and wash 2 white onions with stalks, then slice both stalks and bulbs.

… Peel and chop 1 inch of ginger. Peel and thinly slice 1 garlic clove.

… Boil a little water in the pot of a couscoussier or steamer, place 12 oysters in the upper basket, and take them out once they open. Allow to cool a little, then remove them from the shells, taking care to reserve their water. Place in a dish, drizzle with thick soy sauce, and leave to marinate.

… In a flameproof casserole dish, brown 1 thin slice of bacon on both sides, then remove and set aside.

… In its place put the tomatoes, ginger, sliced onion bulbs, and 2 pinches of Piment d'Espelette or hot paprika and sweat for 3 minutes. Add 3 tablespoons of wine vinegar and deglaze thoroughly, then allow to reduce slightly.

… Add 1½ cups of rinsed mixed red and white quinoa and 3 cups of water. Add the reserved oyster water, stir well, cover, and cook over low heat for 12 minutes.

… In the meantime, in a dry skillet, toast 2 tablespoons of sesame seeds. Cut the browned bacon into small lardons.

… When the quinoa is cooked, add 2 tablespoons of olive oil, the lardons, and the sliced green parts of the onions. Then transfer this mixture to a hot dish.

… Lightly drain the oysters and arrange them on top. Sprinkle with the toasted sesame seeds and serve immediately.

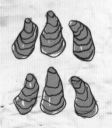

Steamed Fonio with Asparagus and Morels

… Serves 4

Prepare the fonio and morels

… Put 5 ounces of fonio in a sieve and rinse well under running water. Transfer to a bowl, cover well with water, and leave to swell for 20 minutes.

… In the meantime, remove the stems from 7 ounces of fresh morels, then wash the caps in several changes of warm water to get rid of any traces of sand. Dry in a salad spinner. Cut any large mushrooms in half.

… Rinse a bundle of spring onions with stalks, dice the stalks (and set aside), and cut the bulbs into rounds.

… Peel, remove the germ at the center, and finely slice 4 cloves of garlic. Rinse, dry, and chop the leaves of a small bunch of parsley.

Cook the morels and the fonio

… Heat a sauté pan with 3 tablespoons of olive oil. Put in the onion rounds and garlic slices and sweat for 2 minutes, stirring. Add the morels, salt lightly, and cook for an additional 4 minutes.

… In the meantime, heat 1¼ cups of chicken stock (page 10).

… Drain the fonio and add it. Stir well and cook for just 1 minute. Then pour in enough chicken stock to cover, simmer gently (just below a boil) until it is absorbed, then continue to add more: The fonio should cook for about 20 minutes. Then cover the skillet and leave to rest for 10 minutes.

Prepare the asparagus

… While the fonio is cooking, wash and peel 1 bundle of green asparagus, then cut the tips into 4-inch lengths. Heat a sauté pan with a splash of olive oil and cook the spears for 5 to 6 minutes with the lid on.

To finish your dish

… Fluff the fonio grains with a fork and add the onion stalks and chopped parsley.

… Transfer to a dish, arrange the asparagus on top, and, shave ¾ ounce of Parmesan with a vegetable peeler and sprinkle the shavings on top. Serve immediately.

AD— Fonio is an herbaceous plant with small grains. It has been grown in West Africa for centuries, and is now available in specialty grocers, often sold through the fair trade system. It is cooked in a similar way to rice.

PN— A grain rich in carbohydrates, fonio also contains protein but is gluten free. Its nutritional composition is similar to rice, although fonio is richer in minerals.

If fonio cannot be found, quinoa may be substituted; rinse the quinoa well before cooking, but skip the soaking step.

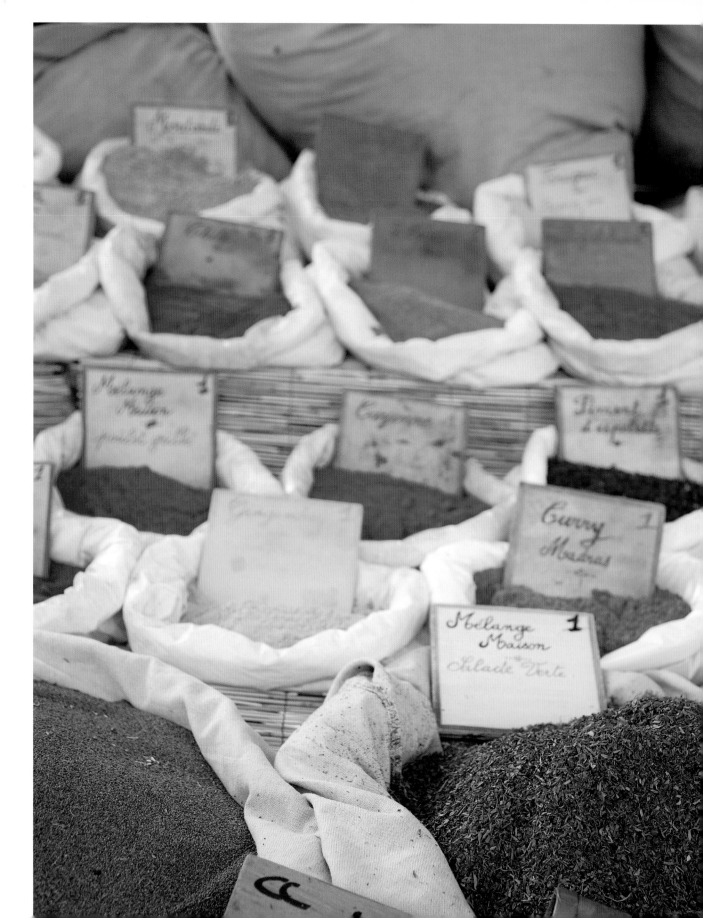

Bulgur, Fresh Harissa, Peppers, and Cucumber

… Serves 4

Prepare the bulgur

… Add 2 cups of bulgur to 2⅓ cups of boiling salted water and cook until all the water is absorbed (approximately 12 minutes). Then add 2 tablespoons of olive oil and mix well. Season with ½ teaspoon of ground cumin, ½ teaspoon of ground coriander, and 1 tablespoon of sherry vinegar. Transfer to a large bowl and refrigerate.

Prepare the fresh harissa

… Pick about 15 leaves from 4 sprigs of cilantro. Pick about 12 leaves from 4 sprigs of mint (set aside the rest of these herbs). Chop them and place in a bowl.

… Peel and crush 1 garlic clove. Chop 1 bird's eye chile very finely.

… Add them to the bowl along with 1 tablespoon of olive oil, the juice of a quarter of a lemon, and some salt. Stir and put somewhere cool.

Prepare the pepper and cucumber salad

… Wash and peel 1 red bell pepper, 1 green bell pepper, and 1 yellow bell pepper with a vegetable peeler, remove the insides, and cut into very small dice (brunoise).

… Wash 1 cucumber and peel it in strips, leaving alternate strips unpeeled (a little green makes it more attractive). Cut in half and remove the seeds. Then cut into fine slivers.

… Combine all these vegetables in a bowl. Chop the remaining cilantro and mint leaves, add to the bowl, and set in a cool place.

To finish your dish

… Dress the pepper and cucumber salad with a drizzle of olive oil, a drizzle of lemon juice, salt, and freshly ground black pepper.

… Arrange the cold bulgur in the center of the dish. Surround it with the pepper and cucumber salad. Serve the harissa in a separate bowl.

AD— A typical Middle Eastern ingredient, bulgur is steamed, dried, and crushed wheat still containing the germ. Its method of production goes back four thousand years. Adapt the herbs to your own taste, using more or less cilantro or mint.

PN— This combination of grains and vegetables is perfectly balanced and rich in carbohydrates and vitamins of all kinds. There's nothing to stop you from adding tomatoes to the salad.

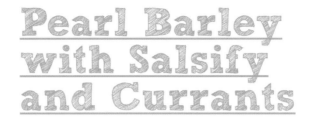

Pearl Barley with Salsify and Currants

AD— Protect your hands with disposable gloves when peeling the salsify; otherwise they will turn black. When peeled the salsify gives off a milk that oxidizes very quickly, which is also why you need lemon water.

PN— Salsify and barley are particularly high in fiber, but have few vitamins and minerals; this is made up for by the currants and onions and their tops, which are rich in nutrients.

… Serves 4

… Soak a small handful of currants in a bowl of water.

… Peel and wash a bundle of salsify, placing the salsify in water with the juice of 1 lemon as you go, then slice at an angle.

… Peel and wash 4 small spring onions with stalks, chop all the tender part of the stalks, and slice the bulbs. Crush 1 garlic clove without peeling it.

… Heat 5 cups of chicken stock (page 10) in a saucepan.

… Heat a splash of olive oil in a flameproof casserole dish, and roll the salsify in it along with the sliced onion bulbs and the garlic clove. Cover the casserole dish with a lid and cook over low heat for 5 minutes, until they are nice and golden.

… Add 1½ cups of pearl barley, stir, and cook for just 1 minute, then add ½ cup of white wine and let it absorb.

… Rinse half a salt-preserved lemon (page 15), cut into small slivers, and add to the casserole dish.

… Drain the currants and add them.

… Stir the mixture well and add a good ladleful of the chicken stock. Continue to cook for 30 minutes, adding more chicken stock as it is absorbed.

… Take the skin off the garlic clove. Add the chopped onion tops, and stir carefully for 1 or 2 minutes. Add salt and freshly ground black pepper to taste.

… Serve in the casserole dish or in a serving dish.

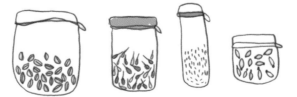

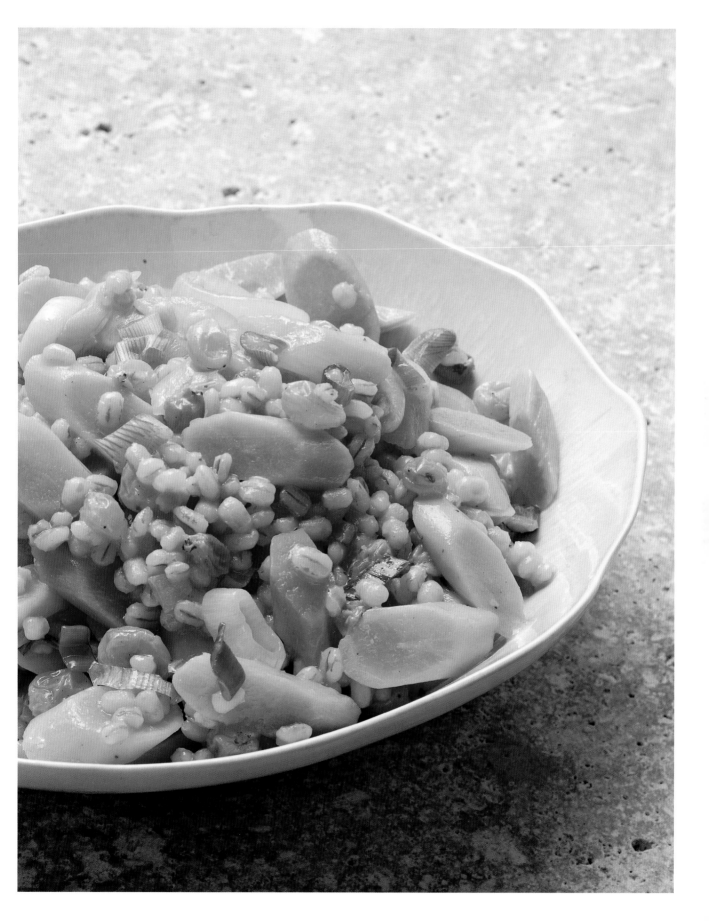

Millet, Porcini, and Smoked Duck

AD— When porcini are not in season, use large white mushrooms and prepare them in the same way, not forgetting to squeeze a little lemon juice over them.

PN— Millet is a cereal with very small seeds that has been cultivated in Africa and Asia for thousands of years. It is rich in carbohydrates but its protein does not contain gluten.

… Serves 4

… Separate all the fat and skin from half a smoked duck breast with a small knife and cut the fat and skin into small dice. Put in a flameproof casserole dish and brown until nice and crisp.

… Then remove most of the melted fat (keep one spoonful) with a tablespoon and throw it away.

… Put 1¼ cups of millet in the casserole dish, stir well, and color slightly. Then pour in 2 cups of chicken stock (page 10). Bring to a boil, cover, then lower the heat and simmer for about 20 minutes.

… In the meantime, thinly slice the duck meat.

… Cut the earthy base off 5 medium-size porcini, wash them briefly, dry the caps, and slice them.

… Pick the leaves off a small bunch of parsley, peel 2 garlic cloves, and chop them all together; set aside.

… When the millet is cooked, take the casserole dish off the heat and leave to rest for 10 minutes.

… In a skillet, heat 1 tablespoon of olive oil and sauté the mushroom slices for 2 to 3 minutes. Add salt and the chopped parsley and garlic. Add freshly ground black pepper.

… Spread out the millet in a flat dish, add the porcini with the parsley and garlic mixture and the slices of duck, then serve.

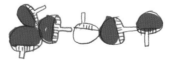

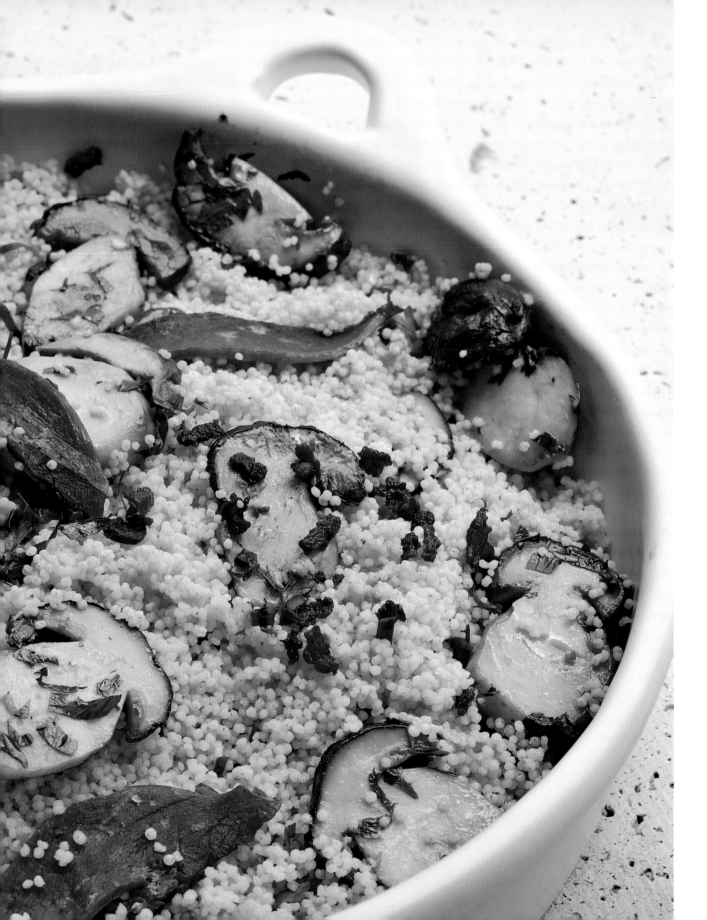

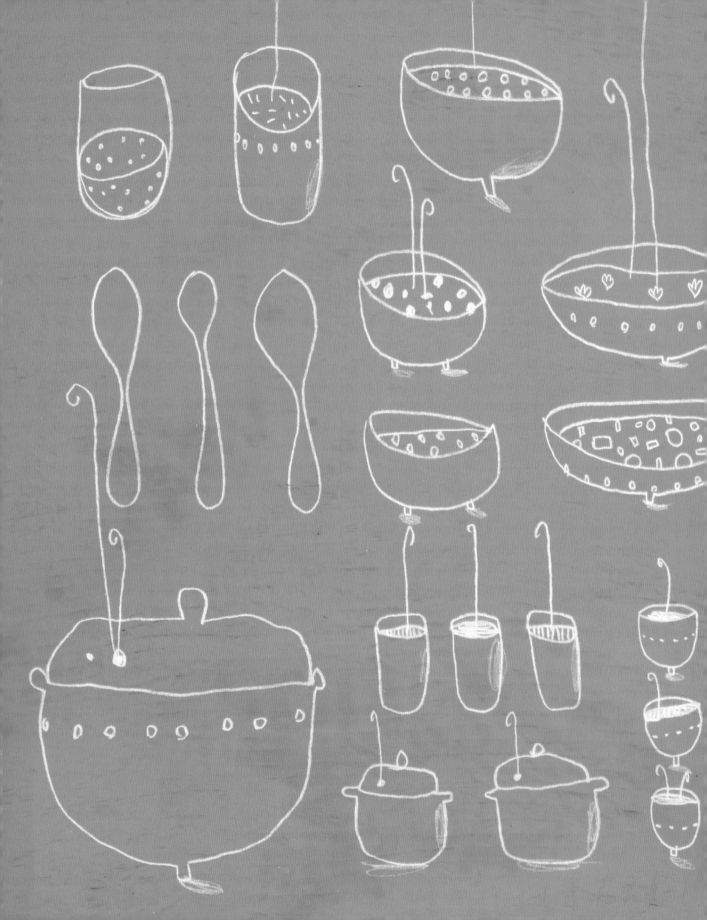

PN— Hot or cold, a soup should always feature on a dinner menu. Soups are an excellent way to eat vegetables. They keep you hydrated, they contribute to a feeling of satiation, and this makes them essential for a healthy nutritional balance.

AD— It's impossible to forget the soups of my childhood made from vegetables from the farm's kitchen garden. They're engraved on my memory, and they still inspire me. These soups find their way onto all my restaurant menus.

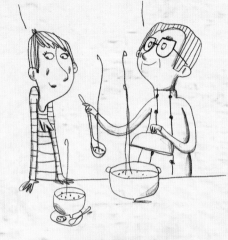

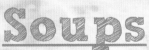

Cucumber and Yogurt Gazpacho with Fresh Mint and a Crisp Garnish

AD— Prepare the gazpacho in advance so that it's nice and cold, or put it in the freezer for 15 to 20 minutes. A useful tip is to cool your soup tureen or soup plates. PN— This gazpacho is rich in calcium thanks to the yogurt and milk, so it's really good for you! As for the tamarind, it is a laxative, which has its uses.

… Serves 4

Prepare the gazpacho

… Peel 2 cucumbers and remove all the seeds. Cut off about a third of one of them and set it aside. Chop the rest into small pieces.

… Halve 1 avocado, remove the pit, and scoop out the flesh with a small spoon.

… Peel and mince 1 garlic clove and 2 inches of ginger.

… Chop the leaves of a small bunch of mint and set aside 2 tablespoonfuls.

… Blend all these ingredients with 1 cup yogurt, ¾ cup of lowfat milk, 5 tablespoons of sherry vinegar, 2 to 3 tablespoons of tamarind puree, 1 pinch of Piment d'Espelette or hot paprika (2 pinches required in total for recipe), 1½ cups of cold water, and 3 tablespoons of olive oil for 1 to 2 minutes.

… Add salt and freshly ground black pepper and keep cold.

Prepare the crisp garnish

… Peel 1 Granny Smith apple. Cut it in half, remove the core, and chop the flesh into very small dice (brunoise), approximately ⅛ inch.

… Cut the reserved piece of cucumber in the same way.

… Put in a large bowl with the reserved chopped mint leaves. Add salt and freshly ground black pepper.

… Pour the soup into a tureen or soup plates. Scatter the crisp garnish over. Then sprinkle 1 pinch of Piment d'Espelette or hot paprika on top. Serve nice and cold.

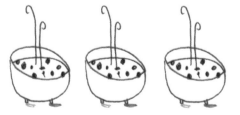

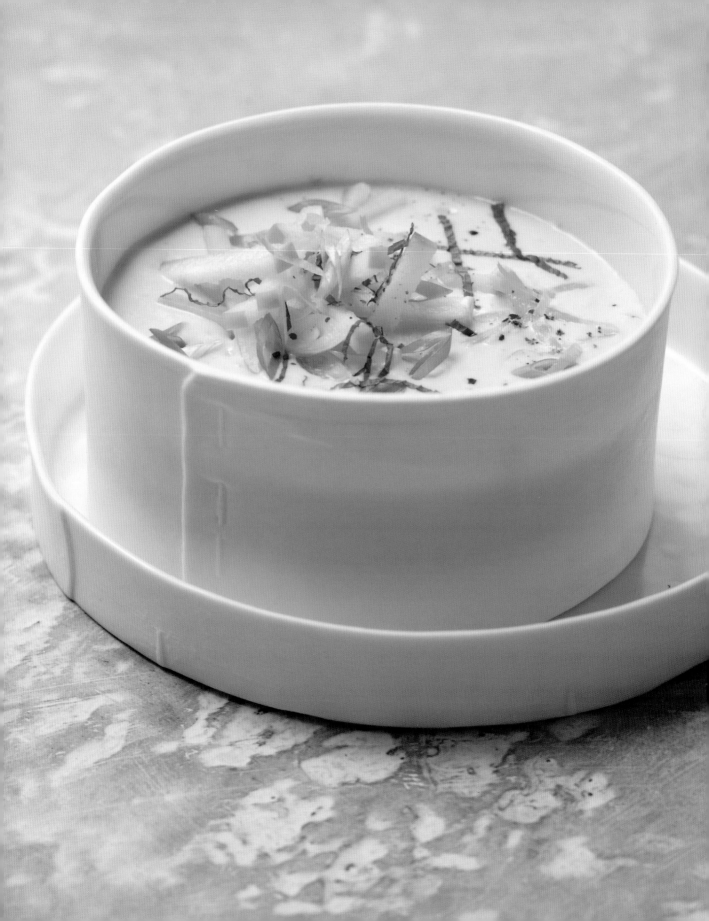

Chilled Lettuce and Watercress Soup with Crisp Vegetables

AD— Take time to pick the leaves from the watercress, because if you leave the stalks on you will find the soup difficult to blend. Putting it in ice water is vital in order to keep the color. Choose field-grown lettuce, which is much better than lettuce grown in a greenhouse.
PN— With the fortifying combination of iron, vitamin C (watercress and fennel), and folate (watercress, lettuce, and fennel), plus a lot of protective carotenoids (fennel and lettuce), this soup has something of a magic potion about it!

... Serves 4

Prepare the lettuce and watercress soup

... Peel 2 heads of lettuce and 4 bunches of watercress, wash in water with a dash of vinegar added, then pluck the leaves from the watercress. Keep 4 small bunches cool on a damp paper towel.

... Fill a large bowl with water and ice cubes. Put a saucepan of salted water on to boil. Immerse all of the remaining watercress and lettuce leaves in the boiling water for 3 minutes.

... Drain with a slotted spoon and refresh in the ice water.

... Drain and blend with a little of the cooking water, adjusting the amount to produce a smooth, creamy texture. Add salt and freshly ground black pepper and, when it has cooled down, refrigerate for at least 2 hours.

Prepare the vegetables

... Wash half a cucumber and half a fennel bulb, and cut into the smallest possible dice (1/16 inch).

... Wash 4 red radishes and remove the tips. Cut 4 fine shavings from one of the radishes with a vegetable peeler. Chop the rest into small dice, like the cucumber and fennel.

... Rinse and dry 1 bunch of chives. Cut off the tips (¾ to 1 inch) and set aside, then chop the rest.

... Put all the diced vegetables and the chopped chives into a bowl.

To finish

... Place 4 soup plates in the freezer to get nice and cold. Drain approximately 4 ounces of fresh soft goat cheese.

... Pour the soup into the bowls. Shape the fresh goat cheese into quenelles with a spoon and place them on top of the soup.

... Dot the top with a radish shaving and a small bunch of the reserved watercress, then arrange the diced vegetables all around. Sprinkle the chive tips on top.

Watercress Velouté with Sorrel

… Serves 4

Prepare the watercress velouté

… Wash 5 bunches of watercress and a small bunch of sorrel carefully in water with a dash of vinegar added. Separate the watercress leaves. Keep about 12 of them cool on a damp paper towel.

… Prepare a bowl of water and ice cubes.

… Heat a saucepan of lightly salted water and immerse the watercress and sorrel when at the boiling point. After 2 minutes, take out the leaves with a slotted spoon (don't drain the cooking water), and plunge them into the ice water to keep them nice and green. Drain in a colander.

… Blend the watercress and sorrel with a small ladle of the cooking water to produce a smooth soup.

… Adjust the seasoning, adding salt and freshly ground black pepper, and refrigerate.

Prepare the ricotta gnocchi

… Pour out the rest of the watercress cooking water, heat fresh water in the same saucepan, and add a little salt.

… Chop 3 sage leaves. In a bowl, mix them with 1 cup of ricotta, 1 tablespoon of all-purpose flour, 1 egg, and 2 pinches of salt. Shape the gnocchi with a teaspoon.

… Immerse them in the salted water, simmering just under a boil, for 4 to 5 minutes. Drain with a slotted spoon and place on paper towels.

To finish

… Melt 3 tablespoons of butter in a skillet, add the gnocchi, and reheat them gently, using a spoon to baste with butter.

… Take the watercress velouté out of the refrigerator, beat in 1 or 2 tablespoons of olive oil, and pour into soup bowls.

… Distribute the gnocchi on top of each bowl of soup and garnish with the reserved watercress leaves that you kept cool. Serve immediately.

AD— You might choose to make the watercress velouté on its own; it's delicious. But gnocchi are not really difficult or time-consuming to make, and they go so well together!
PN— Watercress is a source of minerals and all kinds of vitamins, giving you a real boost. And the ricotta provides a good dose of calcium, too.

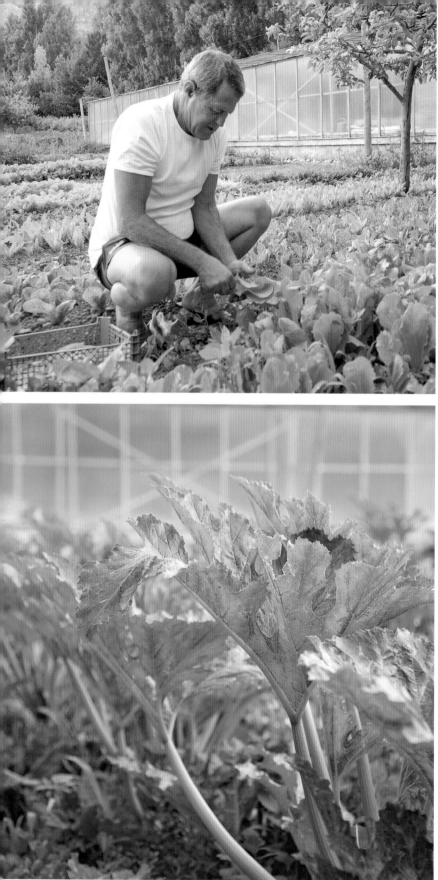

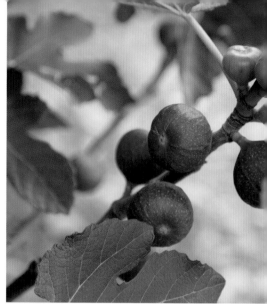

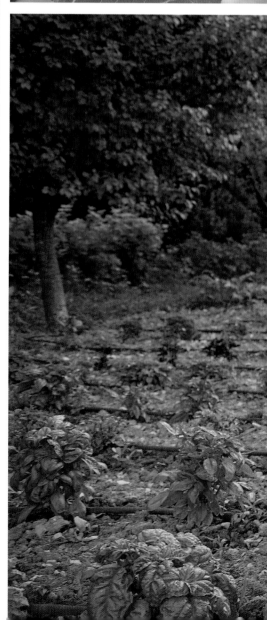

"The kitchen garden at La Bastide de Moustiers has been the proud realm of Gilbert, my gardener, for the last fifteen years. It is an explosion of scents and colors."

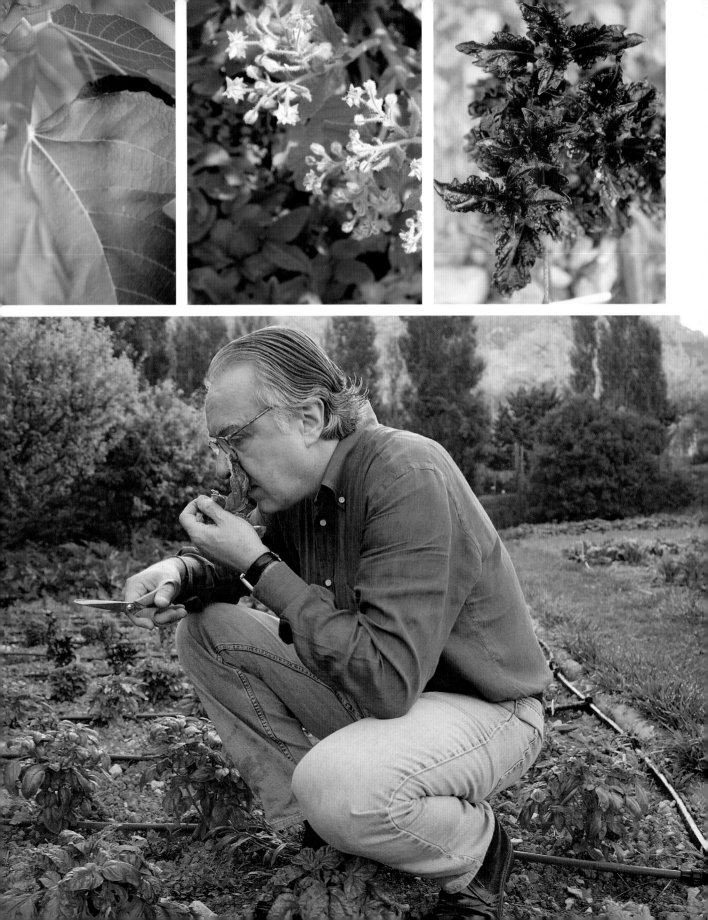

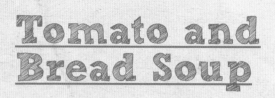

Tomato and Bread Soup

AD— San Marzano tomatoes are a very old variety. They are long, quite plump, fleshy, and firm. They are not easy to find, but they are well worth hunting down. Or look for another tasty variety.

PN— This soup is particularly rich in carbohydrates and fiber thanks to the whole-wheat bread. It is also bursting with antioxidants. You can eat it hot in winter, when you can make it with crushed canned tomatoes or frozen tomatoes.

… Serves 4

Prepare the tomatoes

… Blanch 16 beefsteak tomatoes and 2 San Marzano tomatoes.

… Empty their insides into a small bowl. Strain the juice and set aside.

… Chop the flesh of the beefsteak tomatoes into large cubes and the San Marzano into small dice. Refrigerate in a small bowl.

Make the soup

… Cut 14 ounces of stale whole-wheat bread into large dice and place in a bowl.

… Pour on the reserved tomato juice and 2 tablespoons of red wine vinegar and leave to swell.

… Preheat your oven to 325°F.

… Peel and mince 2 white onions and 4 garlic cloves. Detach about 10 leaves from 2 sprigs of basil and set aside.

… In a flameproof casserole dish with a splash of olive oil, sweat the onions over low heat for 5 minutes without letting them color. Add the garlic, stir for 30 seconds, then add the beefsteak tomatoes and a pinch of salt.

… Cook for 10 minutes, stirring occasionally.

… Add the bread and the rest of the basil and mix well. Cover the casserole dish with a lid and put in the oven for 30 to 40 minutes.

… When the soup is cooked, take the stems off the basil and crush the ingredients with a fork. Check the seasoning and add a little water if the soup is too thick. Allow to cool, then put in the refrigerator.

To serve

… Pour the cold soup into soup plates or a tureen.

… Sprinkle the diced San Marzano tomatoes on top, decorate with 2 ounces of pesto (page 36), and sprinkle with the reserved basil leaves.

Fava Bean Soup

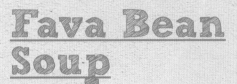

… Serves 4

… Shell 2¼ pounds of small fava beans suitable for eating whole in their pods, and keep the beans and pods separate.

… Pick out any very small beans (smaller than ½ inch) and set aside.

… Wash the pods and chop them as finely as possible with a knife.

… Crush the larger fava beans. Peel and mince 1 large white onion.

… Heat a flameproof casserole dish with a splash of olive oil and sweat the onion for 2 minutes. Add the pods and cook them over fairly high heat for 3 minutes, stirring frequently.

… Then add the large fava beans and cook for just 1 minute.

… Blend, adding 3 cups of chicken stock (page 10) gradually until the soup is smooth.

… Strain through a fine conical strainer, add salt and freshly ground black pepper, and refrigerate for at least 2 hours.

… Break up 4 ounces of finocchiona and chop 4 ounces of fresh goat cheese into small pieces.

… Heat a skillet (without any oil) and cook the finocchiona with 4 sprigs of savory for 1 minute. Add the reserved small fava beans, stir well, and cook for just 1 minute.

… Remove the sprigs of savory and distribute the contents of the skillet in soup bowls or serve in a tureen. Add the pieces of cheese. Pour the fava bean soup on top and serve.

AD— Fava bean pods release a lot of water when you cut them, so it's best to cut them with a large knife rather than chopping them in the food processor. PN— Finocchiona is a Tuscan salami flavored with fennel seeds. If you can't find it, use 4 ounces of good sausage meat and mix with a spoonful of fennel seeds. Fava beans are full of B vitamins, which makes this soup an excellent source.

Frozen Crab and Tomato Soup with Basil Granita

AD— The tomato soup can be prepared the day before. The longer it marinates the better it will be. Don't blend it too much, as this can turn it white, which is not very attractive!

PN— Tomatoes and basil, so lots of the famous lycopene that is good for the arteries and heart, and other carotenoids, vitamins, and minerals by the spoonful! The crab provides protein, so there's no need for any meat or fish in the rest of your meal.

… Serves 4

Make the tomato soup

… Wash 6 large tomatoes, cut into wedges, and place in a bowl with 2 cups of tomato juice (canned), 1 tablespoon of tomato puree, 1 teaspoon of celery salt, 1 teaspoon of ketchup (page 22), 1 tablespoon of sherry vinegar, and 2 tablespoons of olive oil.

… Cut 4 slices of soft crustless bread into small dice and add them. Salt lightly and season with a few drops of Tabasco.

… Refrigerate for as long as possible, up to overnight.

Prepare the basil granita

… Reserve 2 sprigs from 2 bunches of basil.

… Detach all the leaves from the rest and blend with ¾ cup of chicken stock (page 10). Add salt and freshly ground black pepper.

… Pour into a dish and place in the freezer, taking it out and stirring from time to time.

… Also put 4 soup plates in the freezer.

To finish your dish

… Defrost 5 ounces of frozen crabmeat and squeeze firmly to remove the moisture.

… Blend the tomato soup and strain through a conical strainer. Adjust the seasoning and keep cold until it is time to serve.

… Blanch and seed 2 large ripe tomatoes, dice them, and mix with the crabmeat. Add salt and freshly ground black pepper and season with 1 or 2 drops of Tabasco. Place in the middle of each soup plate.

… Chop the leaves of the 2 reserved sprigs of basil.

… Pour the tomato soup around the crab and tomato mixture. Sprinkle the chopped basil over.

… Scrape the basil granita with a fork and place it on top of the crab and tomatoes. Serve immediately.

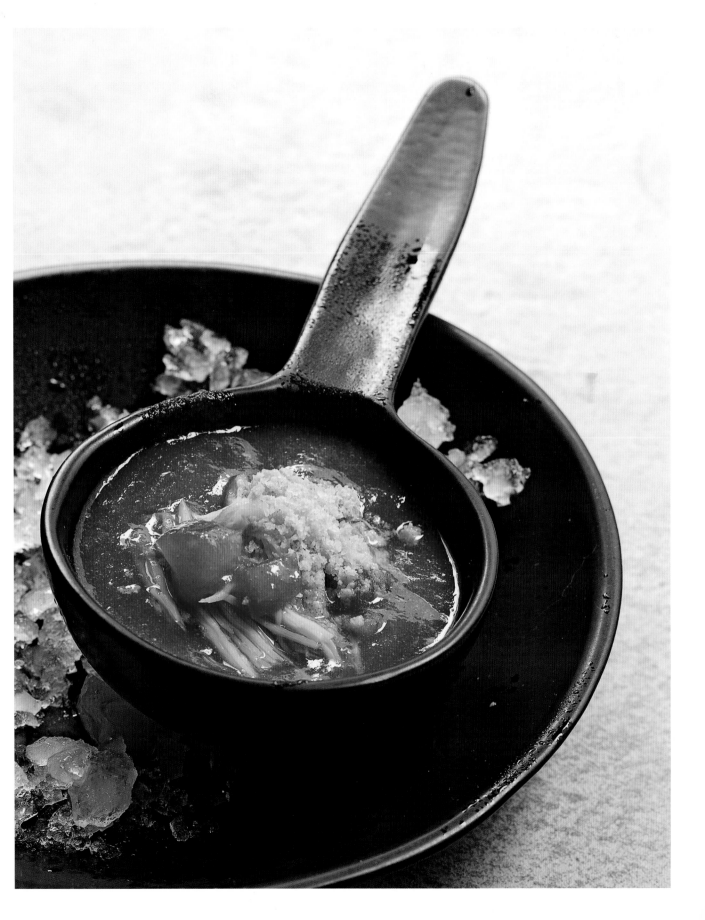

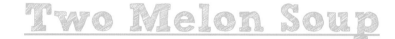
Two Melon Soup

AD— The melon should be nice and ripe. If you are concerned about the fierceness of the bird's eye chile, just put half in to begin with, then taste and adjust according to your liking.

PN— This soup is bursting with carotenoids, which are good for all the body's cells, including the skin cells. It's a good preparation for exposure to the sun.

… Serves 4

… Peel 1 large piece of watermelon (2 pounds) and 1 medium melon, carefully removing all the seeds. Also peel 1 small cucumber and 1 inch of ginger.

… Set aside 2 ounces watermelon, 3½ ounces melon, and 2 ounces cucumber in the refrigerator.

… Cut the rest, and the ginger too, into small chunks and blend to a puree.

… Season with 2 shakes of Tabasco and 2 tablespoons of orange flower water.

… Chop 1 bird's eye chile very finely and add. Keep cold.

… Put 4 bowls (or 4 soup plates) into the freezer to get them nice and cold.

… Chop the reserved watermelon, melon, and cucumber into very small dice (brunoise).

… Chop the leaves of 2 sprigs of cilantro and 2 sprigs of mint.

… Mix all this in a bowl with 2 tablespoons of olive oil. Add salt and keep cold.

… When serving, arrange this garnish in the bottom of the bowls or soup plates. Pour the cold soup on top and serve immediately.

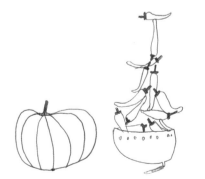

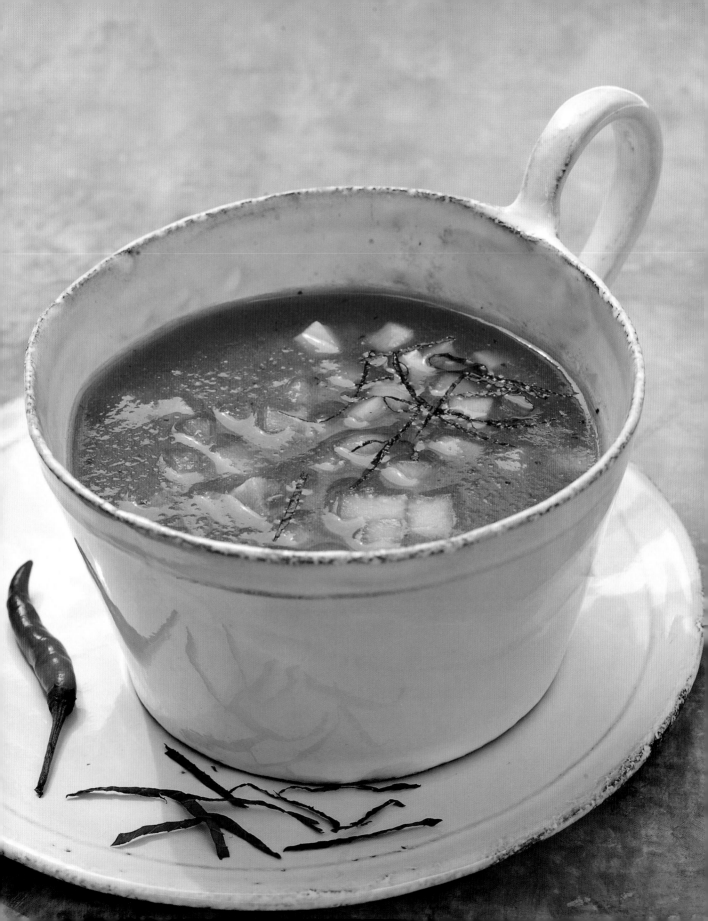

Tomato and Pepper Gazpacho

AD— *There's no need to peel the gazpacho vegetables. Without its garnish, it's perfect for a cold cocktail or as a snack between meals.*
PN— *Whether you serve this gazpacho as a drink or a starter, it provides you with a stack of vitamins, antioxidants, and fiber, with the added bonus of the good fatty acids of a little olive oil. So eat as much as you like!*

... Serves 4

The day before

... Wash 4 very ripe tomatoes (6 required in total for recipe), half a cucumber (1 required for recipe), and 1 green pepper (2 required for recipe). Remove the seeds from the pepper.

... Peel half a garlic clove and 1 pearl onion.

... Cut all these vegetables into cubes and combine in a bowl.

... Pick the leaves from a very small bunch of basil, crush them, and add to the vegetables.

... Cut 2 slices of stale whole-wheat bread into small pieces and put them in a small bowl. Add 5 tablespoons of sherry vinegar and stir until the bread has soaked it up. Add this to the bowl.

... Add 2 tablespoons of olive oil (4 tablespoons required in total) and a little salt. Stir the mixture.

... Cover the bowl with plastic wrap and refrigerate for 12 hours.

On the day

... Pour the contents of the bowl into a blender. Turn it on and add 2 tablespoons of olive oil and 2 cups of water (or more), adjusting the quantity to produce a gazpacho that is not too thick.

... Strain through a conical strainer. Correct the seasoning with salt and freshly ground black pepper and refrigerate for at least 2 hours.

... Blanch, peel, and seed 2 tomatoes, and chop the flesh into small dice. Peel the remaining half a cucumber and 1 green bell pepper with a vegetable peeler and dice similarly.

... Arrange this garnish in the soup plates or a tureen. Pour the gazpacho on top, and serve nice and cold.

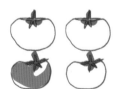

Chilled Broccoli Soup

… Serves 4

… Wash 3 good-sized heads of broccoli. Separate about 10 florets and set aside. Remove the hard part of the base and roughly chop the rest of the broccoli, florets and stalks.

… Heat 3½ cups of chicken stock (page 10). Prepare a large bowl filled with ice cubes.

… Heat a saucepan with a little olive oil, and sauté the broccoli over fairly high heat for 2 minutes. Pour in the boiling chicken stock and simmer for just 10 minutes, until tender.

… Transfer to a bowl and immerse this in the large bowl of ice cubes to cool quickly and preserve the color.

… Then blend until the soup is nice and smooth. Refrigerate.

… Put 4 soup plates in the freezer to cool.

… Peel and halve 16 fresh almonds.

… In a bowl, combine the reserved broccoli florets and half of the almonds. Add salt and freshly ground black pepper and pour a little olive oil onto this garnish.

… Pick the leaves from a very small bunch of chervil. Pour 8 ounces of sheep's curd into a bowl.

… Take the soup plates from the freezer and put the garnish in the middle of each one. Place a quenelle of sheep's curd, shaped with a spoon, on top. Sprinkle a few grains of fine sea salt flakes and freshly ground black pepper over.

… Pour the chilled soup around it. Sprinkle the remaining fresh almonds and the chervil leaves over and serve immediately, very cold.

AD— Use a 2½- or 3-inch circular pastry cutter to help arrange the garnish in the middle of the soup plates. And when fresh almonds are out of season, use sliced almonds. PN— They are forever discovering new nutritional virtues in broccoli. It protects from practically everything! So this is a soup to enjoy as often as you can. If you can't get sheep's curd, use another curd cheese—it will have the same nutritional value.

Fromage blanc or cottage cheese may be used if fresh curd cannot be found.

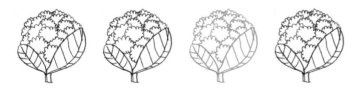

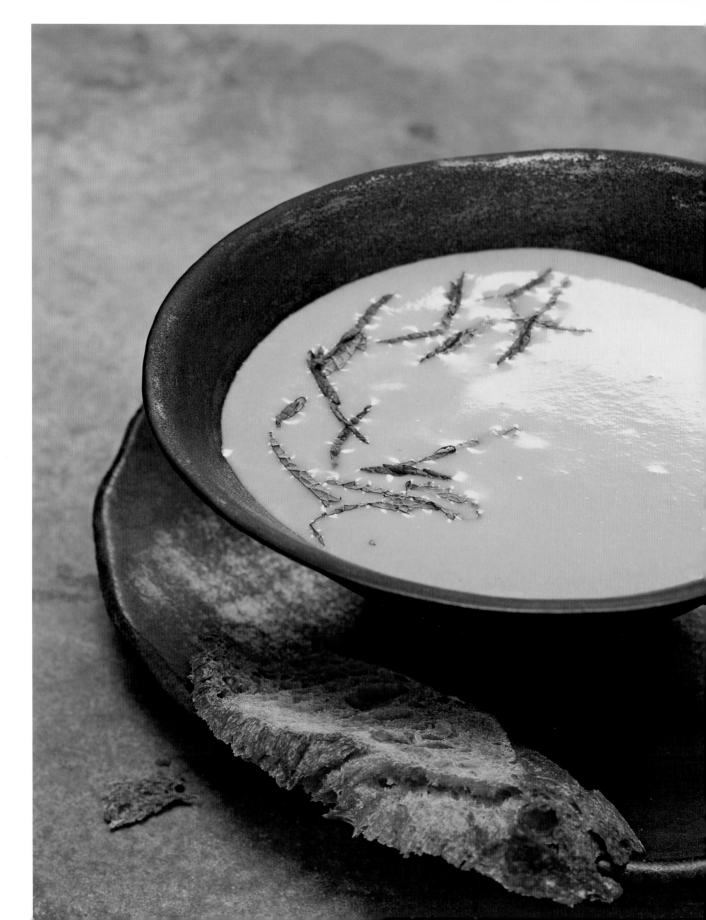

Chilled Cream of Pea Soup

… Serves 4

… Shell 1½ pounds of fresh peas. Select half the pods, choosing the smallest. De-string them like green beans, then wash and chop them.

… Heat a tablespoon of olive oil in a sauté pan, and sweat the chopped pea pods for about 5 minutes.

… Add the peas and 1 teaspoon of sugar and salt lightly. Cook for an additional 3 minutes and add 1 quart of chicken stock (page 10). Bring to a boil, then lower the heat and simmer for 10 minutes.

… Add 1 cup of light cream, then simmer for an additional 10 minutes.

… Prepare ice cubes in a basin and put a large bowl on top.

… Blend the soup to a perfectly uniform and smooth cream.

… Pour it quickly into the iced bowl (to keep the color).

… Taste and adjust the seasoning.

… Refrigerate for at least 2 hours to chill thoroughly. Put your tureen or serving dish in the fridge too.

… When serving, pour the soup into the chilled tureen, and sprinkle with 4 thinly sliced mint leaves and 2 tablespoons of grated pecorino or Parmesan.

AD— If you can get hold of fresh pecorino or Parmesan, crumble the cheese with a fork. Add a few fresh thyme flowers if they're in season. To save time, put the soup in the freezer for 15 to 30 minutes.
PN— The fiber content of this soup is enhanced by the pea pods. Serve this cream soup with slices of toast, then you will have more slow carbohydrates, which is always a good thing!

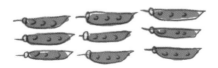

Pureed Wheat and Sheep's Curd Soup

AD— Sheep's curd is a fresh cheese made from ewe's milk. It's a traditional product from the Basque Country.

PN— This soup provides good slow carbohydrates (in the einkorn) and calcium. There's no real need to serve any other cheese with this meal.

Fromage blanc or cottage cheese may be used if fresh curd cannot be found. Spelt may be used in place of the einkorn, but will require 5 minutes of additional cooking time.

... Serves 4

<u>The day before</u>

... Put 8 ounces of einkorn to soak in a bowl of water and keep it cool for 12 hours.

<u>On the day</u>

... Peel and finely slice half a white onion. Peel and remove the central germ sprout from 1 garlic clove. Wash and quarter 1 tomato. Cut 1 thin slice of smoked bacon into small lardons.

... In a flameproof casserole dish, heat 1 tablespoon of olive oil, add the lardons, and brown lightly. Add the onion and garlic clove, cover, and cook gently for 5 minutes. Then add the tomato quarters and 4 sage leaves and cook for 2 to 3 minutes, still over a gentle heat. Finally add a pinch of saffron threads and mix well.

... Drain the einkorn and transfer to the casserole dish. Stir and add 1 quart of chicken stock (page 10). Bring to a boil, salt lightly, then lower the heat and cook gently for 1 hour.

... Drain 5 ounces of sheep's curd in a fine strainer lined with a clean cheesecloth.

... When the einkorn is cooked, take out ¼ cup and keep it hot. Blend the rest until the soup is very smooth. If it's too thick, add a little chicken stock. Check the seasoning and keep hot.

... With a vegetable peeler, shave 1½ ounces of pecorino or Parmesan.

... Pour the soup into a tureen, mold tablespoonfuls of sheep's curd, and add to the top. Sprinkle the reserved einkorn and the cheese shavings on top and serve immediately.

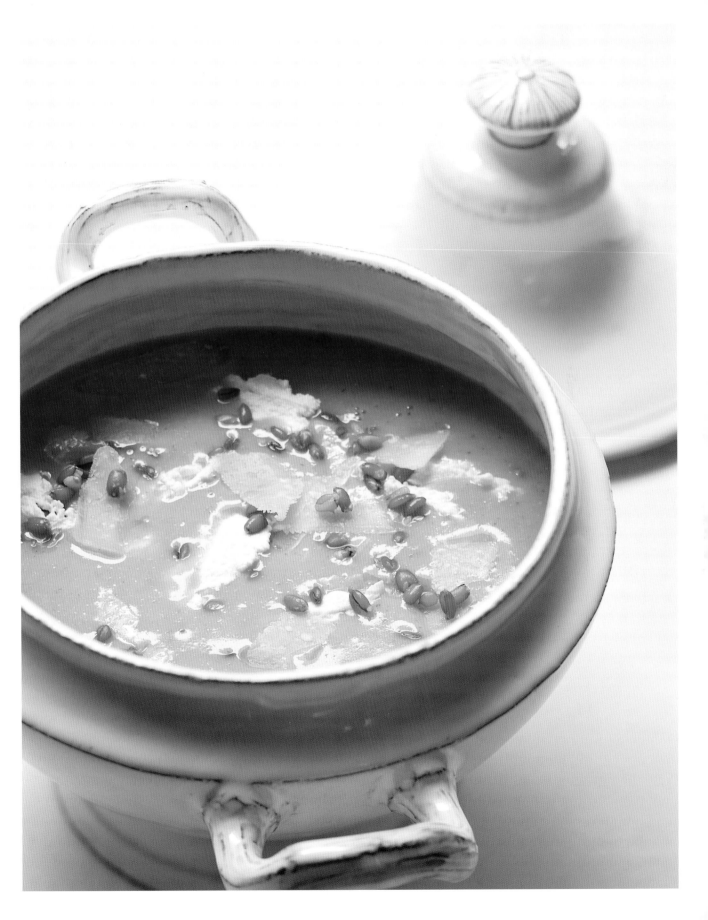

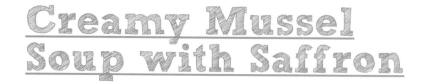

Creamy Mussel Soup with Saffron

AD— If you find your soup a bit too thick after blending, just thin it with a little water. The julienne of raw carrot and fennel adds a nice crunch.

PN— Check the freshness of the mussels and take out any that are open or broken. Shellfish are bursting with minerals, especially iron and magnesium, so this soup is perfect for recharging your batteries.

Bouchot mussels refers to the French technique of growing the mussels on large pilings, or bouchots, driven into the sea. They tend to be smaller than other varieties, but any small mussel will work in this recipe.

… Serves 4

… Clean and scrape 3½ pounds of mussels (use Bouchot mussels if you can get them) or get your fishmonger to do it for you.

… Peel and quarter 1 white onion. Wash and peel 3 or 4 medium potatoes (10 ounces), 1 leek, 1 celery stalk, 2 carrots, and 1 fennel bulb. Crush 1 garlic clove.

… Cut half the fennel and one of the carrots into very fine slivers. Set this julienne aside.

… Thinly slice all the other vegetables.

… Heat a splash of olive oil in a soup pot. Add the sliced vegetables and the garlic.

… Stir, then cover the pot and sweat for 10 minutes. Add ¾ cup of water and cook for an additional 5 minutes.

… When the potatoes are nearly cooked (check with the tip of a knife), add the mussels, then 1¼ cups of white wine, 1 quart of lowfat milk, and 15 threads of saffron. Stir well and simmer until all the mussels have opened.

… Then take the mussels out with a slotted spoon and remove the shells.

… Set aside about 20 of them, and return the others to the pot. Blend with a hand blender until the soup is nice and smooth. Taste and adjust the salt seasoning. Add a generous amount of freshly ground black pepper.

… Place the reserved julienne of vegetables in a (warmed) soup tureen and pour the hot soup on top, add the mussels, and serve.

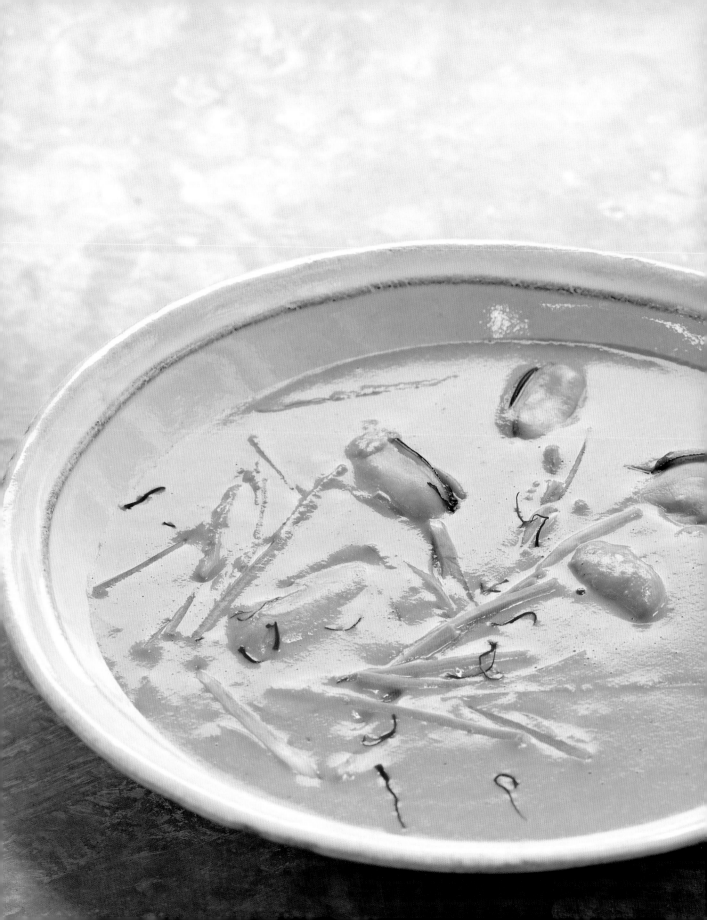

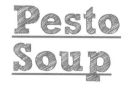

Pesto Soup

AD— A rustic summer soup, this is the great classic of southern French cooking. It may look complicated, but it takes just a little over an hour to make.

PN— An all-around dish that gives you absolutely everything you need. A little cheese and fruit and voilà! Dinner is served.

… Serves 6

… Prepare the pesto (page 36) and keep the basil stems.

… Put 2 cups of fresh hulled white kidney beans in a saucepan with half an onion studded with a clove. Cover well with water (about 1 quart) and bring to just under a boil (simmering).

… Skim off the scum, then add the reserved basil stems, 1 sprig of thyme, and 1 bay leaf. Cook for 30 to 40 minutes and add salt only at the end of the cooking time. Set aside the beans in their liquid.

… While the beans are cooking, wash and cut into slivers 2 cups young fresh stringless green beans. Cut into large sections and immerse in boiling water for 5 minutes (they should still be crunchy), drain, and set aside.

… Blanch and seed 2 tomatoes, then chop the flesh into ⅛-inch dice. Reserve.

… Peel and wash 4 carrots, 4 zucchini (preferably round ones), 1 head of celery, and the white portion of 2 leeks. Cut the carrots, zucchini, and celery into dice and the leek into rounds.

… Dice 3½ ounces of cured ham and soften gently in a large saucepan with a splash of olive oil. Add the carrots, zucchini, celery, and leeks, salt lightly, stir well, cover, and cook for 10 minutes without allowing to color. Drain the kidney beans and add their cooking stock to these vegetables. Boil for 2 minutes, then remove all the vegetables with a slotted spoon and keep hot.

… Add 4 ounces of fresh pasta to the saucepan and cook until al dente.

… Then put the vegetables back and add the kidney beans, the fresh beans, and the diced tomato. Stir, boil briefly, then remove from the heat and check the seasoning.

… Take the leaves off 2 sprigs of basil.

… Pour the hot soup into a tureen. Serve the pesto separately in a sauce boat or add to the soup at the last minute, stirring well. In either case, sprinkle the soup with basil leaves.

Asparagus Soup with Mozzarella and Flakes of Ham

… Serves 4

… Peel and wash 3 bundles of green asparagus. Remove any parts of the base that are too hard. Cut the tips into 2- to 2½-inch lengths and set these aside.

… Cut the rest of the asparagus into rounds.

… Heat 2 cups of chicken stock (page 10).

… Peel and mince 1 white onion and sweat in a sauté pan with a splash of olive oil for 2 minutes.

… Add the asparagus rounds, sweat for an additional 2 minutes, then pour in the boiling chicken stock.

… Stir, add the leaves of a sprig of tarragon, and cook for 10 minutes.

… Blend until the soup is nice and smooth, then check the seasoning.

… Heat a tablespoon of olive oil in a skillet. Put in the reserved asparagus tips and cook for 2 to 3 minutes.

… Cut 4 thin slices of Parma ham into flakes.

… Check the heat of the asparagus soup.

… Cut a ball of mozzarella di bufala into thin slices and spread them over the bottom of a tureen or soup plates. Pour the hot soup on top, then spread the flakes of Parma ham over. Top with the asparagus tips.

… Add a twist of freshly ground black pepper and serve immediately.

AD— If you ever see burrata di bufala, which is even smoother than traditional mozzarella, don't hold back!

PN— Asparagus is fantastically rich in fiber. Blended like this, the fiber is entirely preserved and is very easy to digest.

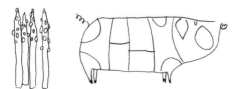

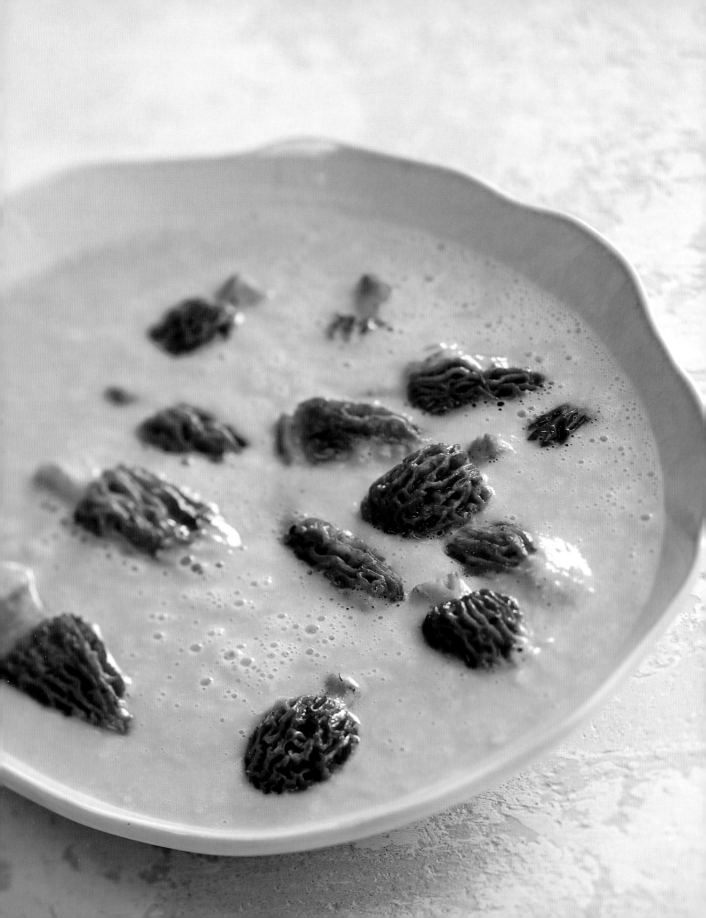

Corn Chowder with Morels

… Serves 4

… Peel and thinly slice 1 white onion. Melt in a saucepan with a splash of olive oil for 3 minutes without letting it color.

… Drain and rinse the contents of a large can of corn and add to the onions. Cook for 5 minutes, stirring.

… Add 1 quart of chicken stock (1½ quarts required in total for recipe) (page 10) and cook gently for 20 minutes.

… While the chowder is cooking, remove the bases of 10 ounces of fresh morels, then wash the caps in several changes of warm water until all traces of sand are gone. Dry in a salad spinner.

… Melt 1½ tablespoons of butter (3 tablespoons required in total for recipe) in a skillet with a drop of olive oil. Roll the morels in this, add salt, and sweat for 3 minutes.

… Pour in 2 cups of chicken stock (page 10) and cook for about 20 minutes, until the morels are nice and soft.

… In the meantime, heat a skillet (without fat), put in 2 ounces of popping corn, cover, and let them pop over high heat.

… When the corn chowder is cooked, blend until perfectly smooth.

… Add the remaining 1½ tablespoons of butter and the morel cooking liquid.

… Check the seasoning and temperature, and emulsify with a hand blender until light and frothy.

… Pour into a tureen (or soup plates) and spread the morels on top.

… Serve the popcorn separately for people to add to their own bowl.

AD— Out of season, use dried morels, rinsing them carefully after soaking. And in the season for fresh corn, make the chowder from 8 to 10 small cobs. Cut off the corn nibs and cook for 30 minutes in salted water before using.

PN— Corn is the only grain that contains antioxidant carotenoids. Rich in carbohydrates, fiber, and magnesium, it is also gluten free.

Shrimp Broth with Lemongrass, Chiles, and Ginger

AD— *This can all be prepared in advance and refrigerated. Take out the bowls containing the garnish an hour in advance to return to room temperature, and reheat the broth gently until boiling hot.*

PN— *This soup is practically a complete meal in itself, and provides your full quota of protein. No need for any fish or meat—all you need to round it off is a starter or side dish of vegetables.*

… Serves 4

Make the soup

… Shell about a third (8 ounces) of 1½ pounds of small shrimp; keep them refrigerated, but don't throw away the heads or shells.

… Cut 1 bird's eye chile and 1 tomato into small chunks. Peel 1 inch of ginger, reserve a third, and cut the rest into pieces. Crush 1 stalk of lemongrass.

… In the blender, combine the remainder of the whole shrimp, the heads and shells, and the pieces of ginger, tomato, and bird's eye chile. Blend for 2 minutes, adding 2 cups of water, and pour into a saucepan, not too big so that the mixture is quite deep. Then add the lemongrass.

… Bring to a boil, add 2 egg whites, and stir well with a whisk. Lower the heat to minimum and allow to simmer for 10 minutes.

… Cover a strainer with a damp dish towel and place it over a large bowl. Ladle in all the mixture gently and gradually so as not to cloud the broth.

… Then close the dish towel by bringing its edges to the middle and squeeze all the liquid into the bowl. Correct the seasoning. This broth should be very clear and fragrant. Keep it hot.

Prepare the garnish

… Wash and trim 2 scallions. Wash and de-string a handful of sugarsnap peas. Cut into fine strips (julienne).

… Cut 1 small bell pepper or sweet chile and the reserved ginger similarly, then combine all these vegetables in a large bowl.

To finish your dish

… Roughly chop the reserved shelled shrimp and season with the juice of a quarter of a lemon and some Piment d'Espelette or hot paprika.

… Mix well and put these chopped ingredients in the bottom of 4 bowls. Add the julienne of vegetables on top.

… Check that the broth is hot, and pour into bowls at the table.

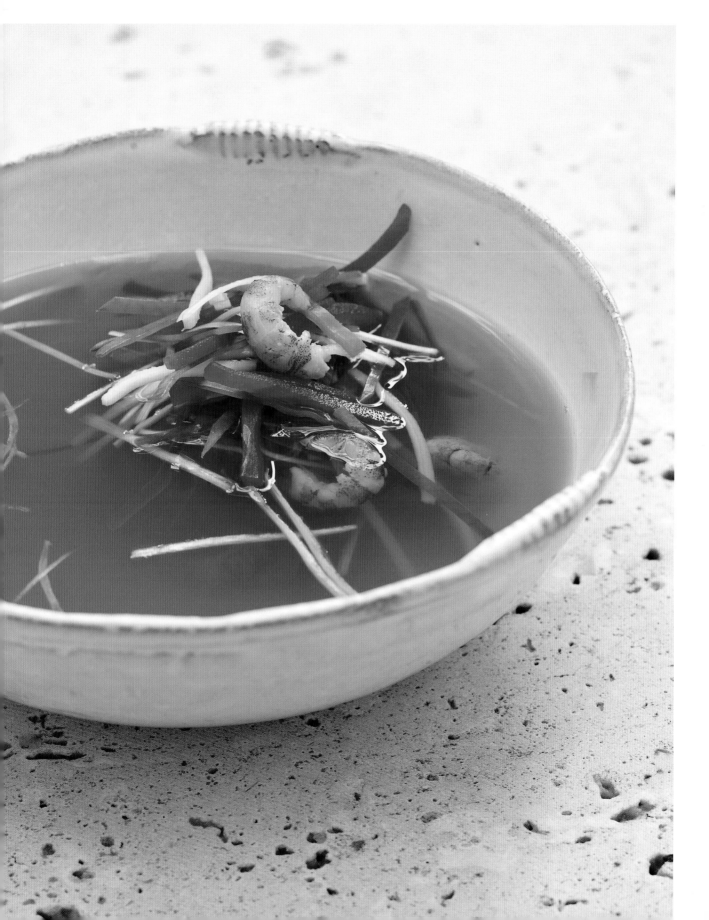

Split Pea Velouté

AD— *Chistorra is a type of sausage from the Basque country, made from pork, ground paprika, and garlic. If you can't get hold of it, you can use chorizo. The split peas will cook in 20 to 30 minutes in a pressure cooker.*

PN— *This velouté will revive your taste for split peas, which have been unjustly overlooked. They're full of minerals, vitamins, and fiber, and they're also a source of good slow carbohydrates.*

… Serves 4

… Soak 1½ cups of split peas for at least 1 hour or, better still, overnight.

… Peel 1 onion, and stud with a clove. Peel and wash 1 carrot and 1 stick of celery and cut into chunks.

… Drain the split peas and put in a saucepan. Add 6 cups of chicken stock (page 10) or water, the onion, carrot, and celery. Cook at a very gentle simmer for 1 hour.

… When the split peas are cooked, heat a skillet with a drop of olive oil and cook 5 ounces of chistorra or other sausage for 2 minutes on each side.

… Cut into thin rounds and keep hot on a paper towel.

… Cut the soft inside of 4 to 5 slices of bread into rounds the same size as the rounds of chistorra. Place them on a baking sheet and put under the broiler until lightly golden.

… Blend the cooked split peas to form a perfectly smooth velouté. If it's too thick, add the necessary amount of water or chicken stock and reheat. Check the seasoning.

… Make a rosette of slices of chistorra and rounds of bread in the center of each soup plate. Froth up the velouté with a hand blender and pour around the chistorra. Serve immediately.

Cream of Parsnip Soup with Bacon

… Serves 4

… Scrape and rinse 1 pound of parsnips and slice thinly. Peel 1 small onion and chop roughly. Peel and wash 1 medium potato and cut into small chunks.

… Pour 2 cups of water and ¾ cup of lowfat milk into a saucepan, then heat.

… Put another saucepan on the heat with a splash of olive oil, and sweat the onion for 1 minute. Add the parsnips and a little salt.

… Pour the hot liquid over the onion and parsnips, turn up the heat, and bring to a boil. Then add the potato and cook for 20 minutes over medium heat, stirring occasionally.

… Blend until the soup is nice and smooth. Keep it hot in its saucepan.

… While the soup is cooking, cut 2 ounces of smoked bacon into tiny lardons (⅛ inch). Put them in a small saucepan and cook over medium heat for 2 to 3 minutes, stirring. Add ¼ cup of light cream and cook over low heat, covered, for 10 minutes.

… Rinse, dry, and chop the leaves of a small bunch of flat-leaf parsley.

… Check the heat and seasoning of the soup.

… Transfer the bacon cream to a soup tureen and pour the parsnip soup over it. Sprinkle with chopped parsley.

AD— Choose small firm white parsnips, because they are more tender and less fibrous. Avoid any that are yellow, soft, or bruised. PN— The parsnip is not particularly rich in vitamins (other than B_9), but parsley makes up for this. On the other hand, parsnip is very rich in fiber. You might be surprised at the bacon and cream, but there's only ½ ounce of bacon and 1 tablespoon of cream per person, so it's not such a lot of fat after all!

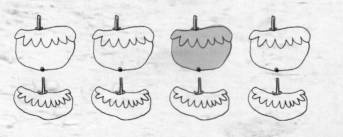

Chestnut Soup with Bacon and Flaked Porcini

AD— You can use frozen chestnuts for this dish if you like. If you do, cook them longer to allow time for them to thaw.

PN— There are carbohydrates, minerals, B vitamins (lots of B₉), and loads of fiber in this soup. Moreover, chestnuts contain no gluten.

… Serves 4

Make the chestnut soup

… Preheat the oven to 250°F. Peel and cut 2 shallots and 3 sticks of celery into large chunks. Peel 3 garlic cloves.

… Heat a flameproof casserole dish and put in 2 slices of bacon ⅛ inch thick. Color well on both sides, then take them out and keep hot.

… Add the chunks of shallot and celery and the whole garlic cloves to the bacon fat. Stir for 1 to 2 minutes.

… Add 2½ pounds of peeled chestnuts to the casserole dish. Sweat for 3 minutes, stirring. Take out about 20 of them and set aside.

… Then add a bay leaf and ½ teaspoon of peppercorns.

… Add 2 quarts of chicken stock (page 10) or water.

… Put the casserole dish in the oven for 45 minutes.

Prepare the mushrooms

… In the meantime, clean 12 ounces of porcini or white mushrooms.

… Slice the caps of 2 firm mushrooms into thin slices and keep cold on a plate covered with plastic wrap.

… Chop the rest into small dice.

To finish your soup

… Blend the soup thoroughly. Taste and adjust the seasoning, adding salt and freshly ground black pepper. Keep hot.

… Cut the two slices of bacon into fine lardons and cut the 20 reserved chestnuts into quarters.

… Heat 1 tablespoon of olive oil in a sauté pan and brown the chestnuts for 2 minutes. Add the diced mushrooms, salt lightly, and cook for an additional 2 to 3 minutes. Add the small lardons, stir, and adjust the seasoning.

… Put this garnish in the middle of each soup plate.

… Pour the hot soup around it. Sprinkle with mushroom slices and serve nice and hot.

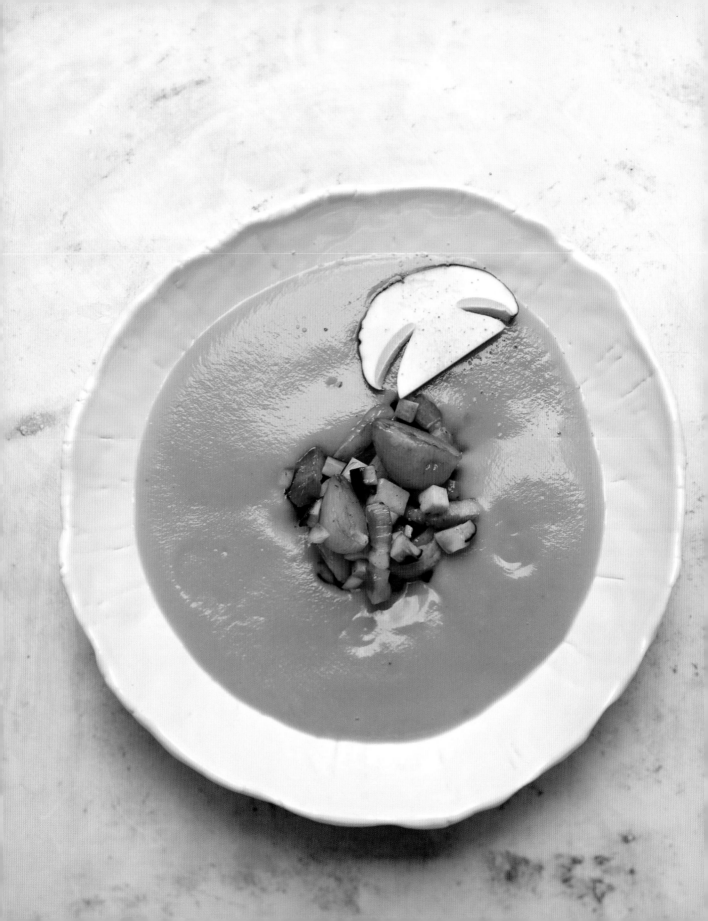

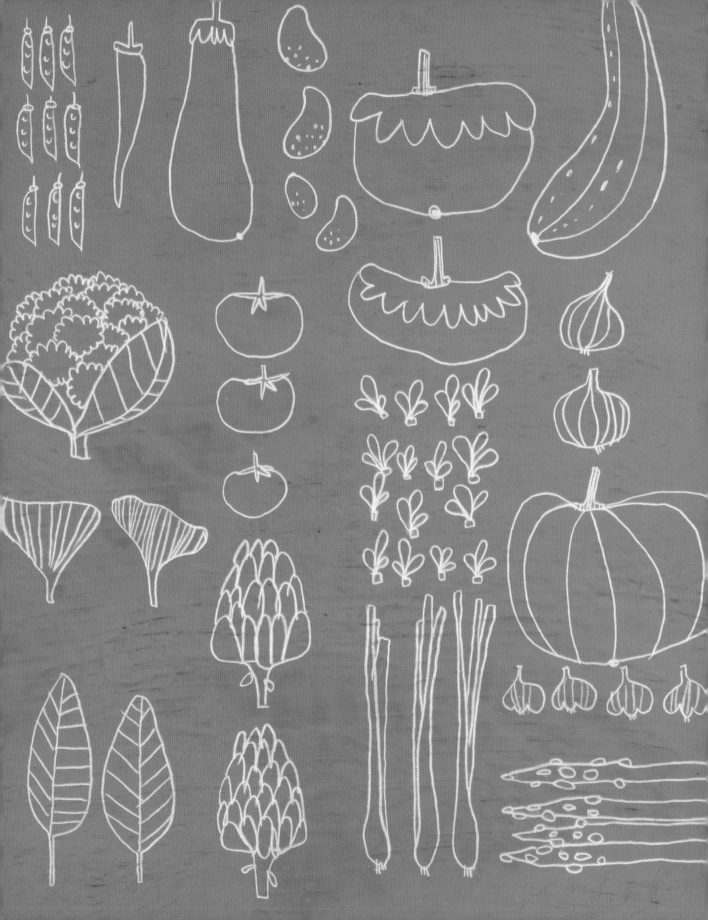

AD— I love vegetables. Their diversity inspires me. So I was pleased to introduce plenty of them, cooked en cocotte, as soon as I arrived at the Louis XV in Monacô. They still reign supreme in my cuisine.

PN— Along with fruit, fresh and dried vegetables are the great protectors of our health because they are rich in fiber, vitamins, minerals, and antioxidants. The more you eat, the better you feel!

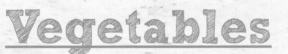

Vegetables

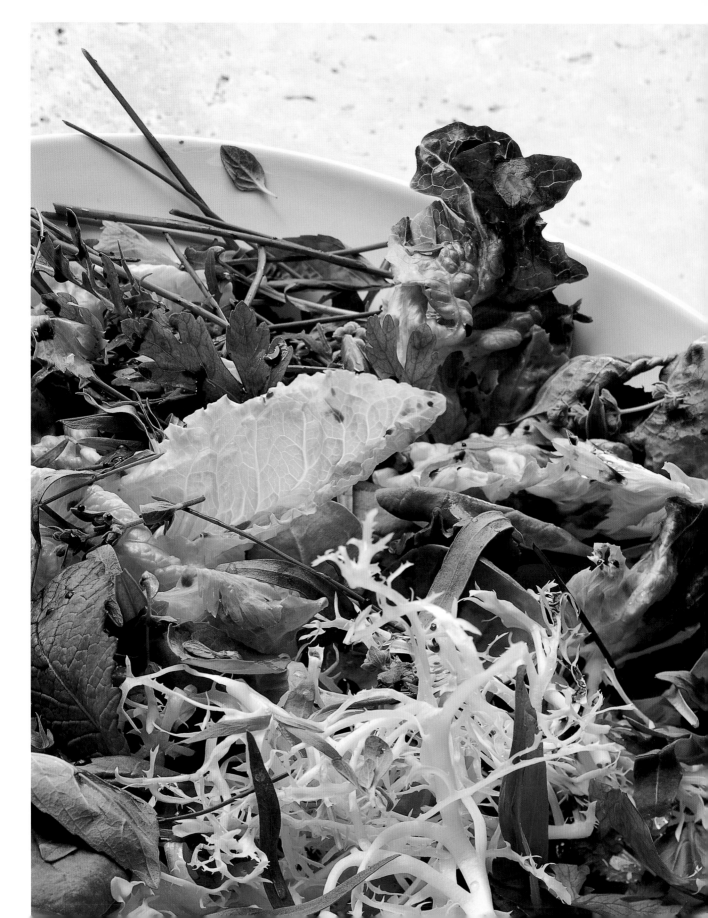

Herb Salad

… Serves 4 to 6

… Separate the leaves from 1 head of frisée lettuce.

… In very cold water, wash 2 ounces of arugula, 2 ounces of baby spinach, 2 ounces of red oakleaf lettuce, 2 ounces of green oakleaf lettuce, 2 ounces of mustard greens, 12 small celery leaves, and 2 ounces of baby romaine lettuce leaves. Dry well.

… Rinse 2 sprigs of marjoram, 2 sprigs of chervil, 2 sprigs of flat-leaf parsley, 2 sprigs of basil, and 2 sprigs of tarragon, dry carefully, then pluck off the leaves.

… Rinse, dry, and cut a very small bunch of chives into 2½- to 3-inch lengths.

… Mix the salad leaves and herbs in a large salad bowl.

… In a bowl, whisk 4 to 6 tablespoons of olive oil with 2 tablespoons of balsamic vinegar and 2 tablespoons of sherry vinegar.

… Salt lightly. Add freshly ground black pepper.

… Keep this vinaigrette separate and only pour into the salad bowl on serving.

AD— This recipe is not set in stone. Adapt it according to the season and to what you can find in the market.

PN— All these herbs are amazingly rich in vitamins, antioxidants, trace elements, and minerals. Eat this salad as often as you like, because it's really good for you.

Fine Ratatouille with Basil

AD— The cooking time depends on the size of the vegetables. The smaller they are, the quicker they cook. You can serve this ratatouille hot, warm, or cold.
PN— Ratatouille is the emblematic dish of the famously healthy Mediterranean diet, bursting as it is with antioxidants of all kinds. This recipe makes quite a lot, so if you have some left over, just freeze it.

… Serves 4 to 6

… Wash 2 purple eggplants, 4 green zucchini, and 2 yellow bell peppers. Cut the eggplants and zucchini into very small cubes. Peel the peppers, remove their seeds, and cut into very small dice (brunoise).

… Blanch 6 tomatoes, quarter them, and remove the insides and seeds. Cut the quarters into small dice.

… Peel and mince 2 white onions.

… Peel 2 garlic cloves and crush well, almost to a puree.

… Heat a large sauté pan with 3 tablespoons of olive oil and sweat the onions, crushed garlic, peppers, and eggplant for 3 to 4 minutes. Add salt and freshly ground black pepper and 2 bay leaves. Stir and cook gently for 5 to 7 minutes.

… Add the tomatoes and zucchini and cook for an additional 5 to 7 minutes. Adjust the seasoning and take the pan off the heat. Take out the bay leaves.

… Take the leaves from a very small bunch of small-leaved basil, add them, stir, and transfer the ratatouille to a serving dish. Sprinkle with a few grains of sea salt.

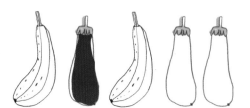

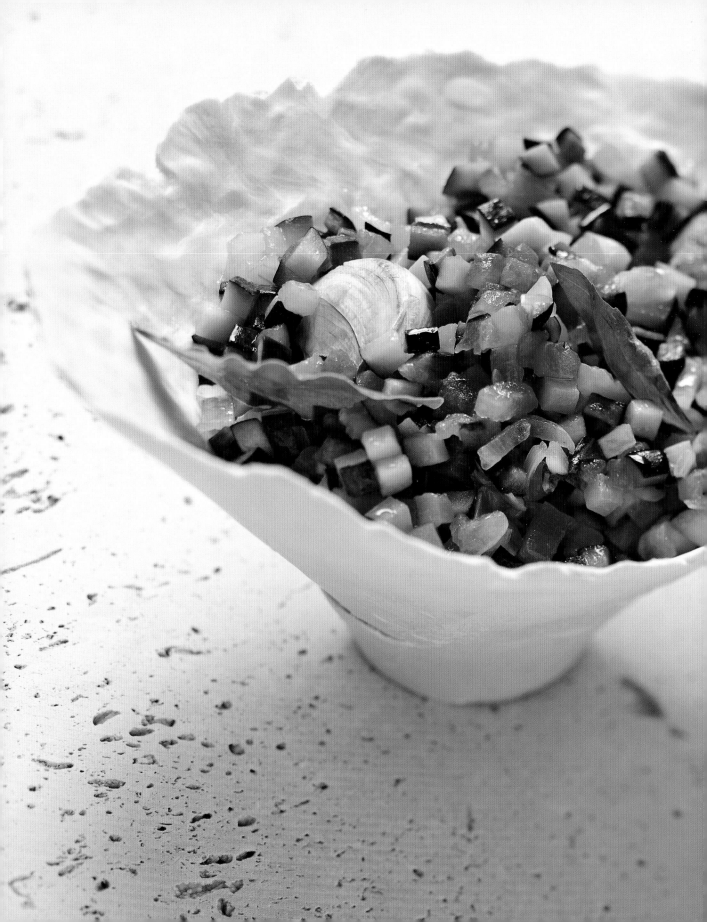

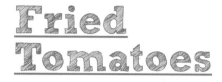

Fried Tomatoes

AD— These fried tomatoes are an excellent accompaniment for roast meat or poultry. But why not eat them on their own, with some bread to soak up the sauce from the bottom of the pan? Or gently push the tomatoes apart, break a few eggs into the spaces, and cook for an extra 2 or 3 minutes.

PN— The more tomatoes are cooked, the better they are for you—not only do their flavors develop but so do their health-giving properties, including lycopene, which is really good for the arteries.

… Serves 4

… Rinse and dry 12 ripe vine tomatoes. Remove the stems and cut in half.

… Peel 2 garlic cloves and cut into thin slices.

… Put a splash of olive oil in a large skillet or sauté pan. Add the tomato halves side by side and close together, cut side down.

… Cook first over medium heat for about 15 minutes, and when they have exuded some juice, sprinkle with the slices of garlic.

… After 15 minutes, lower the heat to minimum and continue to cook, allowing them to reduce and slightly caramelize.

… Add salt and freshly ground black pepper at the end of cooking.

… Rinse and dry 4 sprigs of basil. Take off the leaves, break them up, and add at the end of cooking.

… Transfer the tomatoes to a dish or serve straight from the pan.

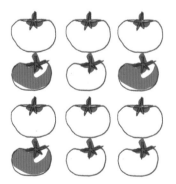

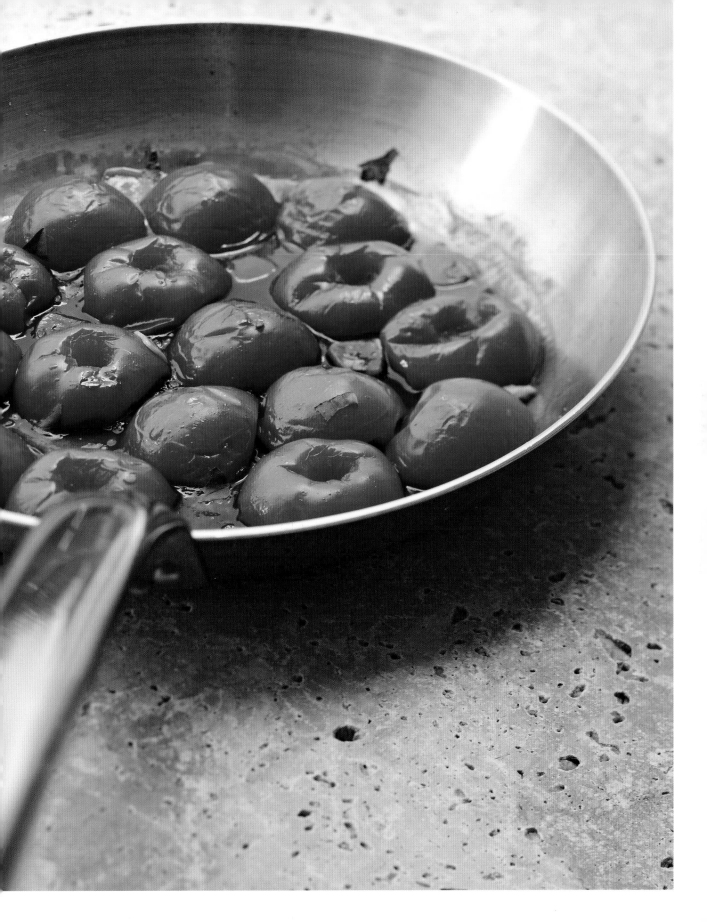

Spring and Summer Vegetables en Cocotte

… Serves 4

Prepare the vegetables

… Peel 4 carrots with tops, 4 turnips with tops, leaving ½ inch of the tops on. Also peel 8 fresh salad onions with stalks. Half peel 12 pink radishes, leaving ½ inch of their tops on too. Cut 4 small young fennel bulbs in half. Peel a bundle of small green asparagus spears and cut the tips into 3-inch lengths (keep the rest of the stalks for a soup). Wash and dry all these vegetables.

… Remove the tough outer leaves from 6 small purple artichokes, peel the stems, halve, and remove the chokes. Set them aside in water with the juice of 1 lemon.

… Take the base off a handful of chanterelles, cut the largest in half, and wash and dry them all carefully.

… Shell 12 fresh almonds and cut in half.

Cook the vegetables

… Heat 1 tablespoon of olive oil in a large flameproof casserole dish. Brown 2 slices of bacon ½ inch thick on each side, then take them out of the pan.

… In their place put the carrots, turnips, onions, radishes, fennel, asparagus, and artichokes.

… Add salt, cover, and cook for 3 minutes. Then add the chanterelles and cook over low heat for an additional 10 minutes, stirring gently from time to time. If the vegetables start to color too quickly at any point, add a few spoonfuls of water.

… While the vegetables are cooking, cut the slices of bacon into small lardons.

… Heat a large saucepan filled with salted water and prepare a large bowl with water and ice cubes.

… Immerse ¾ cup of shelled peas and ¾ cup of shelled fava beans in the boiling water for 3 minutes. Remove with a slotted spoon and drop them into the ice water, then drain and add to the casserole dish when the vegetables are cooked.

… Stir gently. Add a splash of sherry vinegar and stir again gently to deglaze the cooking juices. Finally add the almond halves. Add freshly ground black pepper. Mix again carefully. Serve in the cooking pot or in a serving dish.

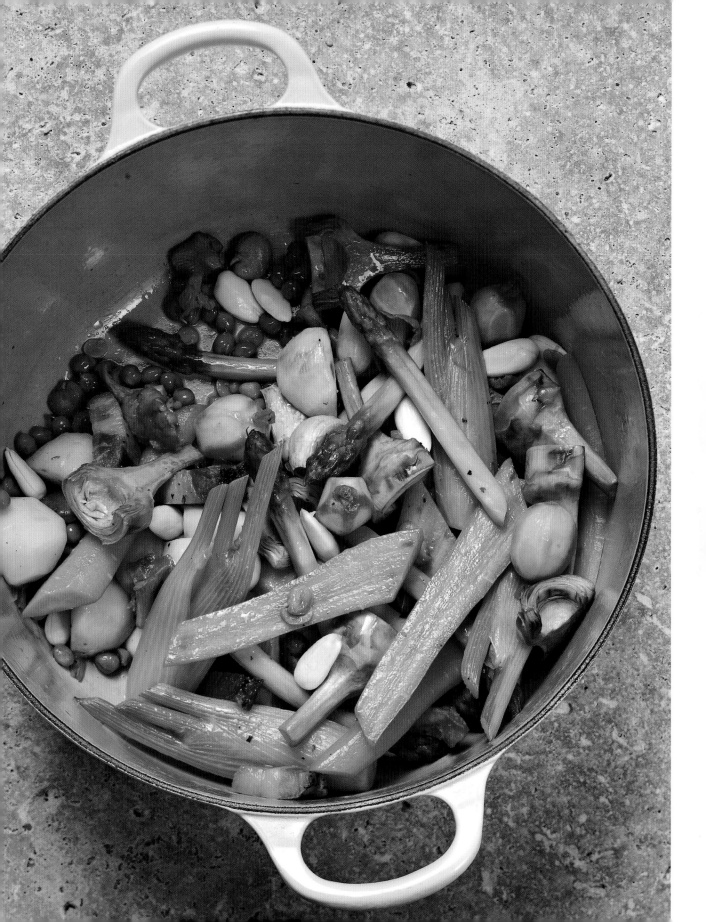

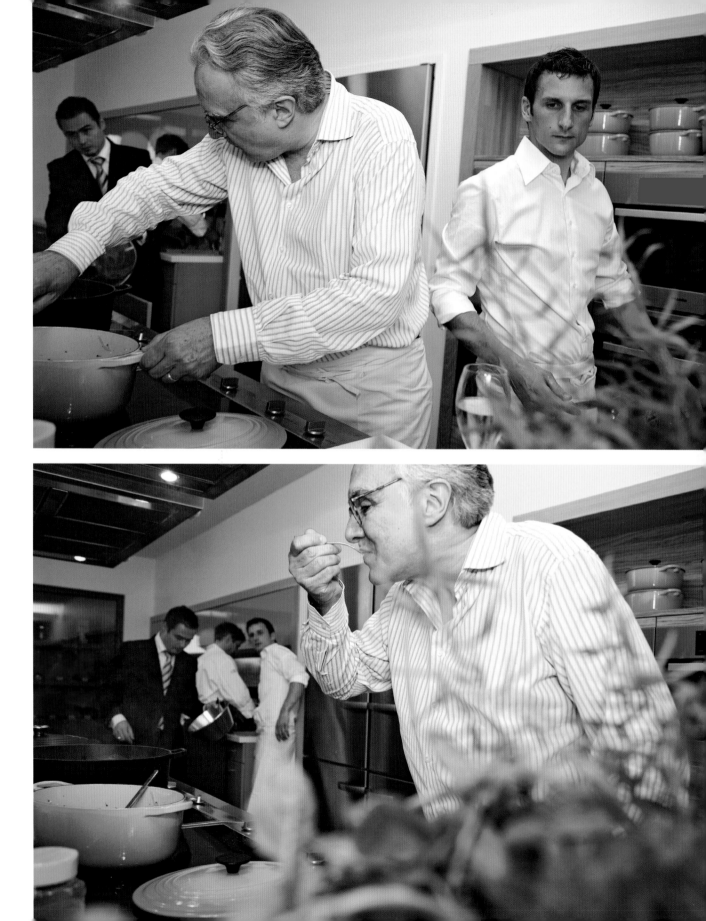

Autumn and Winter Vegetables and Fruits en Cocotte

… Serves 4

Prepare the vegetables

… Peel 4 carrots with tops, 4 stalks of celery, 4 turnips, and 1 red onion, and cut into good-sized chunks.

… Also peel 1 quince, 4 salsifies, 1 apple, and 1 pear, immersing them in water with the juice of 1 lemon as you go.

… Slice the salsify very thinly at an angle, cut the quince into ½-inch cubes, and quarter the apple and pear.

… Rinse 16 large white grapes.

Cook the vegetables

… Heat 3 tablespoons of olive oil in a large flameproof casserole dish and cook 2 slices of bacon ¼ inch thick until browned on both sides, then take them out of the pot and set aside.

… In their place put the apple and pear quarters, color on all sides, and set them aside too.

… Then put the carrots, celery, turnips, onion, quince, salsifies, and a handful of peeled chestnuts (vacuum packed or frozen) into the pot. Add salt and brown lightly for 3 minutes, then add ¾ cup of chicken stock (page 10). Cover the pot and cook over low heat for 10 to 12 minutes.

… In the meantime, cut the slices of bacon into small lardons.

… Check the vegetables with the tip of a knife. When they're all cooked, add the apples, pears, grapes, and lardons. Stir very gently and add a splash of sherry vinegar. Stir again and serve straight from the cooking pot.

AD— The vegetables must be soft enough, but the apples and pears hardly cooked at all. The vinegar adds a welcome touch of acidity to the sweetness of the vegetables and fruit.

PN— An excellent collection of vegetables and fruit with loads of fiber and minerals, but not a lot of vitamin C. An herb salad (page 153) with some cheese would make up for this nicely.

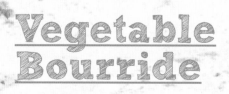

Vegetable Bourride

*AD— The recipe looks long,
but takes only about half an hour,
as you can prepare the vegetables
while cooking the stock. It's all a
matter of organization.*
*PN— A big dish of vegetables,
an original and very nutritious
recipe, Mediterranean in style
and low in fat, this is something
we should all eat more often.*

… Serves 4

Make the stock

… Take the outer leaves off 3 fennel bulbs, dice them, and set the rest of the bulbs aside. Finely dice the white part of 1 small leek, 1 white onion, and 2 garlic cloves.

… Lightly sauté the garlic with a splash of olive oil. Add the leek and onion and cook gently for 5 minutes. Add the diced fennel. Cover and cook for an additional 10 minutes. Add 1 star anise, 4¼ cups of water, 1 sprig of marjoram, and 1 sprig of thyme; add salt, bring to a boil, then simmer gently for 20 minutes.

… Hard boil 2 eggs (10 minutes), then cool and shell them.

Prepare the vegetables

… Remove the tough outer leaves of 4 small purple artichokes, quarter, remove the chokes, and set aside in water with the juice of 1 lemon. Slice 4 carrots with their tops, 4 scallions, and 4 zucchini at an angle.

… Immerse the carrots and fennel bulbs in boiling water and, after 5 minutes, add the zucchini. Cook for an additional 5 minutes, then drain all these vegetables.

… At the same time, cook the artichokes in a sauté pan with a splash of olive oil until tender.

… Peel 1 avocado, cut into quarters, sprinkle with lemon juice, and season with salt.

… Add the carrots, fennel bulbs, zucchini, scallions, and 12 segments of tomato confit (page 16) to the sauté pan with the artichokes, stir, and keep over very low heat.

To finish the vegetable bourride

… Cut up the hard-boiled eggs and crush with a fork.

… Remove the herbs and star anise from the stock and blend. Add the crushed eggs and blend again.

… Reheat the stock and add 9 ounces of haddock fillet. Turn off the heat and leave to poach for 5 minutes, then take out with a slotted spoon.

… Place the vegetables in shallow dishes. Add the avocado quarters. Check the seasoning and the temperature of the stock and give it another burst in the blender to emulsify thoroughly. Pour over the vegetables, nice and hot.

… Flake the haddock and spread it over the vegetables. Serve immediately.

Caponatina with Raisins and Pine Nuts

... Serves 4

... Peel 2 red bell peppers and 2 yellow bell peppers with a vegetable peeler and remove their seeds. Wash 4 zucchini and 3 eggplants. Cut all these vegetables into small cubes (about ¾ inch).

... Peel 2 white onions and cut into thin wedges.

... Soak a good handful of raisins in a bowl of water.

... Preheat your oven to 325°F.

... Sauté the vegetables one after another in a skillet with a splash of olive oil, then combine them in a flameproof casserole dish.

... Toast 3 tablespoons of pine nuts in a dry skillet, add half of them to the casserole dish, and reserve the rest.

... Take the leaves off 2 sprigs of basil. Add the stems to the casserole dish and set the leaves aside.

... Cut 20 pitted black olives into rounds and add to the casserole dish.

... Wash 20 cherry tomatoes, cut them in half, and add to the casserole dish too.

... Rinse and chop 8 salted anchovy fillets, crush 4 garlic cloves, and add these.

... Finish with the well-drained raisins and 2 sprigs of thyme, and stir gently.

... Cover the casserole dish with a lid and put in the oven for 25 minutes.

... When the caponatina is cooked, remove the basil stems and check the seasoning. Add the reserved basil leaves and the rest of the toasted pine nuts. Stir and add a generous twist of freshly ground black pepper.

... Serve straight from the casserole dish or on individual plates.

AD— Don't use too much olive oil for sautéing the vegetables or the caponatina will be too oily. It can be eaten hot or cold. This dish freezes well (that is, it does if you have any left over!).
PN— An improved version of ratatouille, a key dish in the famous Mediterranean diet, which includes antioxidant-rich vegetables, but which here has even more minerals, thanks to the raisins and pine nuts.

Summer Vegetable Gratin with Basil

AD— This gratin is served warm. You can make it in advance, keep it cool, and then reheat gently in the oven at 325°F. But cover it so that the vegetables don't dry out.
PN— The strips of eggplant and zucchini can be broiled or grilled (on a baking sheet, broiler pan, grill, or oven grill pan, depending on what you have). This dish is then low in fat without any loss of its nutritional value.

… Serves 4

Prepare the vegetables

… Wash 4 tomatoes, cut each one into 6 slices, and set aside on a plate.
… Peel 1 small red bell pepper, 1 small yellow bell pepper, and 1 small green bell pepper with a vegetable peeler. Remove all the seeds and the white membranes and cut into strips. Peel 1 white onion and cut similarly. Peel and crush 1 garlic clove. Put all these vegetables together in a bowl.
… Take the leaves off 4 sprigs of basil. Select the small leaves and set aside in the refrigerator. Cut the large leaves with kitchen scissors and keep on a small plate.
… Wash 1 small eggplant, 1 zucchini, and 1 yellow squash. Cut into strips approximately ⅓ inch thick with a mandoline.

Cook the vegetables

… Heat a sauté pan with a splash of olive oil and add the contents of the bowl (peppers, onion, and garlic). Stir and cook, covered, over medium heat for 10 minutes.
… Slip the sliced tomatoes under the vegetables (lifting them with a spatula) and continue to cook for 5 minutes. Then put it all back in the bowl and add the chopped basil.
… Heat a skillet with a splash of olive oil and sauté the eggplant strips for 1 to 2 minutes on each side. Add salt and freshly ground black pepper and place on a hot plate.
… Do the same with the zucchini and squash strips.

Make the gratin

… Preheat the oven to 350°F.
… Arrange a third of the zucchini, squash, and eggplant strips side by side on a dish, alternating the colors.
… Spread half of the tomato-pepper-onion mixture on top.
… Add a second third of the zucchini, squash, and eggplant strips.
… Spread the rest of the tomato-pepper-onion mixture on top.
… Finish with a layer of zucchini, squash, and eggplant, then put in the oven for 15 minutes.
… Allow the dish to cool when it comes out of the oven, then sprinkle with the reserved small basil leaves and a generous twist of freshly ground black pepper.

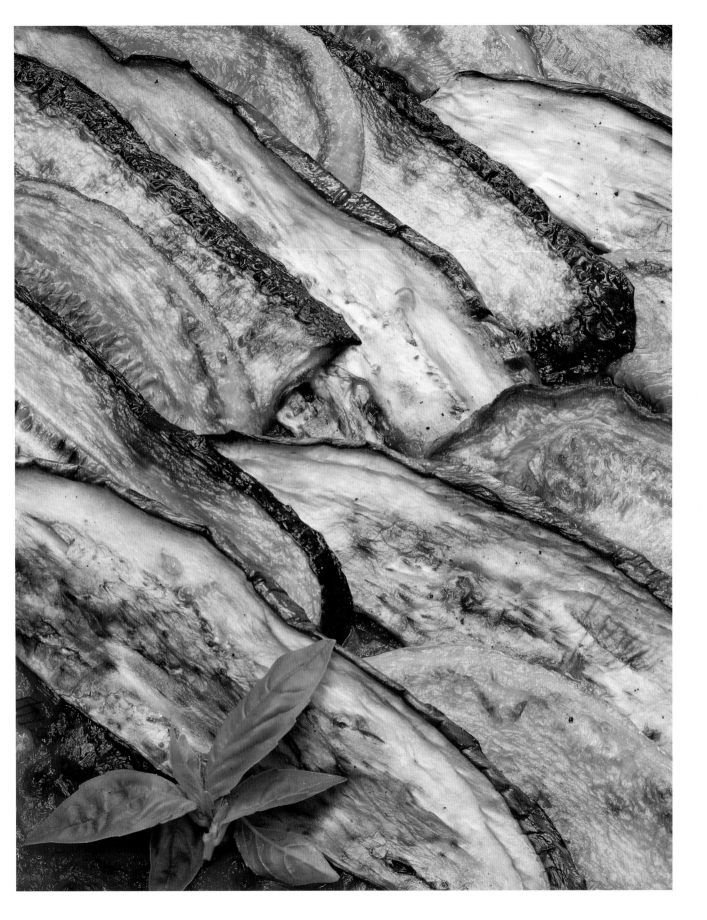

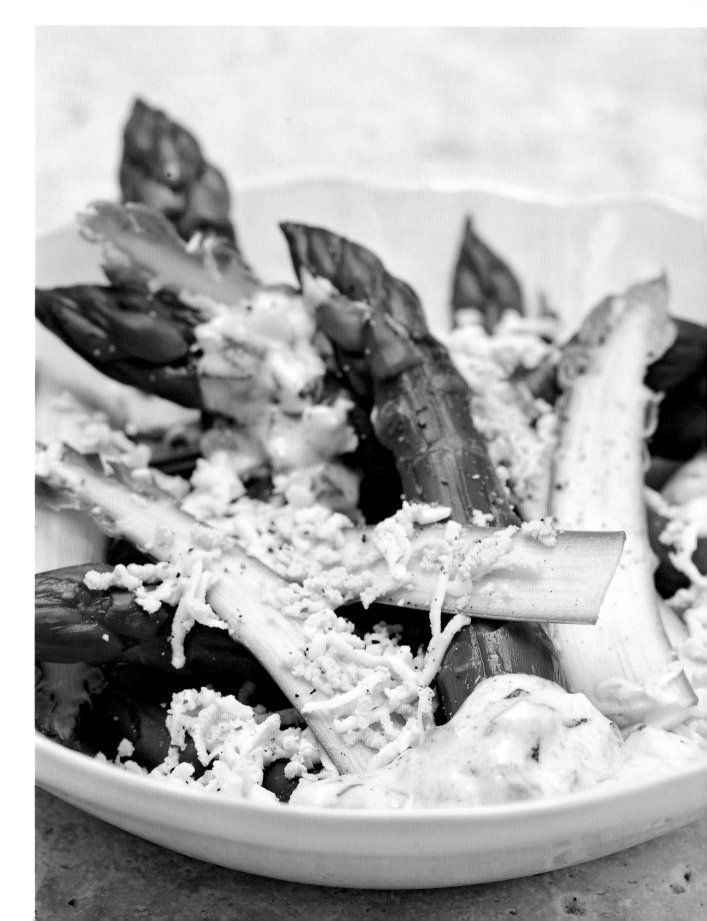

Mimosa Salad with Cooked and Raw Asparagus

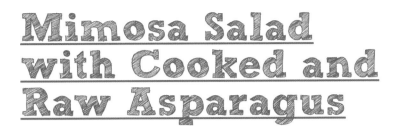

… Serves 4

Prepare the asparagus and eggs

… Peel and wash 2 bundles of green asparagus. Cut the tips into 4-inch lengths. Remove the hard white base and keep the rest.

… Set 4 of the tips aside.

… Plunge all the others in salted boiling water and cook for about 5 minutes (depending on the size). In the meantime, fill a large bowl with water and ice cubes.

… Lift out the asparagus spears with a slotted spoon and cool them in the ice water. Then drain on a dish covered with a dish towel.

… Hard boil 2 eggs (10 minutes) in the boiling water used for the asparagus. Cool and shell them.

… Cut the 4 reserved asparagus tips into fine shavings with a mandoline and place on a small plate.

Make the sauce

… Wash and cut up the leaves of 1 sprig of tarragon, 2 sprigs of parsley, and 2 sprigs of chervil.

… Cut the reserved asparagus stalks into small cubes. Place in a bowl and add, mixing well each time, 4 tablespoons of sherry vinegar, ½ cup Greek-style yogurt, 1 tablespoon of Dijon mustard, 3 tablespoons of olive oil, and the chopped herbs. Season with salt and freshly ground black pepper.

To finish your dish

… Lay the cooked asparagus tips in a serving dish and coat with the sauce.

… Grate the hard-boiled eggs on top with a cheese grater.

… Top with the shaved raw asparagus and serve.

AD— Tie the asparagus spears into small bundles, leaving a long end of string that you can attach to the handle of the saucepan. This way you can take them out easily without damaging them.
PN— Asparagus contains asparagine, a harmless aromatic molecule that can be smelled in the urine after eating. The herbs in the sauce add vitamins, especially vitamin C.

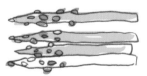

Roasted Asparagus with Black Olives

AD— You can just as easily deglaze with some leftover stock from a daube (page 312) or the juice from a roast beef or chicken instead of the balsamic vinegar. This recipe takes only 30 minutes!

PN— Another simple way to eat asparagus when in season. It's one of the richest vegetables in B vitamins, especially in folate (vitamin B₉), which is often lacking in people's diets. It provides plenty of fiber, too.

… Serves 4

… Peel 2 bundles of asparagus, removing all the hard and fibrous parts of the stems.

… Wash the asparagus, then cut the tips into 3-inch lengths and cut the rest of the stalks in half lengthwise.

… Heat a large sauté pan with 2 tablespoons of olive oil, line up all the asparagus (tips and stalks) side by side, salt very lightly, and cook until tender, turning occasionally. Check to see if they're done with the tip of a knife.

… Using a slotted spoon, place all the asparagus in a serving dish.

… Pour 5 tablespoons of balsamic vinegar into the sauté pan and stir well, scraping the bottom with a spatula. Add 2 tablespoons of pitted black olives (Taggiasche or Niçoise), stir again, and pour over the asparagus.

… With a vegetable peeler, shave 1 ounce of Parmesan on top. Add several twists of freshly ground black pepper and serve immediately.

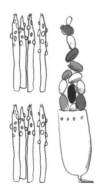

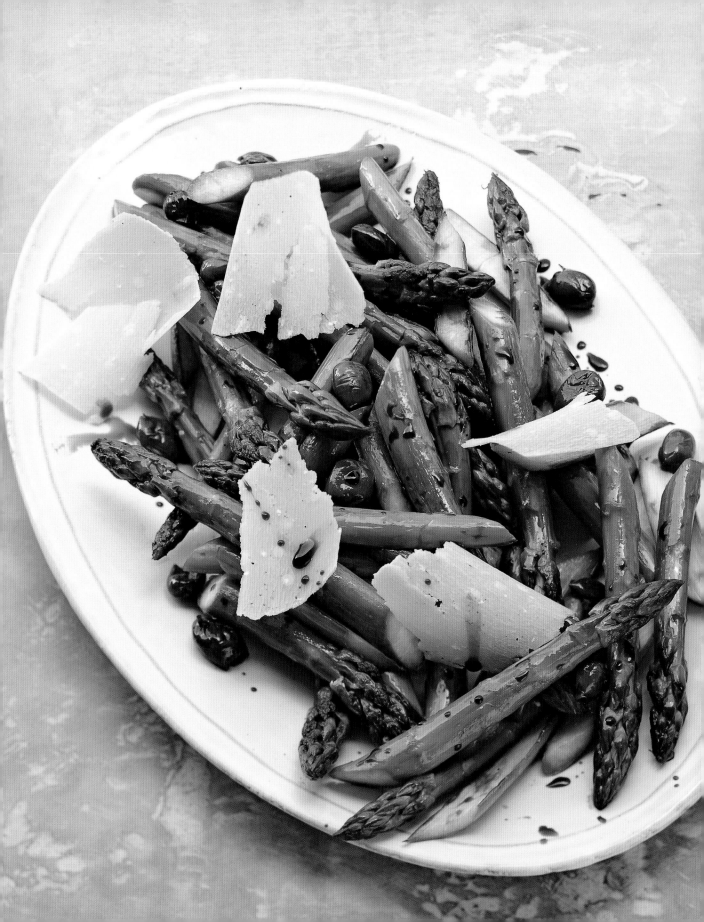

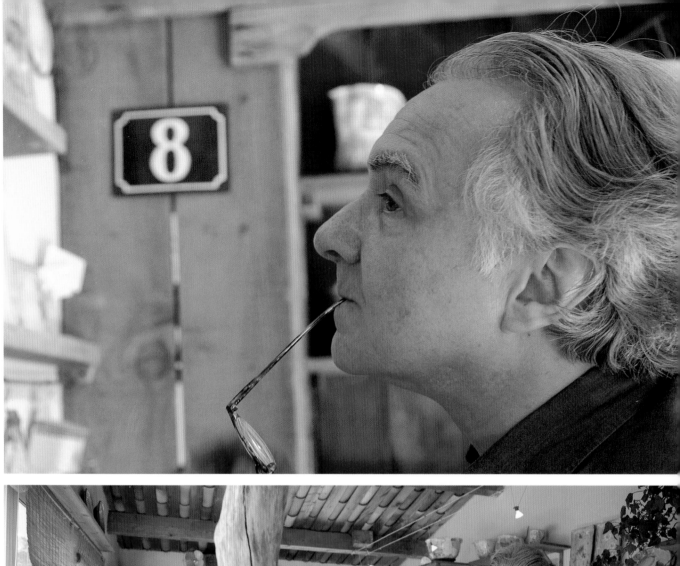

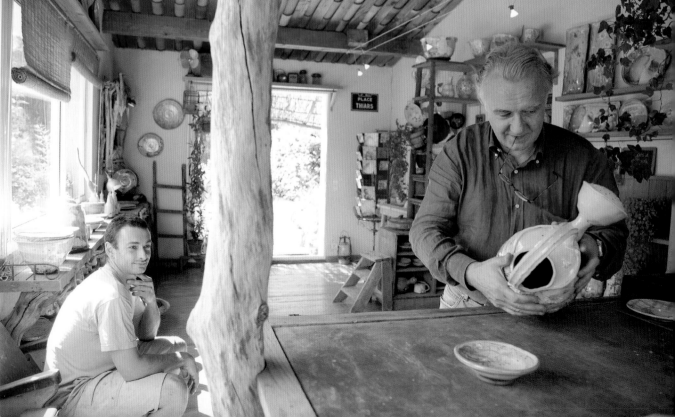

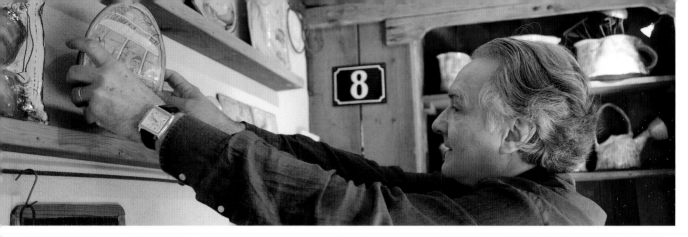

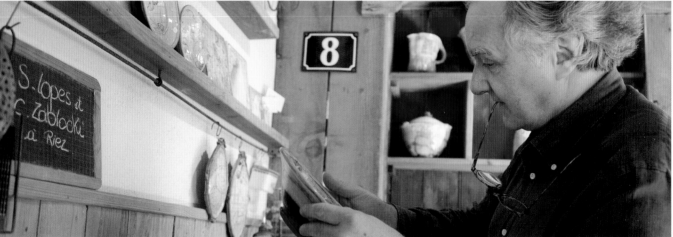

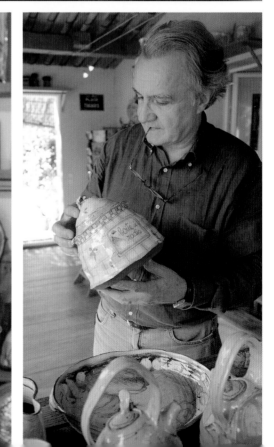

In the pottery studio of Christine Zablocki and Sebastien Lopes, in Riez.

"With their hands and their craft, artists and craftsmen often help me realize my dreams."

Pan-Fried Chanterelles with Almonds and Lemon

AD— Can't get hold of chanterelles? Then use ordinary white mushrooms, quarter them, and cook just once, without draining the first water.

PN— Mushrooms are quite rich in minerals, but they also contain special molecules capable of stimulating our immune system, which makes them a very healthy food. A good reason to put them on the menu frequently.

… Serves 4

… Remove the earthy base of 1¾ pounds of chanterelles, and cut the largest ones in half. Wash all of them several times with plenty of water, then dry in a salad spinner or a dish towel.

… Wash and dry 2 handfuls of baby spinach.

… Peel 12 fresh almonds.

… Rinse half a salt-preserved lemon (page 15) and cut into thin slices.

… Crush 1 clove of garlic confit (page 12).

… Heat a skillet with a splash of olive oil and cook the chanterelles for 1 minute over high heat, adding salt, just long enough for them to release their liquid.

… Drain, wipe your skillet dry with paper towels, and return to the heat with ¾ tablespoon of butter.

… As soon as it has melted, put the chanterelles back in and sauté for 2 or 3 minutes to lightly brown.

… Then add the baby spinach, salt-preserved lemon, garlic confit, and almonds and stir until the baby spinach is just wilted. Add freshly ground black pepper.

… Transfer to a dish or onto individual plates and serve immediately.

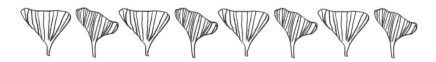

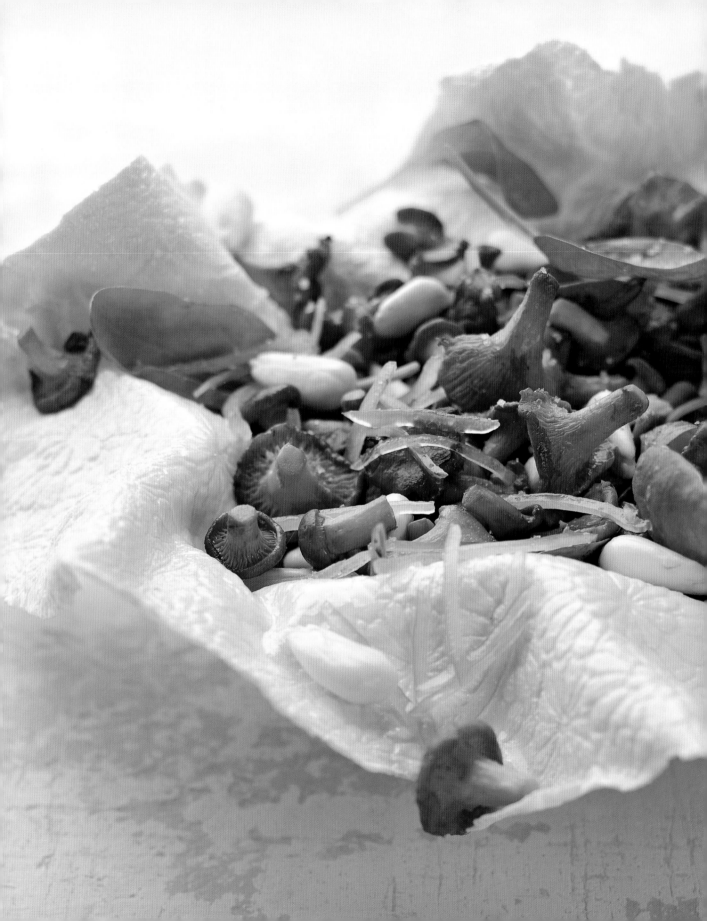

Lightly Spiced Cooked and Raw Summer Vegetables

AD— A fine combination of cooked and raw ingredients—tender and crunchy at the same time. I like this contrast, which wakes up the taste buds.

PN— You can cook the vegetables separately in a smaller sauté pan, but take care not to use too much oil. This dish, which is rich in vitamins, should not be too fatty.

… Serves 4

Prepare the vegetables

… Peel and wash 1 bundle of small fresh spring onions, leaving on 1 inch of their stalks. Wash and de-string 2 handfuls of French beans and 2 handfuls of sugarsnap peas. Cut the French beans in half.

… Peel and wash 2 bundles of asparagus. Cut the tips into 4-inch lengths (keep the rest of the stalks for a soup).

… Clean 1 bundle of pink radishes, keeping ¾ inch of the tops, and wash.

… Cut 4 asparagus tips and 4 radishes into thin slices with a mandoline. Set them aside in a bowl.

Cook the vegetables

… Immerse the French beans and sugarsnap peas in salted boiling water and cook for 3 to 4 minutes. Drain.

… Heat a large sauté pan with a splash of olive oil and put in all the other vegetables. Cook for 2 to 3 minutes, stirring. Pour in a ladle of chicken stock (page 10), salt lightly, and cook for a few minutes more. With a slotted spoon, transfer them to a dish and keep hot.

Prepare the spicy sauce

… Add 2 tablespoons of olive oil to the vegetable cooking stock and stir well. Incorporate 2 pinches of mild curry powder, 1 teaspoon of ground fennel, and 2 pinches of ras al-hanout and mix well.

To finish your dish

… Season the asparagus and radish slices with a splash of olive oil and a little sea salt.

… Combine all the cooked vegetables in a large sauté pan and heat. Pour in a splash of sherry vinegar, then the spicy sauce, and mix again.

… Arrange the vegetables on the serving dish. Then add the slices of radish and asparagus. Serve immediately.

Eggplant and Goat Cheese Clafoutis

… Serves 4

… Wash 3 eggplants and cut in half.

… Cut 4 large slices about ⅛ inch thick from the widest part of one of them, then cut 4 discs 3 inches in diameter from each slice (the size of the pans you are going to use).

… Cut all the rest of the eggplant into very small dice (⅛ inch).

… Peel and mince 2 white onions.

… Heat olive oil in a sauté pan and sweat the onions for 3 minutes. Add the diced eggplant and sauté for 5 minutes.

… Drain in a sieve and allow to cool.

… Preheat the oven to 425°F.

… Peel and mince 1 garlic clove. Chop the leaves from a small bunch of marjoram.

… In a large bowl, mix 2 eggs, ¼ cup of lowfat milk, the garlic, marjoram, and well-drained eggplants. Stir and add salt and freshly ground black pepper.

… Oil four 3-inch round baking pans. Place a disc of eggplant at the bottom of each one. Cut 3 ounces of soft goat cheese into bits and distribute over the eggplant. Pour the egg mixture on top.

… Put in the oven for 6 to 8 minutes.

… Turn the clafoutis out of the pans. Add a twist of freshly ground black pepper and serve warm with an herb salad (page 153).

AD— Perk up these clafoutis with dried eggplant. Cut a few fine rounds, brush with oil, and dry in the oven at 175°F for 1 hour. PN— Drain the eggplant really well to remove as much oil as possible so that these clafoutis are not too high in fat.

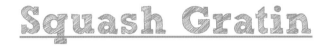
Squash Gratin

AD— In the squash family, you have plenty of choice between pumpkin, butternut squash, and several other varieties. It all depends what you can find in the market. But if you do spot a Muscade de Provence, pounce on it, as it is particularly tasty.

PN— All hard squashes are rich in antioxidant carotenoids: The more orange the flesh, the more they contain. They are best enjoyed in winter, when they are in season.

… Serves 4

… Peel 2¼ pounds of winter squash and cut into cubes.

… Preheat the oven to 450°F.

… In a large ovenproof pot, brown 2 slices of bacon ⅛ inch thick for 5 minutes, turning them over. Add the cubes of squash, 4 garlic cloves (unpeeled but crushed), 1 sprig of rosemary, and a little salt.

… Cover with parchment paper and put in the oven for 30 minutes.

… Lower the oven temperature to 350°F, remove the parchment paper, and cook for an additional 30 minutes.

… In the meantime, heat a dry skillet and toast a handful of dried pumpkin seeds. Cool on paper towels, then crush.

… When the squash is cooked, take the pot out of the oven and turn on the broiler.

… Throw away the rosemary and the peel of the garlic cloves.

… Remove the slices of bacon and cut into small lardons.

… Mash the squash and garlic with a fork and add the lardons. Stir and adjust the seasoning with plenty of freshly ground black pepper.

… Sprinkle the top of the gratin with pumpkin seeds.

… With a vegetable peeler, shave 1 ounce of pecorino or Parmesan cheese into small flakes and sprinkle evenly over the gratin.

… Put under the broiler for about 2 minutes to brown the top. Serve immediately.

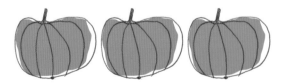

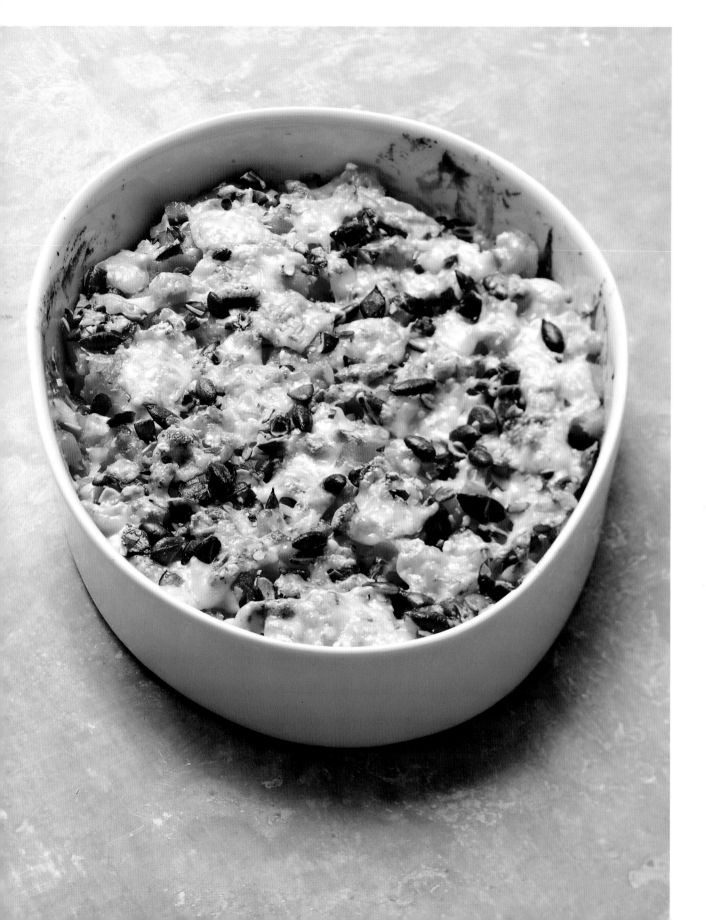

Sweet Onions with Raisins and Corn Couscous

AD— Piment des Landes, a sweet green pepper, tastes very like a green bell pepper. So if you can't get hold of it, you can substitute half of a green pepper.

PN— The onion is not just a food, it's also a medicine. It has a beneficial effect on the digestive and cardiovascular systems, on blood clotting, and is a hypoglycemic and antibacterial agent. There's no gluten in the corn couscous, but there are good vegetable proteins.

Corn couscous can be found online or in specialty baking or health food stores.

… Serves 4

Prepare the onions

… Peel 8 large red onions, then cut them into quarters, and separate the layers.

… Peel and grate 1 inch of ginger. Peel and chop 1 garlic clove.

… In a sauté pan, heat a good splash of olive oil. Add the onions, sweat for 2 to 3 minutes, stirring, then add the ginger and garlic and cook over low heat until the onions are soft.

… Add first 2 pinches of turmeric and 1 teaspoon of ras al-hanout, then ¾ cup of raisins. Mix well and continue to cook for an additional 5 to 6 minutes.

… Pour in ¾ cup of water and cook over low heat, without a lid, for about 10 minutes.

… Cut ½ green bell pepper into thin slices and add at the end of cooking. Keep hot.

Prepare the couscous

… In a measuring cup, measure 1¼ cups of corn couscous. Then put 1¾ cups of water in a saucepan, add salt, and bring to a boil.

… Just as it reaches boiling point, add the couscous, stir well, turn off the heat, and put on the lid. Allow the couscous to swell for 10 minutes. Then fluff with a fork, adding 3 tablespoons of olive oil.

… When the couscous is nice and smooth, season with a pinch of Piment d'Espelette or hot paprika, salt, and freshly ground black pepper.

… Put in a serving dish, add the onions and their garnish on top, and serve immediately.

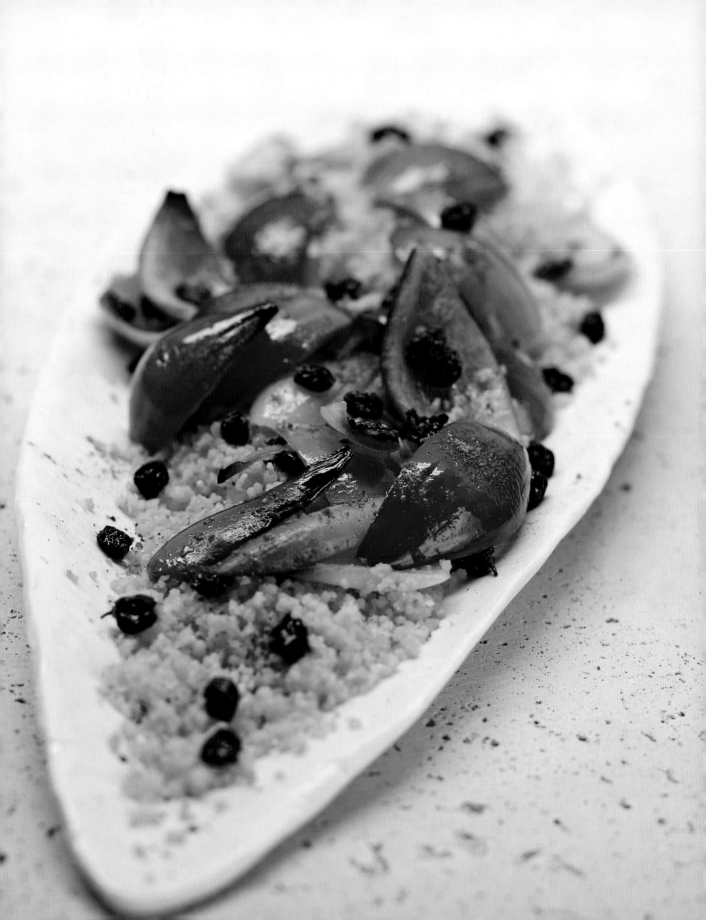

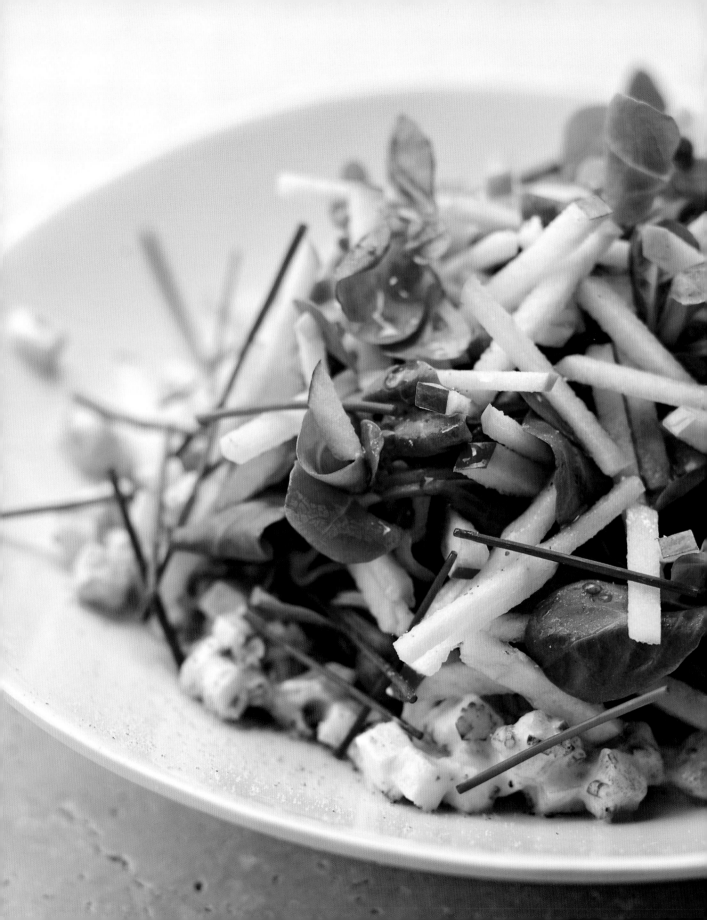

Lamb's Lettuce and Apple Salad

… Serves 4

… Wash 7 ounces of lamb's lettuce in several changes of water and dry it.

… Put in a salad bowl, season with a small splash of olive oil, a little salt, and freshly ground black pepper, and toss well.

… Wash 1 green apple and 1 red apple, but do not peel them. Cut in half, remove the cores, slice thinly with a mandoline, then cut these slices into slivers.

… Add the slivers of apple to the bowl of lamb's lettuce. Mix very gently.

… Cut a small bunch of chives into 2-inch lengths.

… Thin 2 tablespoons of cucumber and apple condiment (page 49) with 1 or 2 tablespoons of Greek-style yogurt to make it nice and liquid.

… Pour onto the bottom of a serving dish or onto individual plates. Pile the lamb's lettuce and apple salad on top, forming a dome. Then arrange the chopped chives around the edge.

AD— This salad goes very well with scallops, halved horizontally and seared for just 30 seconds on each side on a grill or griddle. Or serve the salad with a pan-seared fish fillet.

PN— Lamb's lettuce and apple: two of the best ingredients for your health. Lamb's lettuce is a small nutritional miracle for its richness in carotenoids, vitamins B_9, C, and E, and omega-3s. The apple, thanks to a happy combination of fiber, minerals, and polyphenols, acts on cholesterol, blood sugar, and the digestive system. Nothing but good!

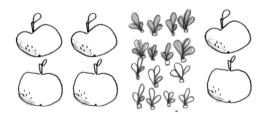

Blanched Asparagus Gratin

AD— You can cook this gratin a few hours in advance and keep it in the fridge. If you do, take it out when you begin to prepare the meal so that it returns to room temperature.

PN— A light combination, rich in B vitamins, carotenoids, and fiber. Both asparagus and mushrooms are well endowed with these nutrients.

… Serves 4

… Put salted water to boil in a large saucepan. Prepare a bowl with water and ice cubes.

… Peel and wash 2 bundles of asparagus and cut off the hard base of the stalks. Tie them in bundles and immerse them in the boiling water for 5 minutes.

… Take them out and cool immediately in the ice water. Then drain on a clean dish towel.

… Quickly wash 10 large mushrooms and cut off the bottom of the base.

… Heat a sauté pan with a splash of olive oil, cut the mushrooms into thin slices, and add to the pan. Add salt and the juice of half a lemon, cover, and sweat for 5 minutes, stirring occasionally.

… Blend the mushrooms, adding ½ cup Greek-style yogurt and 1 tablespoon of grated Parmesan.

… Preheat the oven to 325°F.

… Spread the mushroom puree in a gratin dish, place the asparagus spears side by side on top, sprinkle with 2 tablespoons of grated Parmesan, and put in the oven for 15 minutes. Serve nice and hot.

Artichokes and Fennel à la Barigoule

... Serves 4

Prepare the vegetables

... Remove the tough outer leaves of 12 small artichokes. Cut in half lengthwise and remove the choke. Place them in water with the juice of 1 lemon as you go along.

... Remove the outer leaves of 2 fennel bulbs and cut into 8 wedges. Wash and dry them.

... Peel and wash 1 carrot and 1 small stalk of celery, and cut at an angle into small chunks approximately ¾ inch.

... Peel and thinly slice half a white onion. Cut 1 thin slice of bacon into very small lardons (⅟₁₆ inch).

Cook the artichokes and fennel

... In a flameproof casserole dish, brown the lardons in a teaspoon of olive oil for 1 minute. Then add the pieces of carrot, celery, and onion, 4 garlic cloves, 2 sprigs of thyme, and 2 bay leaves. Stir well and cover the casserole dish with a lid. Cook over low heat for just 3 minutes.

... Add the artichokes and fennel. Add a little salt and freshly ground black pepper. Stir well and cook for an additional 3 minutes.

... Then add ¾ cup of dry white wine. Allow to reduce by half.

... Then pour in 1½ cups of chicken stock (page 10), stir, and cover the casserole dish with a lid. Lower the heat and cook for 8 to 10 minutes, until the artichokes and fennel are tender. Check with the tip of a knife.

... Drain the vegetables, arrange them decoratively on a dish, and keep warm.

... Taste the cooking liquid and correct its seasoning, but also its consistency, and reduce if necessary. Incorporate 2 tablespoons of olive oil, beating vigorously to emulsify, and pour over the vegetables. Add 4 cloves of garlic confit (page 12), season with freshly ground black pepper, and serve.

AD— Always choose artichokes that are fresh and firm, and with a stalk that is green and breaks easily. PN— These vegetables are low in calories and high in fiber and minerals (especially magnesium). Cooking them à la barigoule does nothing to take away from their lightness.

Poached Baby Leeks with Gribiche Sauce

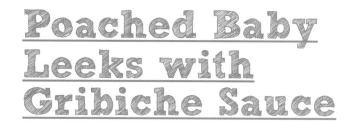

AD— It's perfectly possible to adapt this recipe to other vegetables, such as French beans, asparagus, and even fresh carrots with the tops on or baby turnips— why not? Always choose the freshest possible vegetables and don't overcook them.

PN— Rich in fiber, minerals, carotenoids, and other antioxidants, and vitamin B₉ and vitamin C (especially in the green part), the leek (already praised by Hippocrates) is a vegetable much lauded by nutritionists for its health-giving properties.

… Serves 4

… Prepare a bowl of gribiche sauce (page 48) without grating the hard-boiled eggs over, and keep cool.

… Put salted water to boil in a saucepan. Also prepare a large bowl with water and ice cubes.

… Trim the rootlets at the base of 12 baby leeks and slit their green part lengthwise with 2 or 3 knife cuts.

… Wash in the sink filled with water holding them by the base and shaking them to remove all traces of earth.

… Then tie them into 3 bundles with cooking string and immerse them in boiling water for 12 minutes.

… Check when they are done with the tip of a knife. They should be fairly soft.

… Take them out of the saucepan with a slotted spoon and plunge them in the iced water for just 30 seconds to help keep their color without cooling them too much.

… Drain them, squeeze gently, then arrange in the serving dish and season immediately with salt and freshly ground black pepper.

… Spread the gribiche sauce over.

… Then grate the hard-boiled eggs on top and serve immediately.

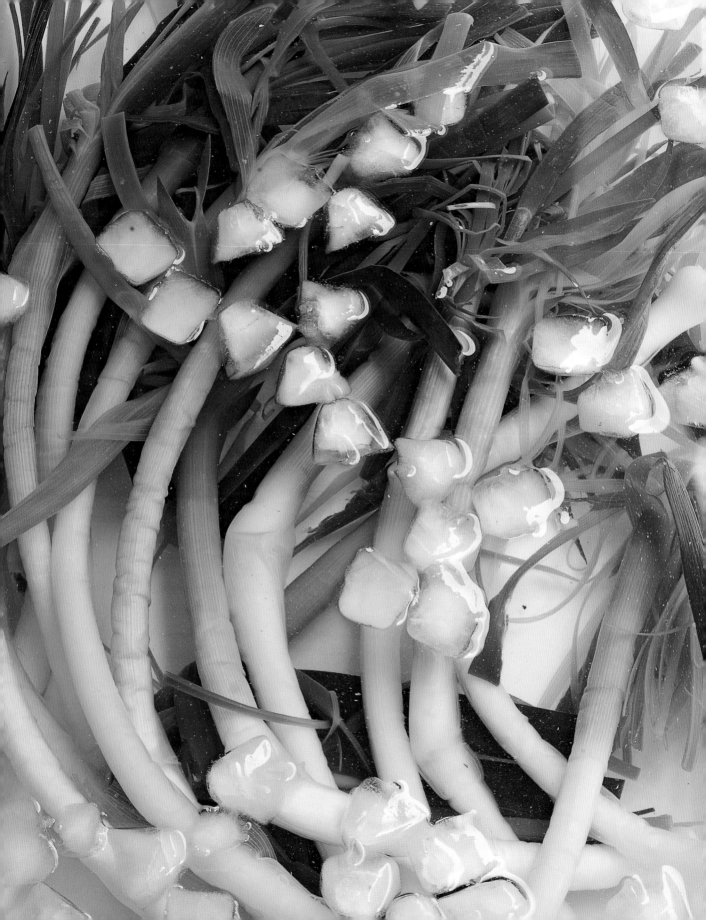

Green Cabbage Salad with Soft-Boiled Egg

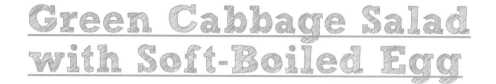

AD— Use walnut bread, if you can get hold of some. Its flavors go very well with those of cabbage marinated in vinegar.

PN— Cabbage has many virtues, due to its fiber and antioxidants, and to the special molecules it contains. It's a very healthy food, and very easy to digest when blanched.

… Serves 4

… Core 1 head of green cabbage. Separate the leaves and wash them. Remove the tougher outer leaves and thinly slice the rest into 2-inch strips.

… Heat a flameproof casserole dish with ¼ cup of wine vinegar.

… Add the sliced cabbage leaves, cook for just 1 minute, stirring, then transfer to a large bowl. Pour ¼ cup of olive oil over and add freshly ground black pepper.

… Leave to marinate for 20 minutes.

… In the meantime, soft boil 3 eggs (6 minutes), cool, and shell them.

… Preheat the oven to 400°F.

… Wash, dry, and cut the leaves off a small bunch of parsley, a small bunch of chervil, and a very small bunch of tarragon.

… Put the soft-boiled eggs in a bowl and crush with a fork.

… Add them to the cabbage when it has sufficiently marinated. Also add the herb leaves.

… When your oven is hot, place 8 thin slices of whole-wheat bread on the rack and toast until crunchy and slightly colored (1 to 2 minutes).

… Put the cabbage in the serving dish. Break up the slices of dried bread and arrange them decoratively on top. Serve right away.

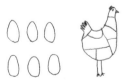

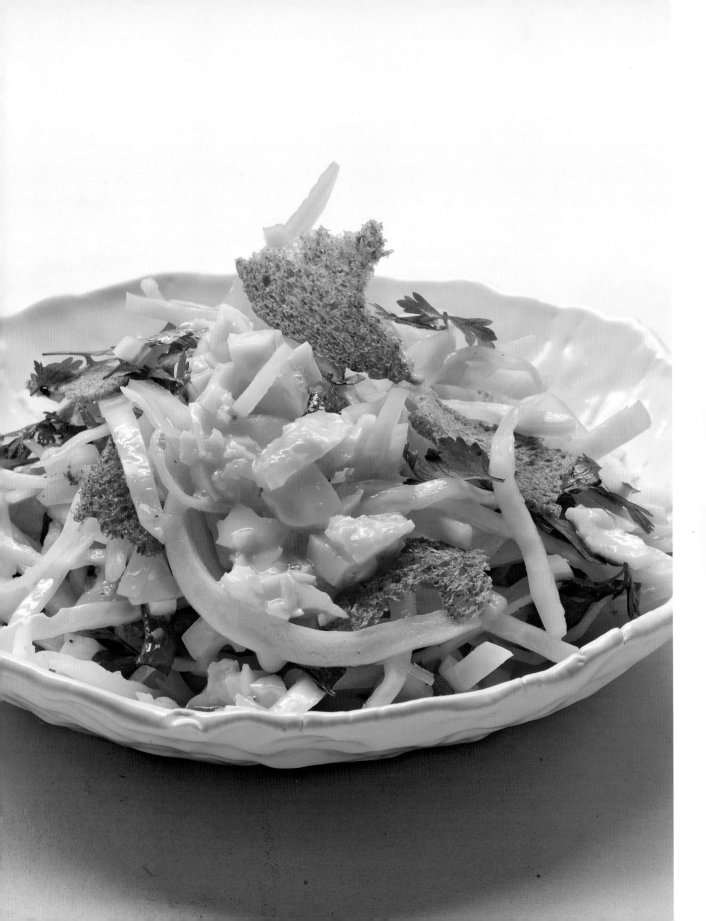

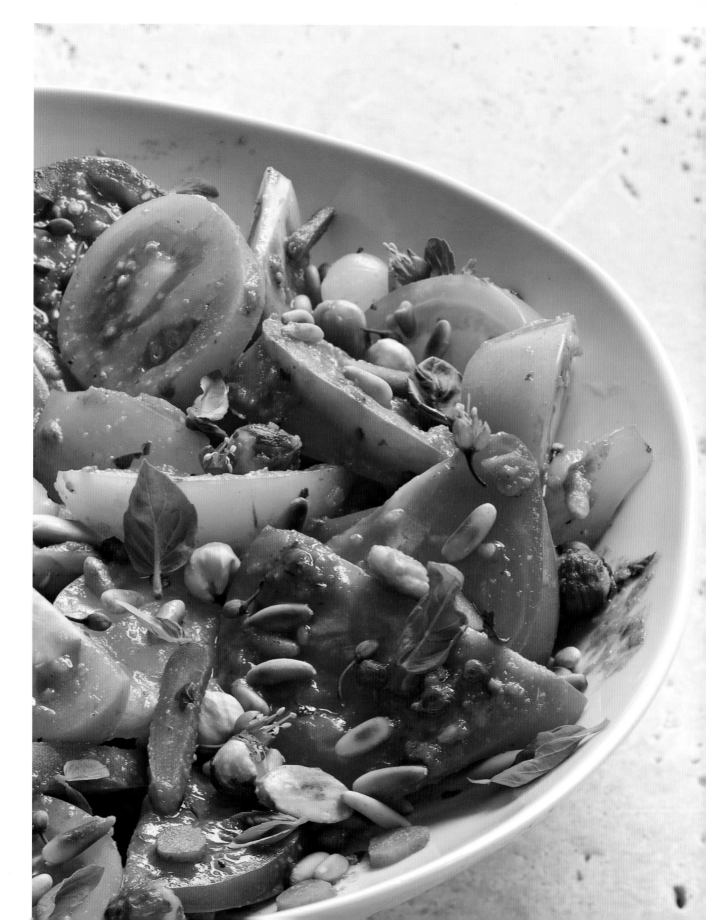

Tomato Salad with Romesco Sauce

... Serves 4

Prepare the Romesco sauce

... Turn on the broiler. Cut 1 small red bell pepper in half, remove the seeds, and place on a baking sheet, skin side up. Peel half a small white onion, slice thinly, and slip it under the pepper. Cut 1 tomato in half, squeeze to remove the seeds, and add it. Then add 4 garlic cloves and 1 slice of stale bread and put the sheet under the broiler.

... Remove the bread as soon as it is toasted, but broil the onion, pepper, garlic, and tomato for 20 minutes.

... In the meantime, heat a dry skillet, add a heaping tablespoon of almonds, a heaping tablespoon of pine nuts, and a heaping tablespoon of hazelnuts. Brown them, then cool them on paper towels. Then crush them.

... Take the sheet out of the oven and remove the skin of the garlic cloves and the tomatoes, but leave the pepper skins on.

... Combine the bread, roasted vegetables, and toasted nuts in the bowl of your food processor and add 2 pinches of Piment d'Espelette or hot paprika and 3 tablespoons of sherry vinegar. Blend until you have an even puree, then add 5 or 6 tablespoons of olive oil. If the sauce is too thick, thin it with a little water.

... Adjust the seasoning and refrigerate.

Prepare the tomato salad

... Wash 6 to 8 ripe tomatoes of different varieties and colors, cut out any hard cores, and quarter but do not seed them. Put them in a salad bowl.

... Cut 5 or 6 gherkins into pieces at an angle, and drain 1 heaping tablespoon of capers and 5 or 6 pickled onions. Take the leaves off 2 sprigs of basil, and rinse and dry a small handful of arugula.

... Pour the Romesco sauce over the tomatoes and stir gently.

... Arrange these seasoned tomatoes in a large serving dish, then add the gherkins, capers, onions, basil, arugula, and perhaps a few garlic or chive flowers. Serve nice and cold.

AD— Vary the tomatoes (green, yellow, black, beefsteak) according to what you can find in the market. Romesco sauce is suitable for making in advance.

PN— Carotenoids and vitamin C in the tomatoes, flavonoids in the peppers and chile, vitamin E in the almonds, pine nuts, and hazelnuts—this is a real potpourri of protective antioxidants!

Provençal-Style Eggplant Cocotte

AD— This Provençal dish is even tastier if you make it the day before. The longer it is kept cold, the better the flavors blend together.

PN— Serve this as a starter or with an aperitif on some lightly toasted slices of country bread, which, with their slow carbohydrates, would balance this dish rather nicely.

… Serves 4

… Wash 6 good-sized eggplants. Half peel them with a vegetable peeler, alternating peel and flesh, then slice into thin rounds (⅛ inch thick).

… Spread them on a baking sheet, sprinkle with plenty of coarse salt, and leave for 30 minutes to draw out the juices.

… Rinse and dry them on paper towels.

… Heat a sauté pan with 1 to 2 spoonfuls of olive oil and cook for 5 minutes on each side, until they are nice and golden.

… Separate the cloves from 1 head of garlic, remove their outer skin, and crush. Take the leaves off 5 sprigs of thyme. Prepare 1 pound of chopped cooked tomatoes (page 21).

… Preheat the oven to 325°F.

… Brush a cast-iron pot with a drop of olive oil. Arrange a layer of eggplant on the bottom, cover thinly with chopped cooked tomatoes, sprinkle a little thyme over, and add 2 garlic cloves. Add a little salt and pepper.

… Continue to make layers of eggplant, tomatoes, thyme, and garlic. Put the pot in the oven for 45 minutes, until the eggplant is nice and soft.

… Then allow the eggplant to cool in its pot. Refrigerate for at least 2 hours. Turn it out onto a dish and keep cold until you are ready to serve.

… Chop the leaves of 3 sprigs of basil and sprinkle over the dish. Sprinkle a few grains of sea salt and add a generous twist of freshly ground black pepper.

Radicchio Cooked on Embers, with Anchovy Tapenade

… Serves 4

… Make 5 ounces of tapenade (page 40).

… Soak 4 whole long heads of radicchio in water with a dash of vinegar. Drain them.

… Cut in half lengthwise, remove the base of the root, and rinse once more. Dry carefully and salt lightly.

… Take 8 sage leaves and insert one into each half radicchio.

… Pour 2 to 3 tablespoons of olive oil into a dish and roll the lettuces in it.

… Crush 4 anchovy fillets in oil with a fork, add to the tapenade, and stir.

… Preheat the oven to 325°F.

… Lay the half radicchios on a barbecue grill, cut side down, and cook over the embers for 3 minutes, taking care that the grate is high enough so that they don't burn.

… Then brush them generously with the anchovy tapenade, place them in a dish, and finish them in the oven at 325°F.

… Transfer immediately to a dish or onto individual plates. Give a few generous twists of freshly ground black pepper and serve right away.

AD— No brazier or barbecue? Then grill your radicchio on a stovetop griddle, taking care not to burn them.

PN— Radicchio is a lettuce that originated in Italy. It's from the chicory family, hence its slight bitterness. It is one of the richest in carotenoids. With the good fatty acids of the tapenade and the omega-3s from the anchovies, this dish will do the trick!

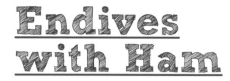

Endives with Ham

AD— Endives are not as bitter as they used to be, and if you remove the core and add a little sugar, they are not bitter at all.
PN— And they are rich in fiber and low in calories. These are their only virtues as, apart from a small amount of carotenoids, they are dreadfully poor in vitamins. If you cook them like this, you will have plenty of calcium and protein, however. Then round off the meal with a good vitamin-rich fruit salad!

… Serves 4

… Wash 10 heads of Belgian endive and cut in half lengthwise. Take out the core, which is the bitter part, but avoid detaching the leaves.

… Heat 2 tablespoons of olive oil in a sauté pan and add the half endives, side by side, cut side down.

… Add 2 garlic cloves, crushed. Add salt and sprinkle with a pinch of superfine sugar.

… Cover and cook gently for 15 minutes.

… Turn the endives over, pour in ½ cup of water, scrape well with a spatula to deglaze the cooking juices, and baste the endives with the liquid. Cook for an additional 5 minutes, basting from time to time.

… While the endives are cooking, crush a handful of shelled walnuts.

… Take out the 4 least attractive half endives and the garlic cloves.

… Blend them, adding 1 cup of lowfat milk and 1 tablespoon of grated Emmental (3 tablespoons required in total for this recipe) until you have a nice thick sauce.

… Correct the seasoning, adding salt to taste and plenty of freshly ground black pepper.

… Turn on the broiler.

… Cut 4 slices of cooked ham in half. Roll a half-endive in each piece of ham and place them in a gratin dish. Pour the endive sauce on top and sprinkle with crushed walnuts and 2 tablespoons of grated Emmental.

… Put under the broiler to brown.

… Serve immediately, nice and hot.

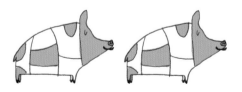

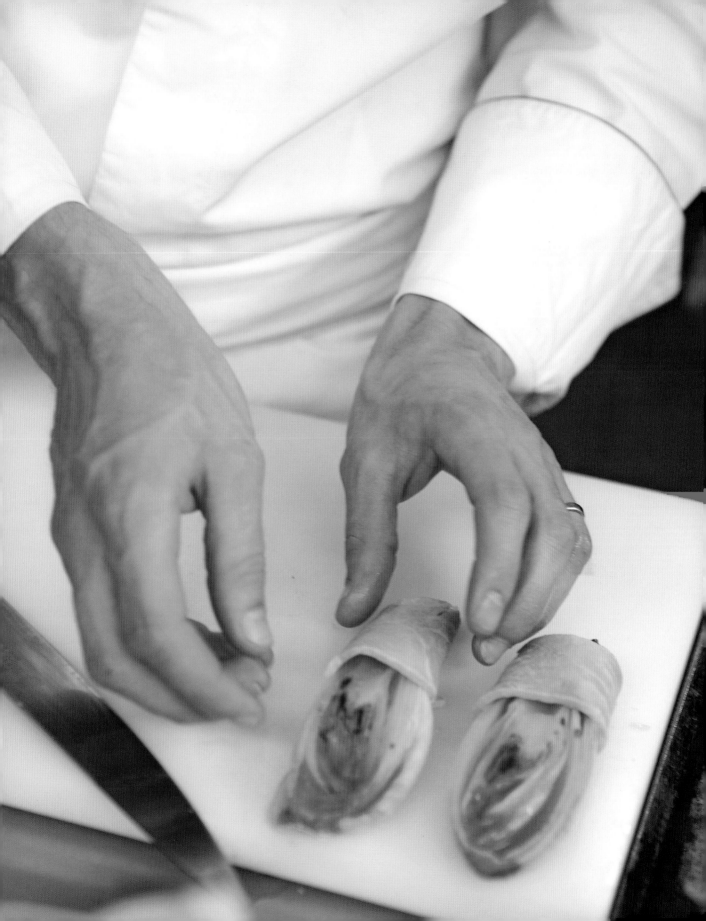

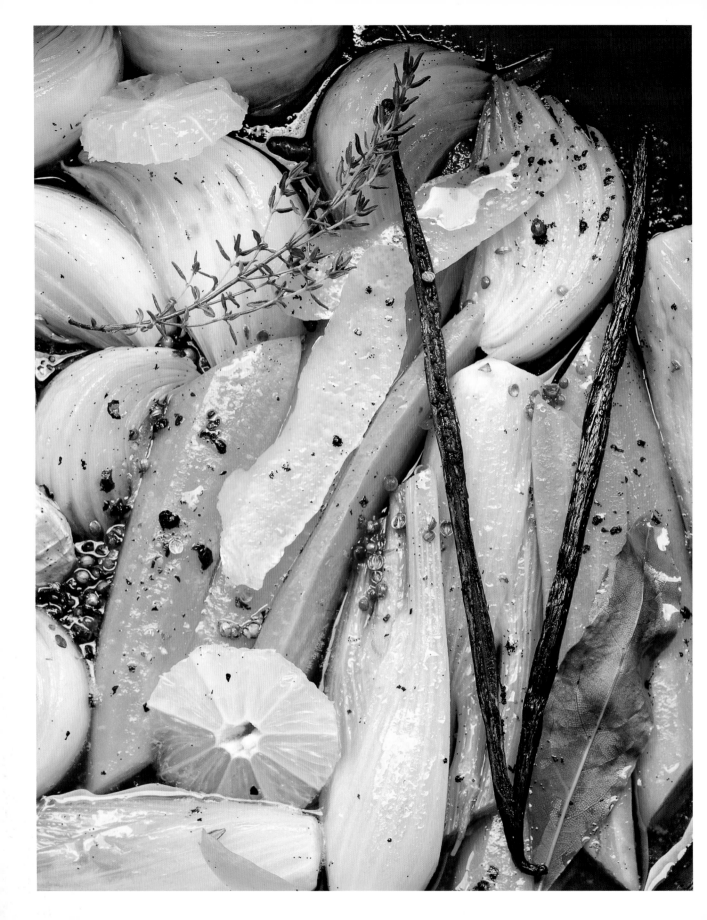

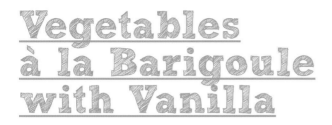

Vegetables à la Barigoule with Vanilla

… Serves 4

<u>Prepare the vegetables</u>

… Peel and wash 4 carrots with tops, keeping ½ inch of the tops, and cut them in half lengthwise. Separate the florets of 1 head of broccoli and wash them. Peel 4 medium white onions. Cut 1 fennel bulb into 8 wedges, and rinse. Peel 4 garlic cloves. Peel and wash 1 bundle of asparagus, cut the tips into 3-inch lengths, and tie in a bundle.

… Plunge the broccoli florets and asparagus in salted boiling water for about 3 minutes. Drain and refresh in ice water.

<u>Cook the rest of the vegetables</u>

… Heat 2 cups of chicken stock (page 10).

… Tie up 10 coriander seeds, 5 peppercorns, 1 bay leaf, 4 sprigs of thyme, and 1 garlic clove in a piece of cheesecloth or an infusion bag.

… Heat a sauté pan with a splash of olive oil. Put in the carrots, onions, fennel, and garlic cloves.

… Split 1 vanilla bean and add it to the hot chicken stock, then pour this into the sauté pan. Then add the bag of aromatic herbs and allow to simmer for 12 to 15 minutes.

<u>To finish your dish</u>

… Take out the vanilla bean and bag of aromatic herbs. Add the broccoli florets and the asparagus tips, then stir gently.

… Lift out all these vegetables with a slotted spoon and keep in a warm dish.

… Reduce the cooking liquid down to 1 cup. Pour in 2 tablespoons of olive oil and a splash of sherry vinegar and stir vigorously. Check the seasoning and pour over the vegetables.

… Add a few grains of sea salt and a few cilantro leaves. Serve hot.

AD— The vegetables should be slightly crunchy. Check with the tip of a knife as you cook them and take any that are cooked sooner out of the sauté pan.

PN— It takes only about 40 minutes to prepare this tasty cocktail of vitamins, minerals, and antioxidants of all kinds, so don't miss out on this dish!

Spinach and Soft-Boiled Eggs

AD— With the garlic clove stuck on a fork, you can lightly flavor the spinach without overwhelming its own flavors. Add the croutons at the very last minute, otherwise they will go soft.

PN— Spinach is exceptionally rich in antioxidant carotenoids. It also contains quite a lot of minerals and vitamins. It can sometimes be high in nitrates, which turn into toxic nitrites. Avoid this by buying very fresh spinach, using it right away, and cooking it quickly, as in this recipe.

… Serves 4

… Remove the stems from 2 pounds of spinach, wash it in several changes of cold water, and drain. Dry in a dish towel.

… Peel 1 garlic clove and stick it on the end of a fork.

… Toast 2 to 3 slices of rye bread then break them up into small pieces.

… Heat some water in a saucepan. When it boils, carefully put in 4 eggs and boil for 6 minutes for a soft boil.

… At the same time, heat 2 tablespoons of olive oil in a large sauté pan. Add the spinach, by the handful, stirring with the fork with the garlic on it. Continue to mix well until it has all wilted. Add salt and freshly ground black pepper. Cook the spinach in batches and transfer into a dish as soon as it is wilted.

… Return it all to the sauté pan, add 2 tablespoons of light cream, and stir.

… Arrange the spinach in a serving dish or on individual plates. Sprinkle the rye bread croutons on top and stir to mix them in.

… Quickly shell the soft-boiled eggs and place them on top of the spinach.

… Poke a knife in the eggs just to open the white and allow the yolk to flow slightly. Serve immediately.

Greek-Style Spring Vegetables and Salad Leaves

… Serves 4

Prepare the vegetables

… Peel and wash 6 small fennel bulbs with tops and 4 small spring onions with stalks, leaving on 2½ inches of stalk, then halve them. Scrape and wash 7 ounces of baby new potatoes. Cut them in half. Peel the cloves of 1 head of garlic, leaving on the inner skin. Cut off the bases of 5 ounces of chanterelles, wash quickly, and pat dry. Shell 14 ounces of baby fava beans.

Cook the vegetables

… Tie up 6 black peppercorns, 15 coriander seeds, half a bay leaf, and a sprig of thyme in a piece of cheesecloth or an infusion bag.

… Heat a drop of olive oil in a sauté pan and sweat the fennel bulbs, onions, potatoes, chanterelles, and garlic cloves in their skins for 2 minutes without coloring. Add salt, pour in ¾ cup dry white wine, and reduce fully.

… Then add 2 cups of chicken stock (page 10), the aromatic herbs, and the zest of 1 lemon.

… Cut a round of parchment paper the shape of the sauté pan and place it over the vegetables. Cook gently for 15 minutes. Add 4 segments of tomato confit (page 16) and the fava beans, stir, and take the sauté pan off the heat immediately.

… Gently lift the vegetables out with a slotted spoon and transfer to a serving dish. Take out the cheesecloth and reduce the sauce by half. Add 3 tablespoons of olive oil and stir well. Correct the seasoning and pour this sauce over the vegetables. Allow to cool.

Prepare the salad leaves

… To cook the salad vegetables, remove the stems from a handful of arugula and a handful of young sorrel or spinach leaves and wash. Pick the leaves off 2 sprigs of cilantro. Combine in a salad bowl and season with a drizzle of olive oil, sea salt, and freshly ground black pepper.

… Arrange the salad in bunches all around the vegetables and serve.

AD— Small fava beans don't need to be cooked. But if you are using larger beans, immerse them in salted boiling water for 3 minutes. PN— Fresh garlic is easy to digest and will not give you bad breath, as long as the central germ sprout has not yet developed in the cloves.

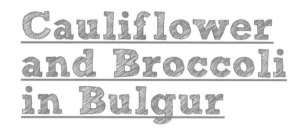

Cauliflower and Broccoli in Bulgur

AD— This recipe can easily be made in advance, but don't store it in the fridge, as the bulgur will lose all its tenderness.

PN— Broccoli has become something of a panacea for nutritionists because it contains molecules that protect us from almost everything. But the cauliflower is not far behind! This combination of the two, plus the carbohydrates in the bulgur, has it all!

… Serves 4

… Wash 1 head of cauliflower and 1 head of broccoli. Separate all the florets and cut them to about ¼ inch with a small knife (keep any leftovers for a soup).

… Measure 1½ cups of fine bulgur into a measuring cup. Then measure 3 cups of water and pour that into a saucepan. Add salt and bring to a boil.

… Gently sprinkle the bulgur into the water, stir, and cook just under a boil for 5 minutes.

… In the meantime, cut the skin of half a salt-preserved lemon (page 15) into small slivers.

… After 5 minutes of cooking, add the cauliflower and broccoli florets, 1 teaspoon of curry powder, 3 pinches of Piment d'Espelette or hot paprika, and the slivers of salted lemon to the saucepan of bulgur. Stir very gently.

… Taste and check the salt seasoning.

… Turn the contents of the saucepan into a serving dish. Serve hot or at room temperature.

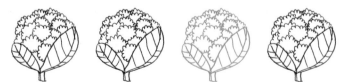

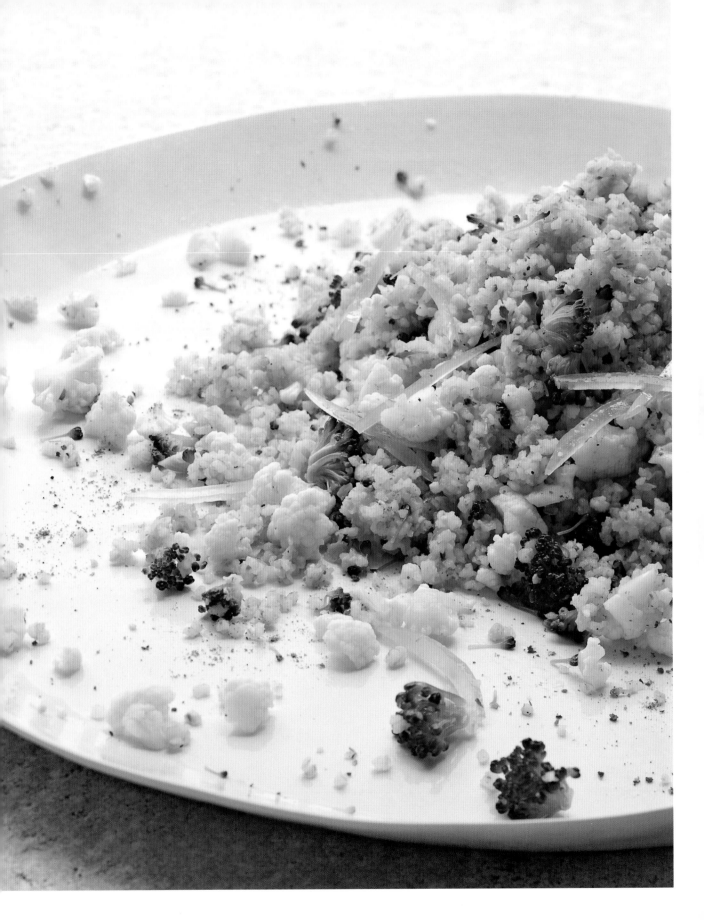

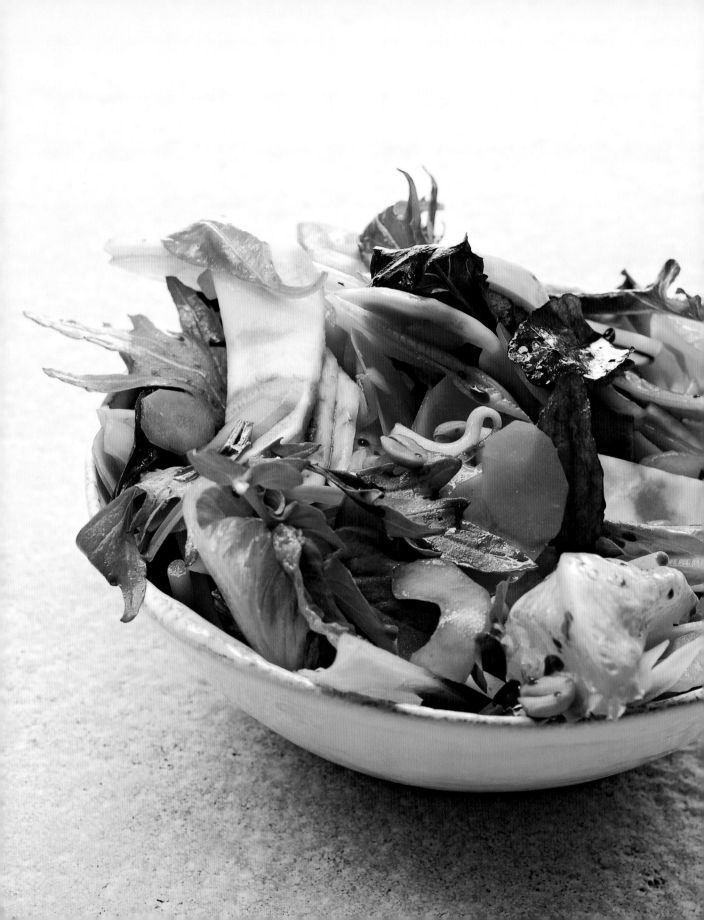

Stir-Fried Vegetables and Salad Greens

… Serves 4

… Wash and peel 2 large carrots, a quarter of a celeriac, and 1 cucumber. Cut into thin slices with a mandoline.

… Wash and dry 1 head of romaine lettuce, 2 handfuls of bean sprouts, and 3 handfuls of mixed salad greens. Finely chop the larger romaine leaves and mix with the bean sprouts and mixed greens in a salad bowl.

… Peel and grate 2 inches of ginger. Chop 2 tablespoons of peanuts. Squeeze the juice of 1 lemon.

… Sauté the carrots, celeriac, and cucumber in a wok with a dash of olive oil for 2 minutes, allowing the vegetables to color lightly. Add the chopped peanuts and stir.

… Then add in the mixture of romaine, salad greens, and bean sprouts. Cook for 1 minute more.

… Add the lemon juice and 5 tablespoons of soy sauce. Stir well as you add them to deglaze the wok.

… Finally, add the grated ginger and stir once more. Add salt and freshly ground black pepper.

… Arrange the vegetable stir-fry in a dish and serve immediately.

AD— You can of course use varieties of lettuce other than romaine. But pick a variety with big crisp leaves.

PN— Cooked quickly like this, the vegetables don't lose any of their vitamins. This is where the wok comes into its own.

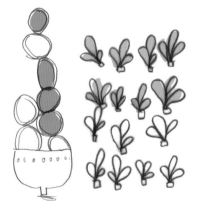

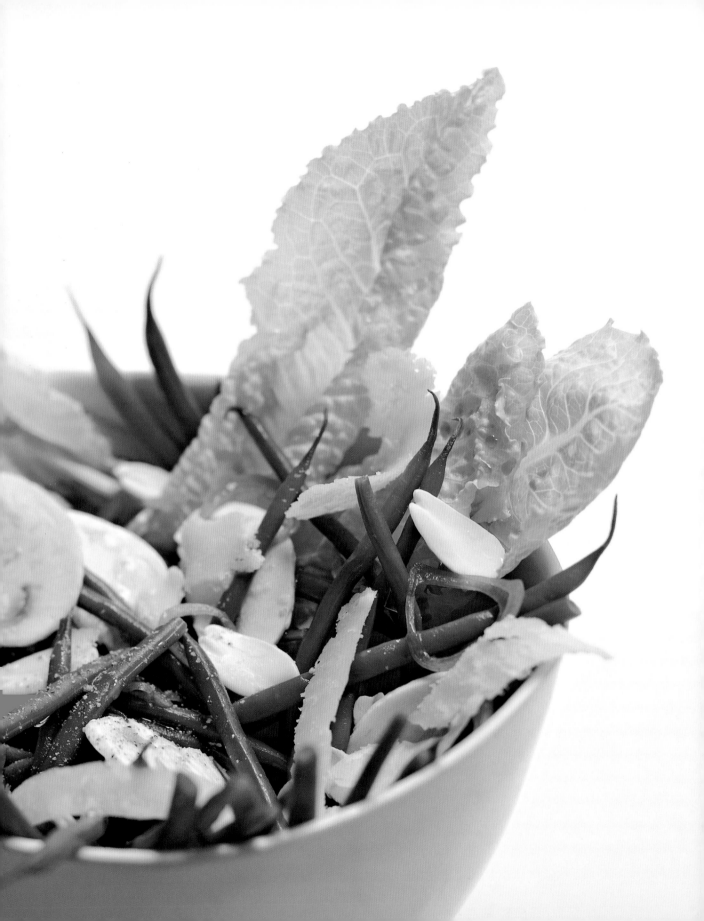

French-Bean Salad

… Serves 4

… Peel 1 shallot and slice into thin rounds. Put them on a small plate, sprinkle with 1 tablespoon of red wine vinegar, and leave to marinate for 30 minutes.

… In the meantime, de-string and wash 8 ounces of French beans, then immerse them in boiling salted water for 5 to 7 minutes, keeping them crunchy.

… Prepare a basin with water and ice cubes. Drain the French beans and refresh immediately in the ice water.

… Cut the base off 3 ounces of small fresh mushrooms. Wash the caps quickly, dry them, and cut into thin slices.

… Rinse and dry the leaves of 1 romaine lettuce heart.

… Shell 12 fresh almonds and cut them in half.

… Squeeze the juice of 1 lemon and pour into a salad bowl. Add a pinch of salt, stir, then add 3 to 4 tablespoons of olive oil.

… Place the French beans, mushrooms, romaine lettuce leaves, and almonds in the salad bowl and toss gently.

… Sprinkle the shallot rounds on top. Then, with a vegetable peeler, shave 1 ounce of Parmesan over the top.

… Finish with a generous twist of freshly ground black pepper.

AD— If chanterelles are in season, use small ones rather than white mushrooms: They are delicious raw. And when fresh almonds are not in season, you can make do with sliced almonds.

PN— French beans are rich in vitamins (especially folates), minerals, carotenoids, and fiber. Don't cook them too much so as to avoid destroying their vitamins, which are fragile!

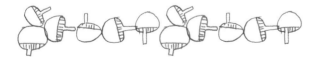

Celery and Apple Salad

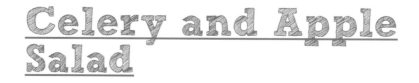

AD— *If you want to add a touch of sophistication to this salad, grate a little black truffle into it. The caramelized walnuts add a pleasant little note of sweetness.*
PN— *Since ancient times, celery has had a reputation of being an aphrodisiac; the Romans ate it in large quantities for this reason. Although the effect has never been verified scientifically, the vegetable does contain a substance similar to testosterone.*

… Serves 4

Prepare the caramelized walnuts

… Preheat the oven to 250°F. Pour ¼ cup of superfine sugar and ¼ cup water into a saucepan and bring to a boil. Season with a pinch of salt and a tiny pinch of cayenne pepper. Take the saucepan off the heat.

… Separate 12 shelled walnuts in two and soak them in this syrup for 20 minutes.

… Cover a baking sheet with parchment paper. Drain the walnuts and spread them on top. Bake for 35 minutes, until they are lightly caramelized, then cool on a plate.

Prepare the yogurt sauce

… In a bowl, mix ½ cup of plain yogurt and 1 egg yolk. Add 1 tablespoon of Dijon mustard, the juice of 1 lemon, and 1 tablespoon of vinegar. Then gradually incorporate 3 tablespoons of soy oil, beating as you go. Add salt and freshly ground black pepper. Keep cool.

Prepare the salad

… Wash 2 Granny Smith apples and 2 Red Delicious apples, cut them in half without peeling, and remove the cores. Then cut them into small slivers.

… Peel and wash 4 stalks of celery and half a celeriac. Cut the celery into thin slices with a mandoline and the celeriac into thin slivers.

… Separate the leaves from 1 romaine lettuce heart, wash and dry, then line a salad bowl with them.

… Crush half of the caramelized walnuts.

… In a large bowl, combine the slivers of apple, celery, and celeriac and the crushed walnuts, add the yogurt sauce, and toss gently. Add to the salad bowl. Sprinkle the rest of the caramelized walnuts on top and serve.

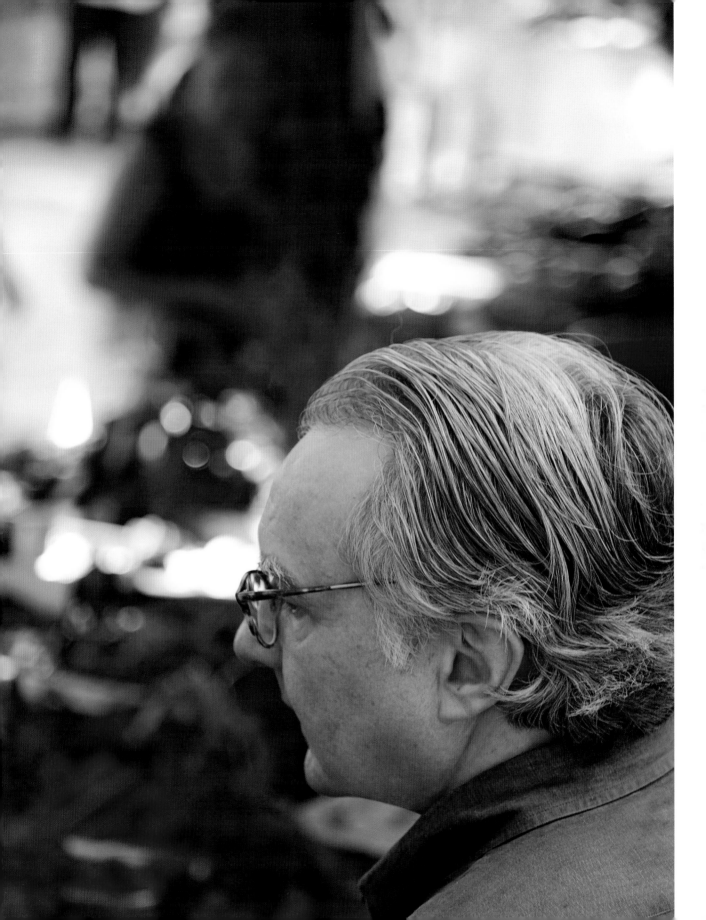

"Markets have a life of their own: a whole world of aromas, textures, and shapes created at dawn."

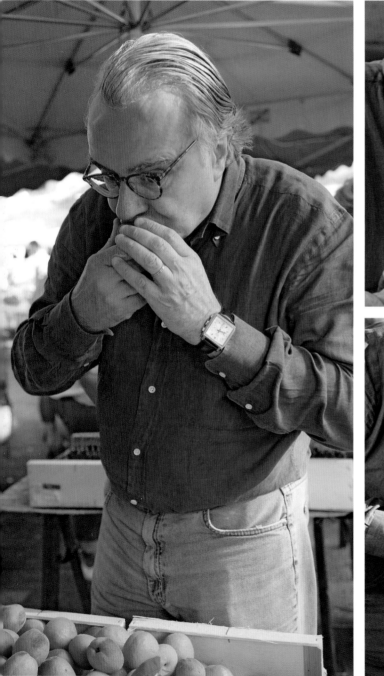

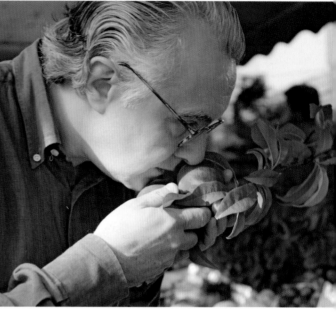

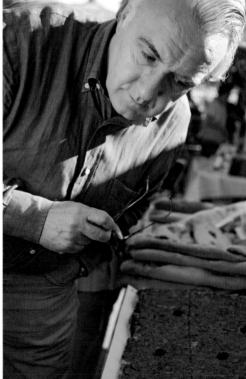

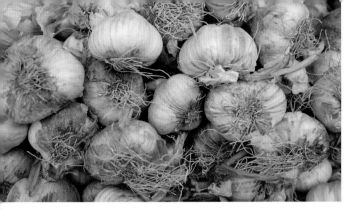

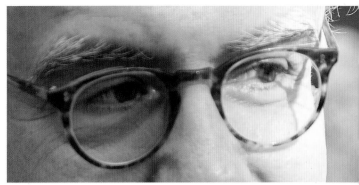

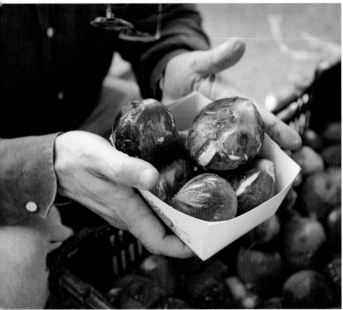

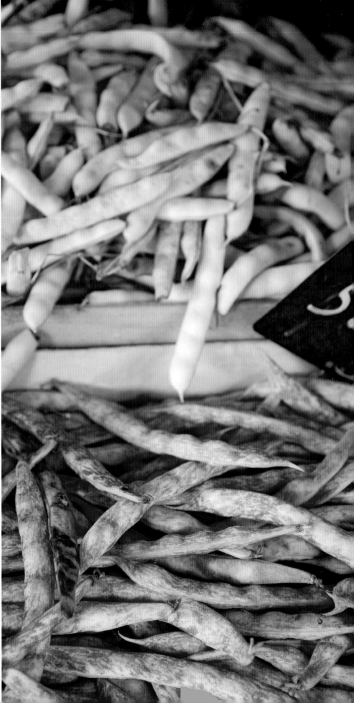

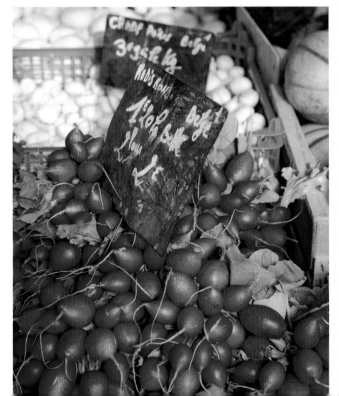

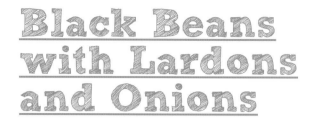

Black Beans with Lardons and Onions

AD— If you can't get hold of pancetta, substitute slices of lean bacon. And if you want to save time, cook the beans the day before, keep them in the fridge, and reheat them gently.

PN— The beans and pancetta provide enough protein, so you don't need any other meat in this meal. Start with a vegetable salad and finish with a little cheese and some fruit.

… Serves 4

… Soak 1 cup of dried black beans in water for 12 hours.

… Drain and put in a saucepan.

… Add 3 cups of chicken stock (page 10), 1 sprig of thyme (3 sprigs required in total for the recipe), and 1 garlic clove and cook gently for 40 to 45 minutes, until the beans are soft without being reduced to a puree.

… Salt lightly (add only once the beans are cooked).

… While the beans are cooking, cut 3 slices of pancetta into lardons (approximately 1 inch). Peel 4 carrots with tops and 3 small white onions with stalks. Remove the top of the onion stalks, thinly slice the stalks, and set them aside.

… Slice the onions into rounds and slice the carrots at an angle into small pieces.

… When the beans are cooked, drain them and keep their cooking liquid.

… In a flameproof casserole dish with a drop of olive oil, sweat the pancetta lardons, the onion rounds, and the pieces of carrot with the leaves of the remaining 2 sprigs of thyme for 3 minutes, without letting them color too much.

… Add the beans and stir.

… Then add a good ladleful of their cooking liquid and 5 tablespoons of balsamic vinegar, mix well, and cook for just 2 minutes.

… Then add the sliced onion stalks and stir. Taste and adjust the seasoning.

… Serve in the casserole dish.

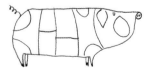

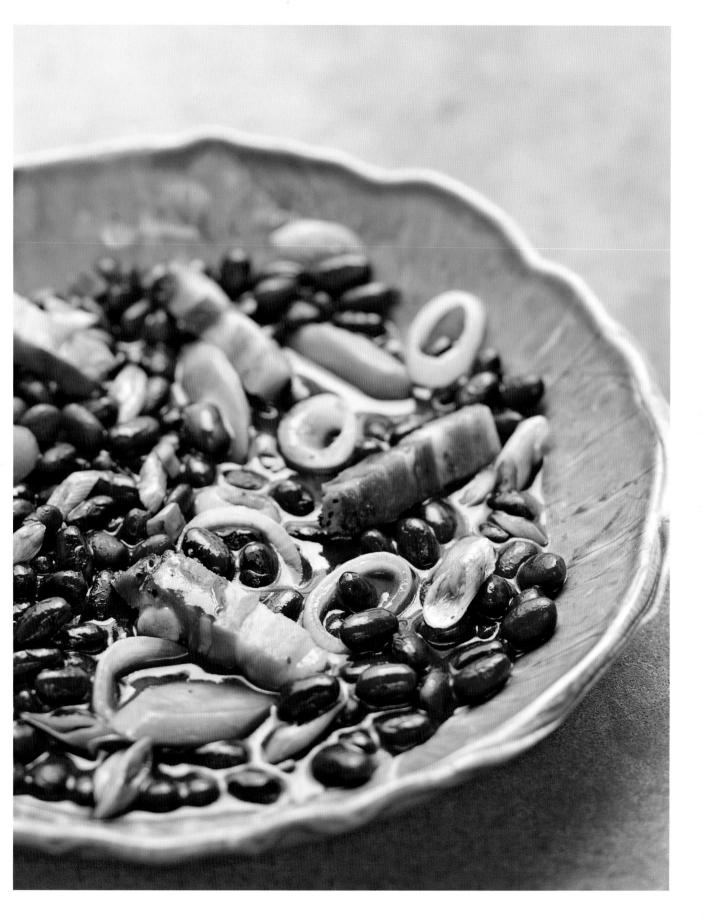

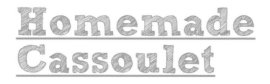

Homemade Cassoulet

AD— This cassoulet takes about an hour to prepare, and the beans need to be soaked overnight. You can make it a day in advance, keep it in the fridge, and finish cooking it before the meal, and it will taste even better.

PN— Contrary to what many people think, cassoulet is a genuinely healthy dish. It contains fiber and slow carbohydrates, and the fatty acid composition of goose fat is similar to that of olive oil.

… Serves 8

<u>The day before</u>

… Soak 2 pounds of white navy beans.

<u>On the day, prepare the aromatic vegetables</u>

… Cut 2 carrots and 1 stalk of celery into small dice. Peel 3 onions; cut 2 of them in the same way and stud the other with 1 clove.

<u>Cook the beans</u>

… Put the drained beans in a saucepan and add 4 times their volume of water. Heat gently, take the saucepan off the heat as soon as it starts to boil, and drain.

… Return the beans to their saucepan and pour in boiling water to cover. Add 1 bouquet garni (2 bunches required in total for the recipe), the clove-studded onion, and half of the carrot and celery dice. Cook for 1 hour over low heat, until the beans are soft. Add salt only at the end of cooking.

<u>Cook the meat</u>

… In the meantime, melt 1 tablespoon of goose fat (5 tablespoons required in total for the recipe) in a flameproof casserole dish and brown 4 duck confit legs and 1½ pounds of lamb shoulder trimmed of its fat. Drain them on paper towels.

… Put the onion dice and the rest of the carrot and celery dice in the casserole dish and sweat for 2 to 3 minutes. Return the meat to the casserole dish, add water to cover, and pop in another bouquet garni and 6 crushed garlic cloves. Cook at just under a boil for 45 minutes. Strain the cooking liquid through a fine-mesh sieve and set aside.

<u>Prepare the cassoulet</u>

… Heat the oven to 325°F. Chop 6 garlic cloves. When the beans are cooked, drain and return them to the saucepan with this garlic and the reserved liquid from the meat. Check the seasoning.

… Cut the lamb shoulder into pieces and cut the duck legs in half. Arrange them on a dish. Pour over the beans with their cooking liquid; the liquid should just cover them. Spread ¼ cup of melted goose fat on top. Sprinkle the cassoulet with dried bread crumbs and put in the oven for 1 hour. Serve in its dish, nice and hot.

Chickpea and Lentil Salad with Hummus Sauce

… Serves 4

The day before

… Soak 1¼ cups of dried chickpeas.

On the day

… Peel 2 onions and 2 carrots and cut into chunks.

… Drain the chickpeas and put them in a saucepan with 1 bay leaf (2 required in total for the recipe) and half the onions and carrots. Cover well with water and cook for 1½ hours. Add salt only at the end of cooking.

… In another saucepan filled with water, cook ½ cup of red lentils similarly with the rest of the onions and carrots and another bay leaf for 30 minutes. Leave to cool in their cooking water.

… Peel and mince 1 garlic clove.

… Take out approximately two thirds of the chickpeas with a slotted spoon. Blend them with the garlic and 1 or 2 ladles of their cooking liquid until you have a smooth cream. Add the juice of half a lemon, 1 teaspoon of ground cumin, 1 teaspoon of ras al-hanout, and 2 pinches of paprika and blend a little more to incorporate well. Taste the hummus and correct its seasoning with salt and freshly ground black pepper.

… Rinse and dry 1½ ounces of bean sprouts and put in a salad bowl. Drain the lentils and the rest of the chickpeas and add them. Season with 2 to 3 tablespoons of olive oil, 1 tablespoon of sherry vinegar, salt, and freshly ground black pepper.

… Detach the leaves from 3 sprigs of mint.

… Spoon the hummus into the center of a round dish. Spread the chickpea-lentil-bean sprout salad all around. Sprinkle the mint leaves on top.

AD— Hummus is a great classic of Lebanese cooking. Make it with sufficient liquid so that rather than the usual puree you have a softer cream that will mix well with the salad.

PN— Chickpeas are the most useful of all the pulses, not only because they're rich in carbohydrates, proteins, and minerals, but also because they contain antioxidants: carotenoids and vitamin E.

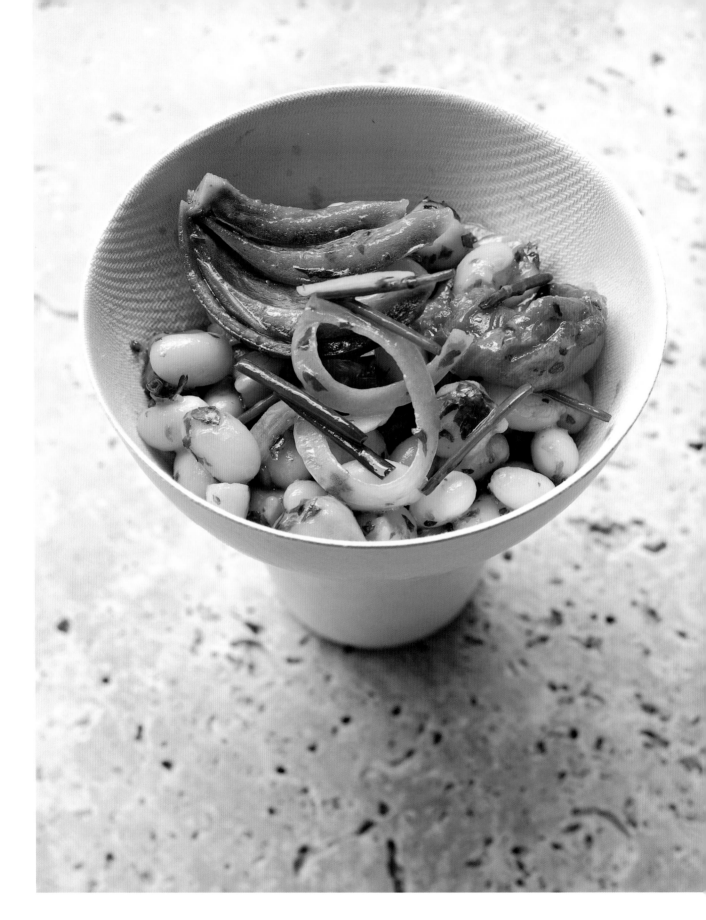

White Kidney Bean and Chickpea Salad with Herb Pesto

… Serves 4

Prepare the white kidney beans and chickpeas

… The day before, soak ¾ cup of white kidney beans and ¾ cup of chickpeas.

… On the day, peel 2 red onions, blanch and seed 2 nice ripe tomatoes, and cut them all into wedges.

… Drain the beans and chickpeas and put in a saucepan. Add the onions and tomatoes, 2 sprigs of thyme, 1 bay leaf, 4 crushed garlic cloves, and 1 quart of chicken stock (page 10). Cook gently for 45 minutes, until the beans are soft. Salt lightly once they are cooked.

Prepare the herb pesto

… Wash, dry, and separate the leaves from a very small bunch of chervil, a very small bunch of flat-leaf parsley, and a very small bunch of basil.

… Blend them, gradually adding 6 tablespoons of olive oil and 2 spoonfuls of the bean cooking liquid. Add salt and freshly ground black pepper.

To finish the salad

… Cut a very small bunch of chives into 1-inch lengths.

… Cut 8 segments of tomato confit (page 16) in half.

… Peel and thinly slice 1 pearl onion.

… Drain the white kidney beans and chickpeas and place them in a bowl. Add the onion, tomato confit segments, herb pesto, and chives and mix well.

… Transfer to a dish and serve warm or cold.

AD— If you are serving this salad cold, don't put it in the fridge, as that would make it unpleasantly hard. Why not serve it with squid, simply grilled, with a dash of lemon?

PN— Carbohydrates, vegetable protein, fiber, vitamins, minerals, antioxidants; this dish is nutritionally very rich in a way that would be good to see more of.

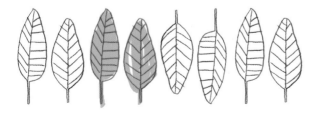

White Kidney Bean Ragout with Cockles

AD— When fresh white beans are out of season, use dried navy beans (about 2 ounces per person). Put them to soak the day before and cook them for a little longer.

PN— With its slow carbohydrates and fiber, plus vegetable and animal protein, this is a complete and well-balanced dish. There is no need to serve meat or fish in this meal. A green salad, a little cheese, some fruit, and you're there!

... Serves 4

Prepare the beans

... Shell 2 pounds of fresh white kidney beans. Put them in a large saucepan and cover well with water. When it boils, lower the heat and skim several times.

... Add 1 carrot, 1 onion cut in half, 1 sage leaf, and a small sprig of rosemary. Cook gently for 30 to 40 minutes; the beans should be soft. Add salt only at the end of cooking. Take out the vegetables and allow the beans to cool in their cooking liquid.

Prepare the cockles

... Meanwhile, rinse 2 pounds of cockles well. Slice 2 shallots thinly and sweat in a large sauté pan with a splash of olive oil for 3 minutes. Add the cockles and 1 cup of white wine, stir, and cover. When all the cockles are open, transfer them to a large bowl. Remove just one shell from a few of them and the whole shell from all the rest.

... Strain the cooking liquid through a fine-mesh strainer and set aside.

Prepare the white kidney bean ragout

... Cut 8 segments of tomato confit (page 16) into strips. Set aside 5 tablespoons of the cockle liquid in a bowl. Pour the rest into a large sauté pan with a splash of olive oil and reduce by half. Add the drained beans, the strips of tomato confit, and 1 tablespoon of capers. Cook gently until the beans are nicely coated with the cooking liquid. Check the seasoning.

... Pour 2 tablespoons of olive oil into the bowl of cockle liquid, beating as you go, then add a splash of lemon juice and some freshly ground black pepper.

To finish your dish

... Slice 1 shallot into thin rounds. Completely peel and remove the inner membranes from 1 lemon and chop the flesh into small dice. Chop the leaves from a small bunch of parsley. Add all this to the sauté pan of the beans along with the shelled cockles. Check the seasoning for salt and freshly ground black pepper.

... Arrange the cockles still in their shells on top. Drizzle with the sauce and serve in the sauté pan or in a dish.

Lentil Salad with Vinegar Mushrooms

… Serves 4

… Rinse 2 cups of green lentils, put in a large saucepan, and cover well with water.

… Peel 1 large carrot and 1 onion, cut in two, and add them.

… Cook gently for 30 minutes and add salt only at the end of cooking.

… Leave the lentils to cool in their cooking water.

… Take out the carrot and onion and cut into small dice (brunoise). Place them in a small bowl.

… While the lentils are cooking, rinse 3 ounces of enoki mushrooms and remove their stems.

… Set aside about 20 of the mushrooms in a bowl.

… Pour 1 quart of water and ½ cup of white wine vinegar into a saucepan and bring to a boil. Immerse the rest of the enoki mushrooms for 3 minutes, then drain.

… Rinse and dry a very small bunch of parsley, take off the leaves, and chop them.

… When the lentils are cooked, drain and put them in a salad bowl or deep dish.

… Add the carrot and onion brunoise, the chopped parsley, and the vinegared enoki mushrooms.

… Season with a splash of olive oil, and of sherry vinegar, add salt and some freshly ground black pepper, and stir delicately so as not to damage the mushrooms.

… Pour just a splash of olive oil onto the reserved raw enoki mushrooms, add salt and freshly ground black pepper, and arrange them on top of the lentils.

AD— The botanical name for enoki is Flammulina ("little flame") velutipes ("velvet foot"). In Europe, it is the Collybia mushroom, which is found growing wild on elms. The enoki is cultivated widely in Japan and exported. If you can't get hold of any, use small button mushrooms for this recipe.
PN— Lentils, rich in slow carbohydrates, protein, fiber, B vitamins, and minerals (including some iron and magnesium), are an excellent food to have regularly on the menu.

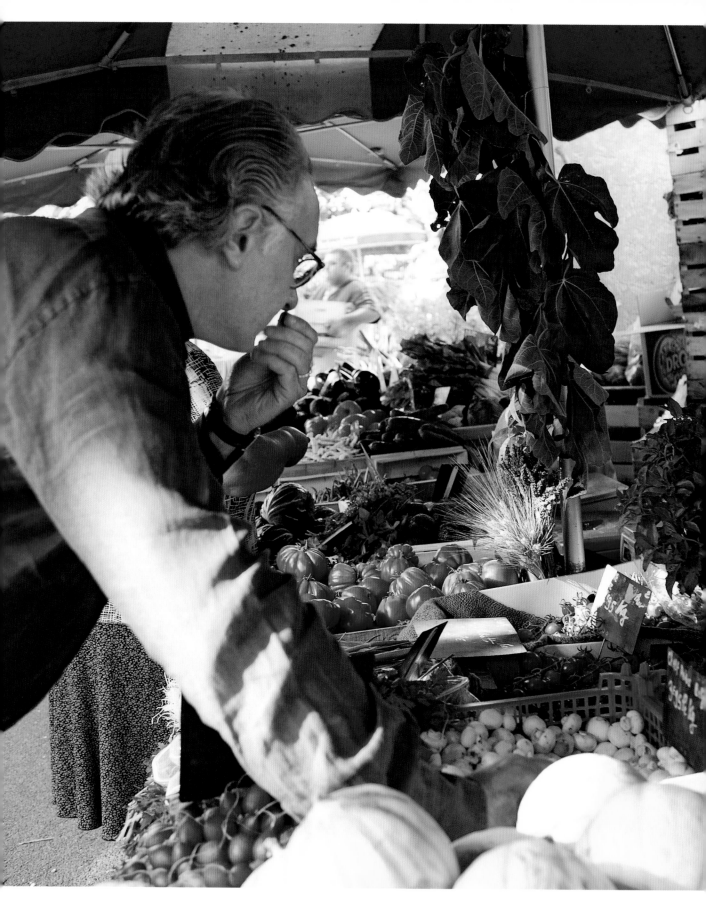

Salad of Yellow Soybeans and Mushrooms

… Serves 4

… Boil 2 cups of salted water in a saucepan.

… Sprinkle 10 ounces of dried yellow soybeans into it.

… Cover with a lid and simmer for 20 minutes.

… Meanwhile, remove the stems from 10 ounces of mushrooms, and wash and slice thinly.

… Peel and mince 2 fresh spring onions with stalks.

… Wash and dry a small bunch of flat-leaf parsley and separate the leaves.

… Peel and chop 1 garlic clove.

… Combine all this in a salad bowl.

… Cut the zest of half a salt-preserved lemon (page 15) into strips and add them, too.

… Then add 1 teaspoon of curry powder and 3 tablespoons of olive oil.

… Finish the seasoning with 3 pinches of salt and the juice of 1 lemon and mix.

… Add the cooked soybeans, mix well, and serve right away.

AD— When in season, use very small chanterelles instead of white mushrooms. Enoki mushrooms will also do nicely.

PN— Dadou (which is what they call the soybean in China) is the only bean whose proteins contain all the essential amino acids. And it is very rich in them. So there's no need for meat or fish in this meal; you already have enough, and plenty of minerals and fiber, too. With the mushrooms, this is a terrifically healthy dish.

—————

Dried yellow soybeans are available in health food stores and online.

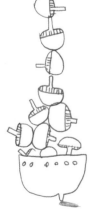

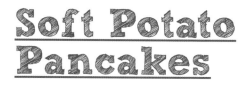

Soft Potato Pancakes

AD— The potatoes must be peeled when they are hot. Let them cool slightly so you don't burn yourself, or wrap your hand in a clean dish towel.

PN— A nice herb salad (page 153) would go very well with these potato pancakes, making it practically a complete dish. Potatoes and eggs provide protein. Follow with a yogurt or other dairy product (but not cheese, as the cream is already high in fat) and some fruit.

… Serves 4

… Thoroughly wash 3 large potatoes (1½ pounds), but don't peel them yet.

… Cook them in salted boiling water until they are soft through the middle. Check with a knife.

… Drain and peel them.

… Mash with a potato masher or fork and put in a large bowl.

… First add ½ cup of flour, then 3 whole eggs, then 3½ ounces of crème fraîche.

… When it is all fully incorporated, beat 3 egg whites into stiff peaks and fold them in gradually to keep the mixture light. Add salt and freshly ground black pepper.

… Heat a nonstick skillet with a drop of olive oil. With a small ladle or large spoon, pour the batter into several places in the skillet to form small, not necessarily regular pancakes.

… Cook for 2 minutes on each side.

… Cook in batches if all the batter does not fit in your skillet in one go.

… Arrange the pancakes on a serving dish and serve immediately.

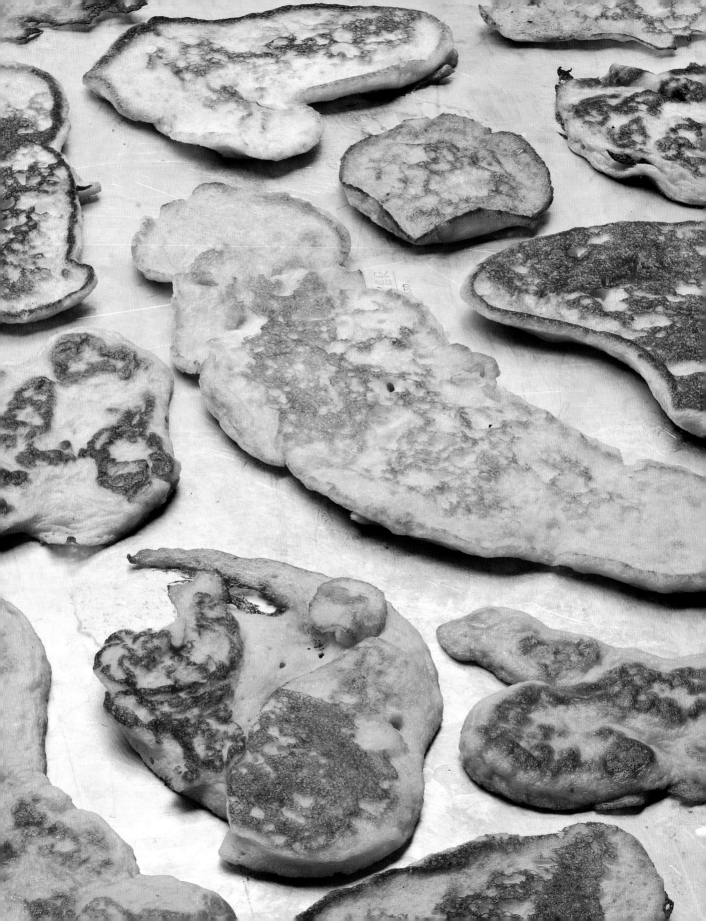

Fork-Crushed Potatoes

AD— You can serve these just as they are, or add a few leaves of basil marinated in olive oil (spread them on a plate and brush them with olive oil), or a scattering of black olives. Better still, grate some truffle on top—a nice way to combine sophisticated and rustic ingredients.

PN— Carbohydrates and unsaturated fatty acids from the olive oil—can there be anything better? Serve these potatoes with a nice slice of cured ham and a salad. Finish with yogurt and some fruit and you have a simple, beautifully balanced dinner.

… Serves 4

… Thoroughly wash 8 potatoes to get rid of any traces of earth, and brush if necessary.

… Put them in a saucepan and cover well with water. Add 1 tablespoon of coarse salt.

… Cook the potatoes at a low boil for 20 minutes or so. Check when they are done with a fine knife; the blade should glide easily into the flesh.

… Put a dish or individual plates to warm.

… Drain the potatoes and lay them on paper towels. Peel them right away, while still hot, holding them with a fork and protecting your hand with a paper towel folded in four.

… Place 2 potatoes on each plate and crush with a fork. Pour on a splash of olive oil, and sprinkle a pinch of sea salt over. And sit down to eat them right away; they should be eaten nice and hot!

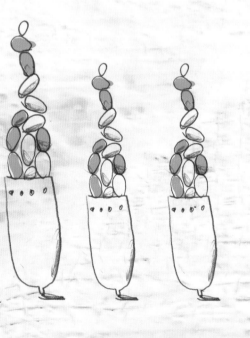

Potatoes Baked Loosely in Foil

… Serves 4

… Rub 2 pounds of small potatoes in a bowl with coarse salt and a glass of water to remove some bits of skin, but do not peel.

… Preheat the oven to maximum, 500°F.

… Take 4 ovenproof cereal bowls. Cut 4 large pieces of aluminium foil and put each one in a bowl, taking care not to pierce the bottom with your fingernails.

… Distribute the potatoes among the bowls. Take 4 garlic cloves and 4 sprigs of thyme or rosemary and pop one of each in each bowl.

… Add 1 tablespoon of water and 1 teaspoon of olive oil.

… Gather together the corners of the aluminium foil to form a tall parcel, and seal tightly.

… Bake for 30 to 35 minutes.

… Serve the bowls straight out of the oven as they are. Diners can season their own potatoes with sea salt and freshly ground black pepper.

AD— The King Edward potato is an English variety dating from 1902 that had fallen out of fashion but is being revived. Its skin is marbled with red, and its white flesh is very fine. But you can also use other small potatoes.
PN— Cooked like this, you can eat these potatoes as they are, nice and low in fat. But if you want to serve them with salted butter (not tons!), they're even better.

Roasted Potato Wedges

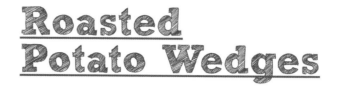

AD— You can use flavorings other than garlic, such as paprika, chili powder, or whatever you fancy. You can also add the leaves from a small bunch of chervil once they are cooked.

PN— The herb salad (page 153), a slice of cold meat, a cheese, or yogurt and a piece of fruit and there you are! A really well-balanced meal, quickly prepared, with no headaches.

… Serves 4

… Thoroughly clean 2 pounds of medium potatoes by brushing them under running water; do not peel.

… Cut each lengthwise into four or six wedges and put in a large bowl as you go.

… Add 3 or 4 unpeeled garlic cloves, 1 sprig of thyme, and 1 sprig of rosemary.

… Add 3 tablespoons of olive oil and a little salt.

… Then, with nice clean hands, mix well until all the potato wedges are coated in oil.

… Spread them out in a large baking dish.

… Set the oven to 400°F (do not preheat) and put in the dish for about 30 minutes. Stir the potatoes from time to time. When cooked they should be nice and golden, but check with the tip of a knife anyway.

… Add 10 segments of tomato confit (page 16) to the cooked potatoes, mix, and return to the oven for just 5 minutes to heat through. Serve in the baking dish.

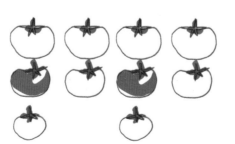

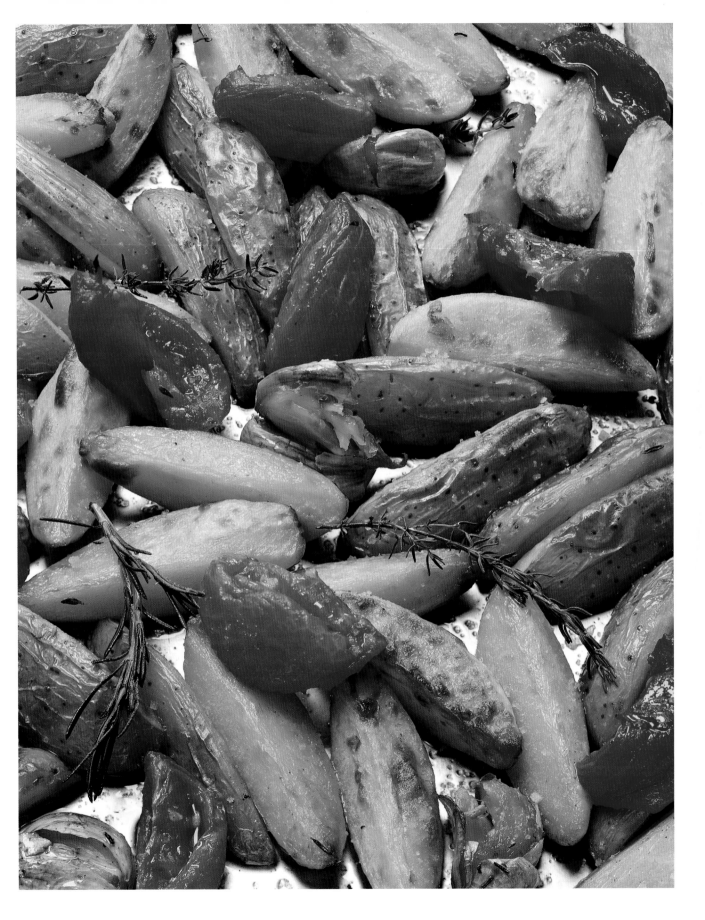

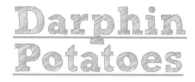

Darphin Potatoes

*AD— Variations: Add 1 or 2
chopped onions or chopped herbs,
or grated carrots, celery, or zucchini,
to the potatoes when seasoning.
PN— A nonstick pan in good
condition is essential for this dish!
Otherwise you will have to use
too much olive oil and your
Darphin potatoes will not be as
low in fat as these. Serve them with
a green salad and a slice of ham or
other cold meat. With yogurt and
fruit to follow, you have a quick,
easy, balanced meal.*

… Serves 4

… Peel, wash, and dry 2 pounds of potatoes and grate finely.

… Squeeze them between your hands and spread them on a clean dish towel.
   Add salt and freshly ground black pepper.

… Mix well with your hands so that they are seasoned evenly.

… Heat a large nonstick skillet with 1 tablespoon of olive oil, add the potatoes, and
   press down with a spatula to form an evenly thick pancake.

… Cook for about 15 minutes over medium heat.

… Place a large round dish over the skillet and turn it over so that the potato cake is
   in the dish.

… Brush your skillet with olive oil and slide the potatoes back in. Cook for an
   additional 12 to 15 minutes, still over medium heat.

… Transfer the Darphin potatoes back to the round dish. Add a generous twist of
   freshly ground black pepper and serve.

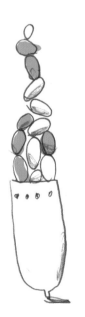

Baked Potatoes and Tomatoes

… Serves 4

… Preheat the oven to 425°F.

… Wash 10 new potatoes the size of an egg, rubbing them with a brush.

… Cut into quarters lengthwise, rinse, then dry them very carefully with a dish towel or paper towels.

… Rinse and dry 5 nice ripe tomatoes. Remove any hard cores and cut into large wedges.

… Oil a baking sheet and put in the potatoes and 5 garlic cloves (unpeeled).

… Distribute the tomatoes in between and over the potatoes.

… Add 2 or 3 tablespoons of olive oil and a little salt, then mix it all with a spatula (or better still, use your hands).

… Put the sheet in the oven and cook for about 40 minutes; the potatoes will absorb the juice of the tomatoes. Stir from time to time, so that the juice is well distributed.

… Check the potatoes with the tip of a knife to see if they are tender.

… Sprinkle the potatoes with thyme flowers and oregano flowers and cook for an additional 5 minutes.

… Serve straight from the sheet after carefully scraping up the pan juices with a spatula. And add a generous twist of freshly ground black pepper.

AD— Thyme flowers are perfect for this dish, but they're not always easy to find, so use thyme leaves that are as fresh and tender as possible. The acidity of the tomato goes wonderfully well with the sweetness of the potato. PN— The carbohydrates from the potato and the lycopene in the cooked tomatoes give you energy and antioxidants. Serve with grilled meat or grilled or poached fish.

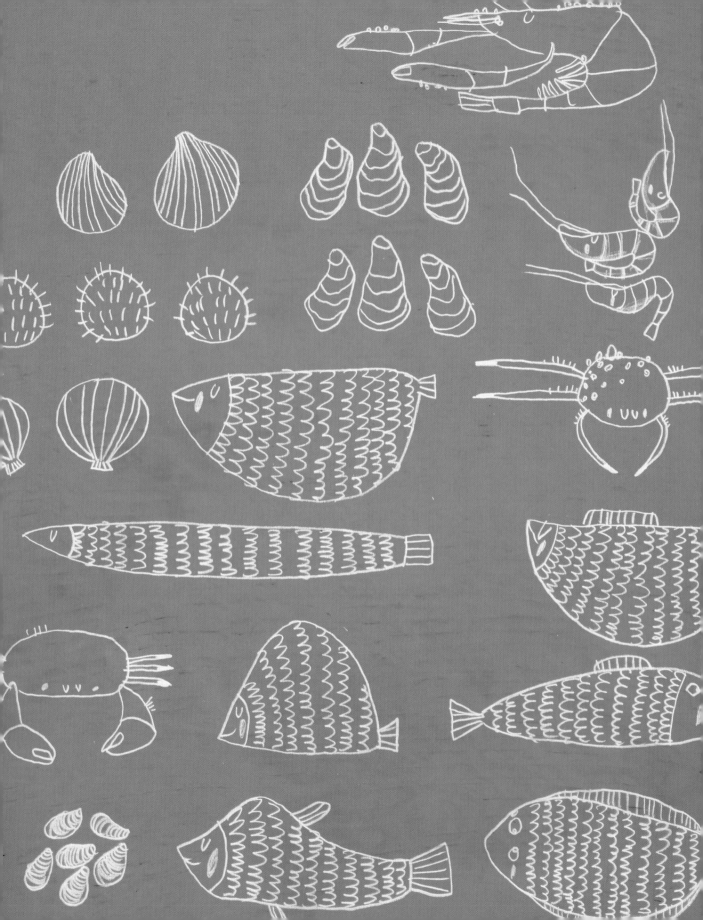

AD— *Shellfish, crustaceans, and fish— the sea offers me a superb variety of easy-to-cook produce all year round. The important thing is to treat it with respect and cook it very lightly.*

PN— *Some of this seafood contains precious omega-3s, and it all contains iodine, which is essential for life, and protein. Nutritional guidelines advise us to eat seafood at least three times a week.*

Sea

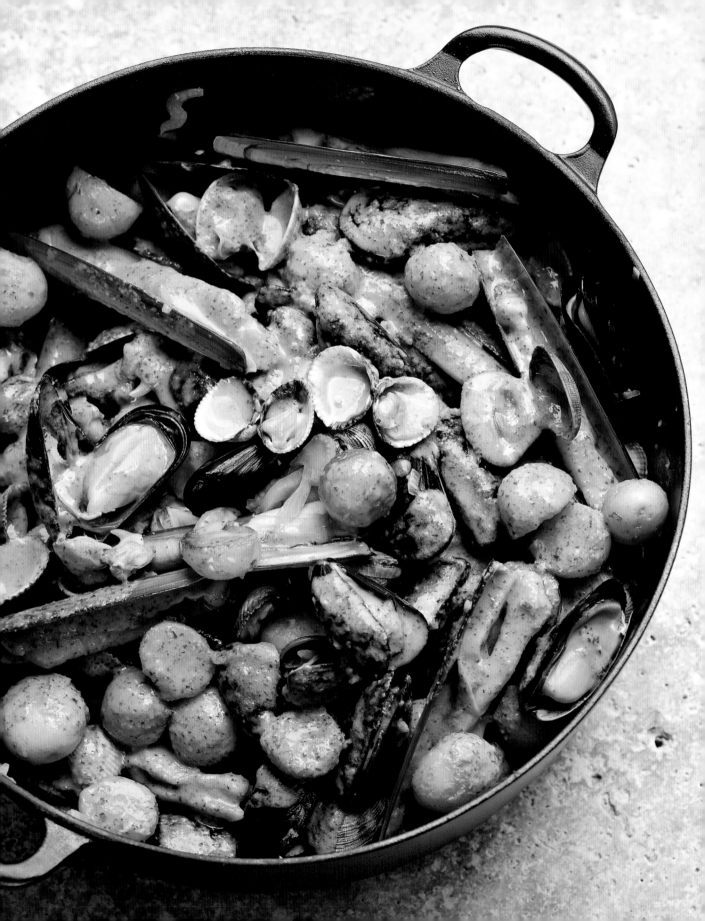

Shellfish and Potatoes à la Marinière

… Serves 4

… Wash 1½ pounds of bouchot or other small mussels, 1½ pounds of cockles, 1½ pounds of half-shell clams, and a handful of razor clams in several changes of fresh water, removing any whose shell is damaged or open.

… Rub 1¼ pounds of baby new potatoes with coarse salt to take off their skin, rinse, and cook in salted water for about 15 minutes.

… In the meantime, peel and mince 2 shallots and 1 fennel bulb.

… Peel 4 garlic cloves, chop two of them, and crush the other two.

… Wash and dry a bunch of parsley and take off the leaves. Reserve about 20 whole leaves, chop the rest, and set them all aside.

… Heat a large flameproof casserole dish with 2 tablespoons of olive oil and 1½ tablespoons of butter. Add the shallots, fennel, chopped garlic and the crushed garlic cloves, and cook for 3 minutes.

… Put all the well-drained shellfish in the casserole dish, pour in ¾ cup of dry white wine, cover the casserole dish with a lid, turn up the heat, and cook quickly for 4 to 5 minutes, stirring regularly so that all the shellfish open.

… Take the casserole dish off the heat. Lift out the shellfish and whole squashed garlic cloves with a slotted spoon and keep warm in a dish.

… Pour what is left in the casserole dish into the bowl of your food processor. Add the chopped parsley and blend until the mixture is nice and smooth and coats the back of a spoon.

… Pour this sauce into the casserole dish, return the shellfish and garlic cloves, then drain the potatoes and add them. Stir until everything is coated in the parsley sauce.

… Add several twists of freshly ground black pepper, add the whole parsley leaves, and serve straight from the casserole dish.

AD— It's not a bad idea to buy the shellfish the day before and soak them in a basin of water with a handful of coarse salt away from the light. They will then release all their sand. This will save you time, as all you then have to do is rinse them in fresh water before cooking. PN— This is an excellent complete dish, giving you a whole lot of minerals (shellfish are brimming with them), as well as protein, and carbohydrates thanks to the potatoes. Charlotte potatoes are perfect, but if you cannot find these, any small, firm, waxy potato, such as fingerlings or baby Yukon golds, will work in this recipe.

Scallops in Cream of Watercress

AD— Avruga is smoked herring roe. Cook the velouté at the last minute because if you keep it hot while you are preparing the scallops, it will darken.

PN— Watercress and spinach have the most minerals, antioxidants, and vitamins of any green vegetables. The combination of iron and folic acid (vitamin B₉), in which watercress is rich, makes it a kind of natural tonic. With the iodine from the scallops, this dish is a nutritional feast!

… Serves 4

… Have your fishmonger prepare 12 scallops, asking him to detach the white meat and remove the coral.

… Take the leaves off 2 bunches of watercress, stem 2 handfuls of spinach, and wash and dry them.

… Keep aside a few watercress leaves to decorate your dish.

… Peel 1 garlic clove.

… Cut the scallops horizontally into four.

… Season them with the juice of half a lemon and a splash of olive oil and arrange them in soup plates.

… Then add the contents of a small jar of Avruga or salmon roe and the reserved watercress leaves.

… Brush 4 slices of walnut bread with a little olive oil. Toast them lightly under the broiler, cut them in half, and arrange them in a small basket.

… Bring a saucepan of salted water to a boil. Immerse the watercress, spinach, and garlic, stir well, and cook until the leaves can be crushed between your fingers.

… Remove with a slotted spoon and blend immediately, adding 2 tablespoons of crème fraîche and a little cooking water; the broth should be nice and smooth, the consistency of a velouté.

… Add salt and freshly ground black pepper and reheat.

… Put the basket of bread and the plates with the scallops on the table. Pour the boiling velouté over them; its heat will cook them.

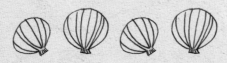

Crab, Cucumber, Mango, and Papaya

... Serves 4

Prepare the crab salad

... Defrost and drain 10 ounces of frozen crabmeat.

... Mince 1 garlic clove, 2 mint leaves, and the leaves of 2 sprigs of cilantro. Peel and grate 2 inches of ginger.

... Combine all this in a bowl, add 1 tablespoon of crème fraîche and 1 tablespoon of ketchup (page 22), and stir. Grate a little zest from 1 unwaxed lime and 1 unwaxed lemon and add this. Squeeze the juice of these citrus fruits and mix it in well.

... Season with salt, freshly ground black pepper, and Piment d'Espelette or hot paprika. Refrigerate the crab salad.

Prepare the fruit and vegetables

... Wash and peel 1 bunch of scallions. Peel 1 red bell pepper, 1 medium cucumber, 1 mango, and 1 papaya.

... Cut the vegetables into thin slivers and the fruit into thin slices. Put them in a bowl.

... Chop 4 basil leaves, 2 mint leaves, and the leaves of a sprig of cilantro. Add them to the bowl.

... Season with salt and freshly ground black pepper, toss, and keep cold.

Arrange your salad

... Arrange the cold crab salad in the middle of the dish.

... Spread the fruit and vegetable salad all around it.

... Decorate with a few cherry tomatoes. Serve nice and cold.

AD— For a more attractive presentation, place a 3-inch pastry cutter in the center of each plate and fill to three-quarters with crab salad. Arrange the vegetables and fruit around it and pop a few cherry tomatoes on the crab.

PN— An explosive cocktail of minerals, vitamins, and antioxidants, this salad is a complete dish. For the crabmeat, you can also use cooked crab claws.

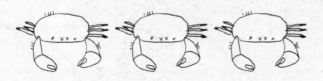

Grilled Langoustines with Lemon

AD— This takes only 2 minutes to cook, otherwise your langoustines will be too hard and dry. Serve with a nutcracker, so that everyone can open the claws without damaging their teeth.

PN— It would be hard to make anything simpler and lighter! Adapt the quantity of langoustines according to the size of the ones available. If they are large, four per person will be enough. Like all crustaceans, langoustines are full of iodine and minerals.

… Serves 4

… Split 24 medium langoustines in half lengthwise. Remove the black vein and also the sand sac in the head (or get your fishmonger to do it for you!).

… Turn on the broiler.

… Trim, wash, and finely chop 2 scallions.

… Take the leaves from about 10 sprigs of lemon thyme.

… Cut 1 unwaxed lemon in half.

… Line up the half langoustines side by side, head to tail, in a broiler pan or on a baking sheet.

… Sprinkle the chopped scallions and thyme leaves over.

… Broil for 2 minutes.

… When you take them out of the oven, grate a little lemon zest over and drizzle with a splash of olive oil and lemon juice. Sprinkle a little sea salt and Piment d'Espelette or hot paprika on top and serve immediately.

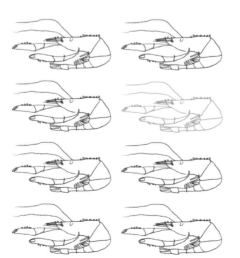

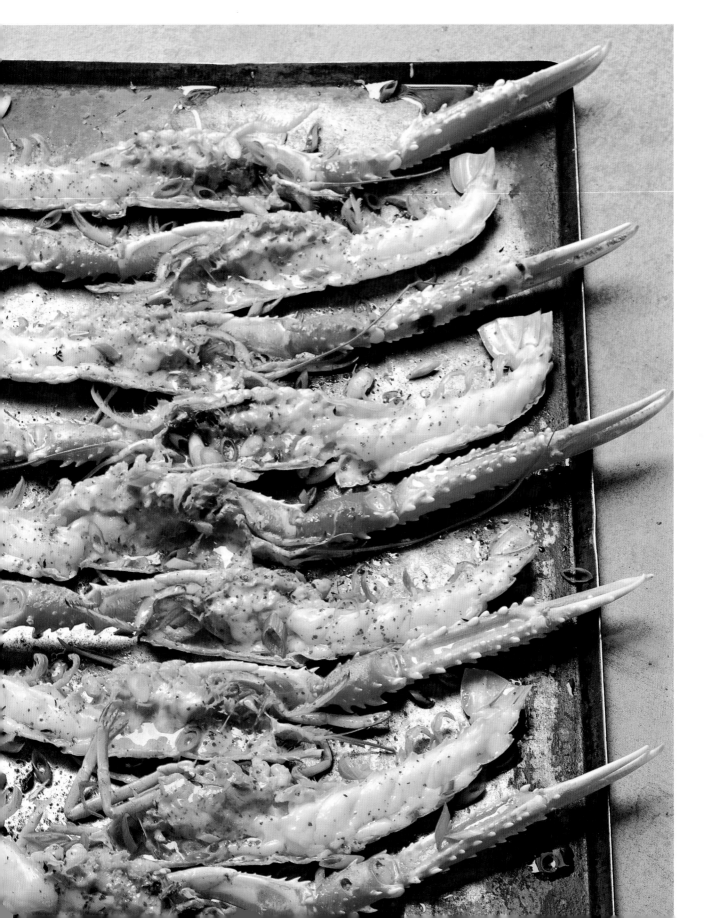

Scallops with Green Cabbage

AD— A fine marriage of land and sea! Take care not to add too much salt to the cabbage at the beginning of the cooking, as the haddock takes care of this. Better to season to taste afterward.

PN— Scallops are ultra-lean, and full of iodine and minerals! If they are very big (and people's appetites normal), three per person will be pretty much sufficient in terms of protein.

… Serves 4

… Get your fishmonger to prepare 16 scallops, asking him to detach the white flesh and get rid of the coral.

… Separate the leaves and wash 1 head of green cabbage and immerse in boiling salted water for 2 minutes. Drain well and slice thinly.

… Peel and wash 1 carrot, 1 onion, 2 stalks of celery, and 1 small leek (take off any green part that is not tender) and cut all these vegetables into small dice (brunoise). Cut 4 ounces of haddock fillet similarly.

… Heat a flameproof casserole dish with 2 tablespoons of olive oil and sweat the vegetables for 2 to 3 minutes.

… Add the cabbage and cook gently for an additional 2 minutes, stirring.

… Add 2 juniper berries and ¾ cup of chicken stock (page 10), cover, and cook gently for 30 minutes, stirring occasionally.

… Then add the haddock, stir, then place the scallops on top of the cabbage. Cover the casserole dish with a lid and cook for just 3 minutes over very low heat.

… Taste and adjust the seasoning.

… Arrange the cabbage mixture in the serving dish, then place the scallops in the center. Drizzle with the cooking liquid.

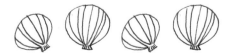

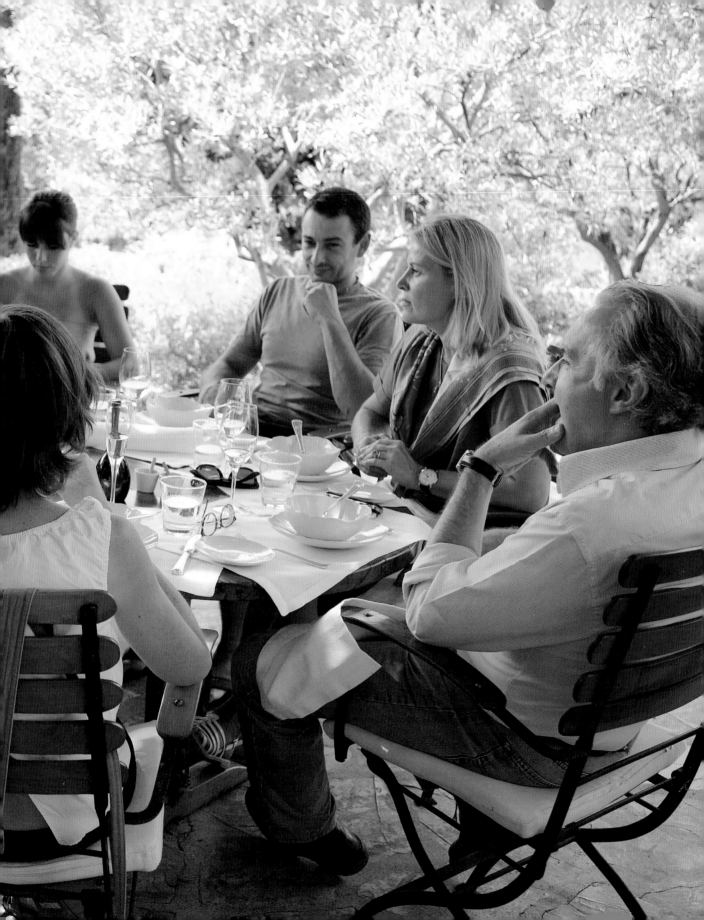

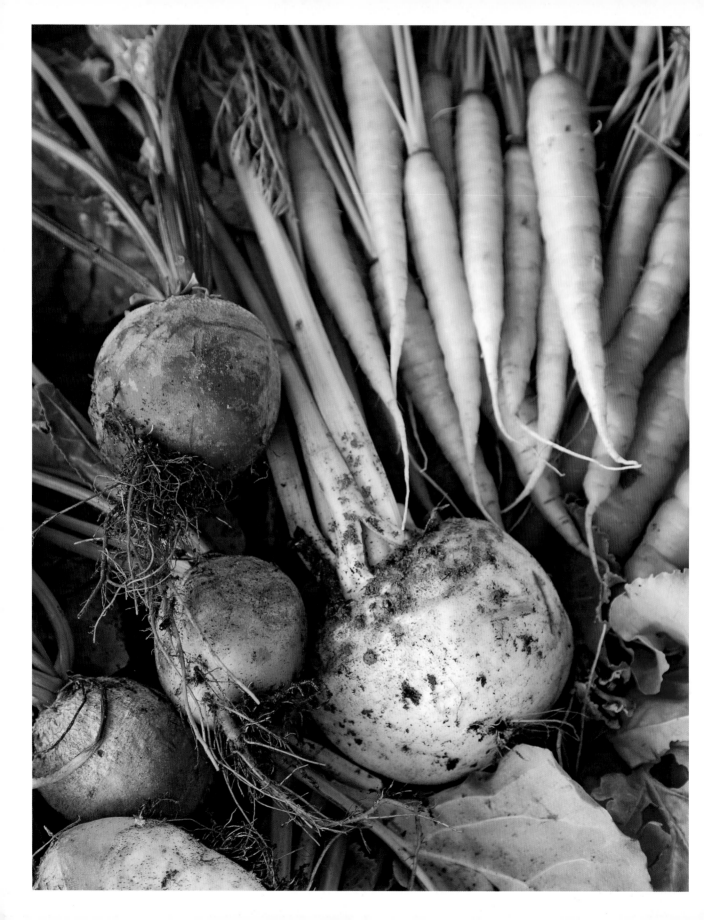

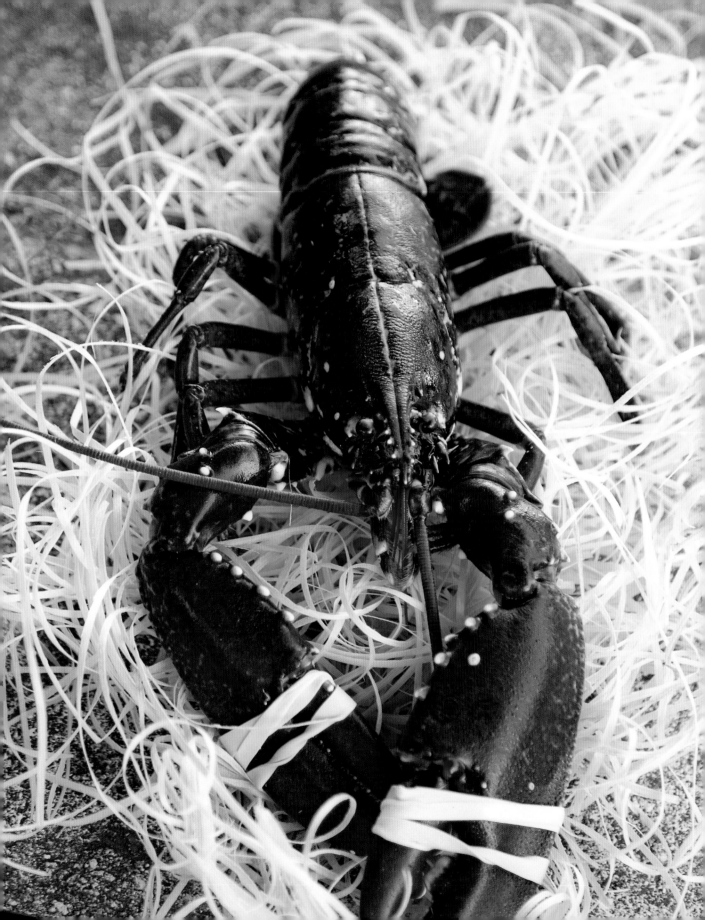

Poached Lobster with Vegetable Macedonia

AD— The lobster must of course be alive, its claws firmly closed with elastic bands. After plunging it in boiling water, keep the lid on the cooking pot to avoid splashes. PN— The flesh of the lobster is particularly low in fat but rich in protein. The vegetables are low in calories but full of vitamins and dressed with a yogurt sauce. This is a luxury dish but one that's really low in fat.

… Serves 4

… Peel and wash 2 carrots with tops and 3 turnips with tops. Wash and de-string 2 handfuls of French beans. Cut these vegetables into very small dice (brunoise).

… Shell a handful of fresh peas.

… Heat salted water in a saucepan and prepare a bowl of water and ice cubes.

… Immerse all the vegetables in the boiling water for 4 minutes, then drain and plunge them in the ice water. Drain once more, put in a large bowl, and set aside.

… Pour 3 quarts of water and 1¾ cups of white wine into a large cooking pot. Add 10 black peppercorns and bring to a boil. Plunge a 1½-pound lobster into the liquid, put on the lid, and cook for 5 minutes once it returns to a boil.

… Take the lobster out and, as soon as it's not burning hot, shell the tail, elbows, and claws. Remove the black intestinal vein. Take the sand sac from the head and collect the coral.

… Cut the shell of the head and tail in half lengthwise. Rinse and dry them.

… Cut up the meat and add it to the bowl of vegetables.

… Trim, wash, and finely chop 2 scallions and put them in a bowl. Add the lobster coral, ½ cup Greek-style yogurt, the juice of an unwaxed lemon, a little of its grated zest, and a pinch of Piment d'Espelette or hot paprika. Taste and correct the seasoning with salt and freshly ground black pepper.

… Pour this sauce into the bowl of vegetables and lobster. Stir gently, then distribute this mixture into the shells of the half tails and half heads.

… Arrange on a dish and keep cold until serving.

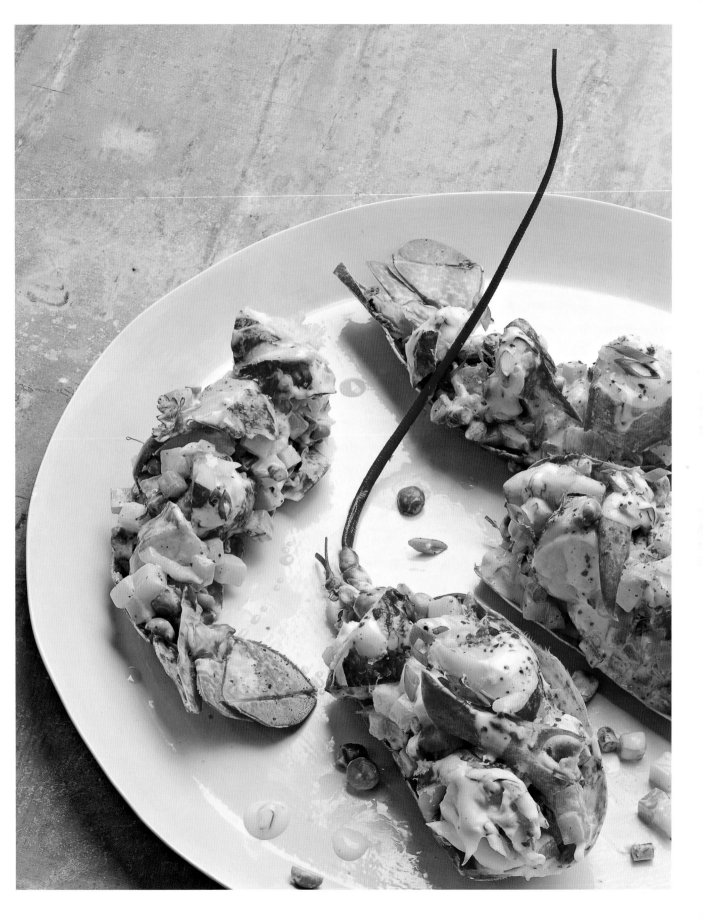

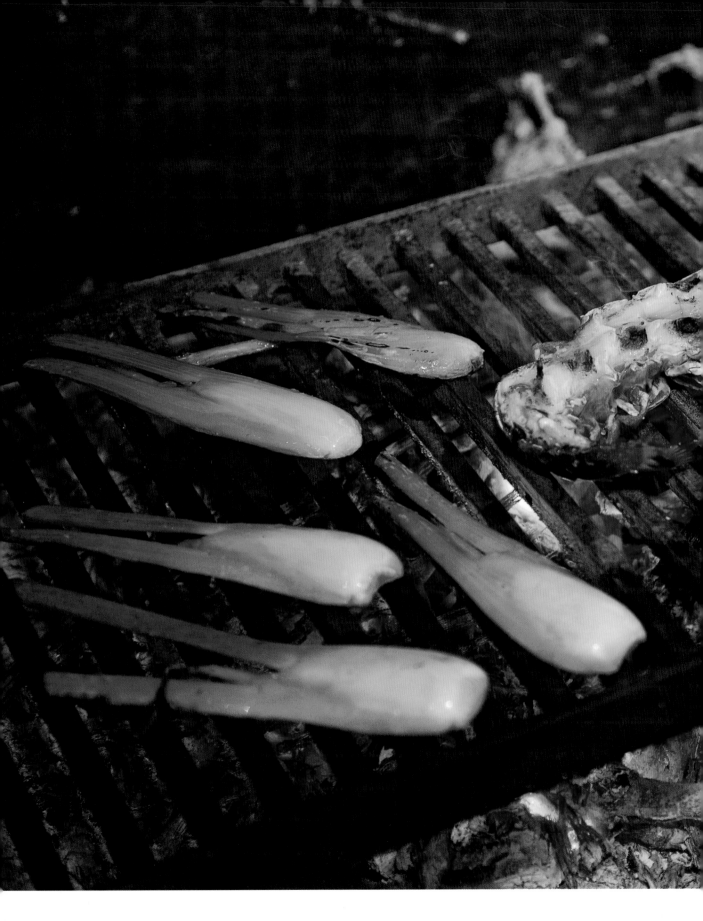

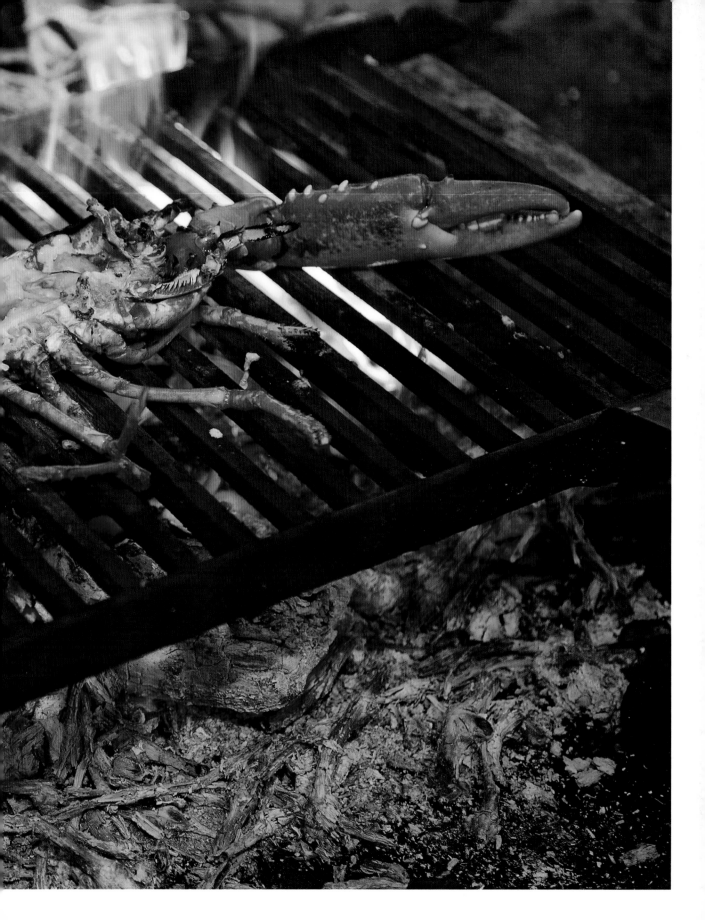

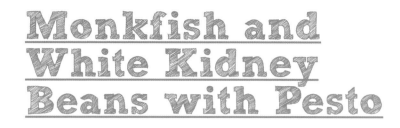
Monkfish and White Kidney Beans with Pesto

AD— Monkfish is a large fish, native to the Atlantic and Mediterranean. It is commonly sold without the head because it is very large and scary looking. Hence its other names: "frog-fish" and "sea devil."

PN— In winter, use dried haricot beans (don't forget to soak them overnight). Their nutritional qualities are the same as fresh: loads of minerals and fiber plus good slow carbohydrates. Monkfish is lean, and the pesto is full of beneficial nutrients—what more could you ask for?

… Serves 4

… Shell 1¾ pounds of fresh white kidney beans. Peel 1 white onion and 2 carrots, and cut into chunks.

… Combine all these vegetables in a saucepan with 1 bouquet garni and cover well with water.

… Cook gently for 45 minutes, skimming regularly. Add salt only at the end of cooking.

… In the meantime, prepare 2 ounces of pesto (page 36).

… Put 4 pieces of monkfish tail each weighing 4 ounces in a sauté pan. Pour a ladleful of the bean cooking water into the sauté pan and cook the monkfish gently for about 10 minutes.

… Cut 4 piquillo pimientos (see note, opposite) into strips. Chop the leaves from 2 sprigs of basil.

… Drain the beans. Add to them three quarters of the pesto, ¾ cup of light cream, and the chopped basil and stir gently to coat well.

… Transfer to the serving dish or onto individual plates.

… Place the monkfish on top. Drizzle the rest of the pesto in a line all around. Add the strips of piquillo pimientos. Serve hot.

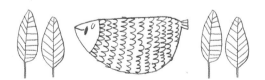

Poached Cod with Piquillo Coulis

... Serves 4

<u>Prepare the cod</u>

... Sprinkle some coarse salt in a dish, lay a cod fillet weighing about 1½ pounds on top, and cover with more coarse salt.

... Leave to marinate for 15 minutes. Then rinse and cut into four equal pieces.

<u>Prepare the piquillo coulis</u>

... In the meantime, peel and mince 1 white onion, then cut up 4 piquillos pimientos (12 required in total for the recipe).

... In a sauté pan with a splash of olive oil, sweat the onion for 3 minutes without allowing it to color. Add 9 ounces of chopped cooked tomatoes (page 21) and the chopped piquillos and cook over low heat for 5 minutes. Take the saucepan off the heat, pour in ½ cup of light cream, and stir. Then blend it all to obtain a nice smooth coulis. Check the seasoning and keep warm.

<u>Grill the lettuce and piquillos</u>

... Rinse and dry 4 small heads of Boston lettuces and cut in half lengthwise. Broil for just 1 minute on each side. Do the same with the remaining 8 piquillo pimientos.

<u>To finish your dish</u>

... In a saucepan, bring to a boil 3 cups of lowfat milk with 2 garlic cloves squashed but left whole, 1 sprig of thyme, and 1 bay leaf, then turn off the heat.

... Immerse the cod fillets and cook until you can insert a toothpick without meeting any resistance.

... Drain on paper towels and arrange in the serving dish or on individual plates.

... Coat with piquillo coulis. Arrange the grilled lettuce and piquillos all around, alternating the colors. Sprinkle with a few grains of sea salt and 1 pinch of Piment d'Espelette or hot paprika. Serve immediately.

AD— Piquillo pimientos are one of the gems of Basque gastronomy. You can buy them canned or in jars. Drain well before using.
PN— Piquillos are members of the pepper family. They provide not only a good dose of carotenoids, which are good for the heart and skin, but also vitamin C. This is a useful dish in winter when these nutrients are harder to come by.

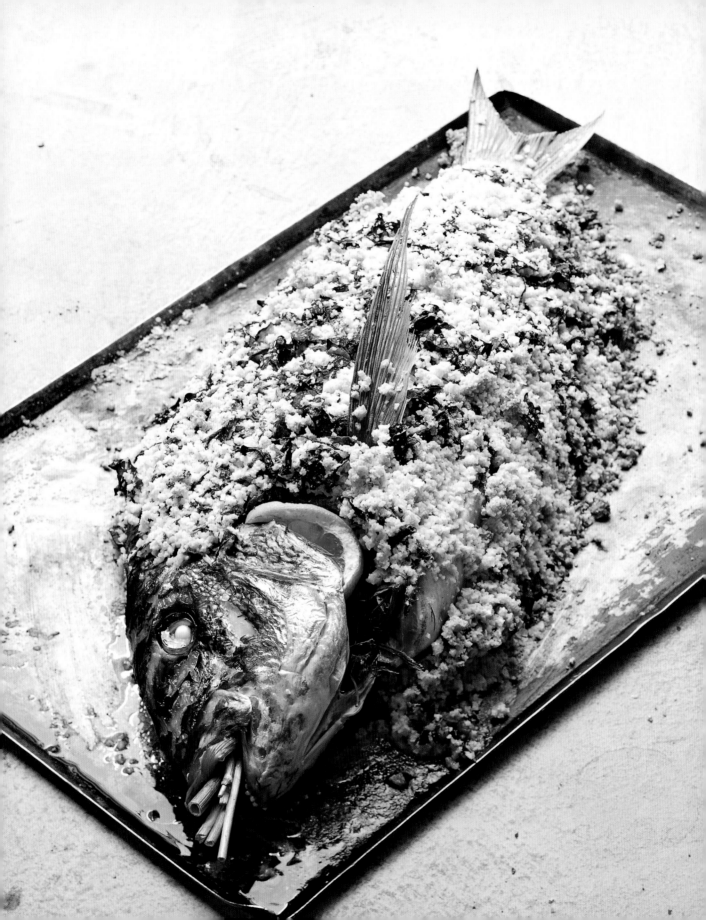

Gilthead Bream in Salt and Seaweed Crust with Dill Sauce

… Serves 4

… Have your fishmonger prepare a 3½-pound sea bream, asking him to gut it through the gills and trim the fins on the back, which are very prickly, but definitely not to scale it.

Cook the bream

… Preheat your oven to 350°F.

… Cut an unwaxed lemon into slices. Detach the leaves from a bunch of dill and set aside for the sauce.

… Through the head, stuff the bream with the dill stems, lemon slices, and 2 sprigs of dried fennel.

… In a large salad bowl, combine 2 pounds of coarse gray sea salt, 7 ounces of multicolored seaweed, and the whites of 3 eggs. Stir vigorously to mix thoroughly. Then spread the mixture over the bream.

… Transfer to an ovenproof dish and put in the oven for 30 minutes.

Prepare the dill sauce

… While the bream is cooking, chop the dill leaves. Peel and mince 1 shallot.

… Put the shallot in a small saucepan with 6 tablespoons of water and 6 tablespoons of vinegar and reduce by two thirds.

… Beating, gradually incorporate 4½ tablespoons of cold butter in small pieces into this hot reduction. Then add 1 tablespoon of crème fraîche, then the chopped dill. Allow to cool a little and then beat in 7 ounces of fat-free fromage blanc. Taste and adjust the seasoning with salt and freshly ground black pepper.

To finish your dish

… When you take it out of the oven, allow the bream to rest for 20 minutes.

… Then break the crust, remove all the salt, and take out the fillets.

… Arrange them on a serving dish or on individual plates, coat with the dill sauce, and serve immediately.

AD— You can also serve the bream still in its crust and break it at the table. If so, try a decoration with a piece of pastry. And serve the sauce separately in a sauce boat.

PN— There are different varieties of dorade or bream, all in the same family. The gilthead sea bream is a particularly fine fish. Known as daurade royale in France, it is a very lean fish.

Cod with Slow-Cooked Endives and Oranges

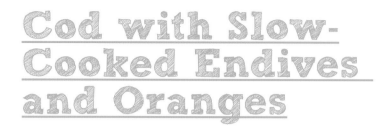

AD— I always choose endives that are nice and firm and white. There's no real need to wash them; just take off the outer leaves and remove the hard core at the base if you are not keen on their slight bitterness.

PN— The endive gives you beneficial fiber but few vitamins. Luckily the fresh orange added at the last minute provides vitamin C. Cod is a very lean fish, and this is a surprisingly low-fat dish!

... Serves 4

... Peel and thinly slice 3 shallots and 10 heads of Belgain endive (12 in total required for the recipe).

... Separate the leaves from 2 more endives and cut off the white lower part of the leaves. Set the tips aside on a plate.

... Squeeze the juice of 2 oranges (4 in total required for the recipe) and set aside in a glass. Remove the skin and inner membrane of 2 more oranges, keeping the segments on a plate.

... Heat a flameproof casserole dish with a splash of olive oil. Sweat the shallots with 2 pinches of mignonette pepper (see page 30) until they are translucent. Then add the sliced endives and cook for an additional 2 minutes. Add salt.

... Pour in the orange juice and stir well. Cook gently until the liquid is very reduced. The endives should be very tender.

... Heat a splash of olive oil in a nonstick skillet. Cook 4 cod steaks each weighing about 4 ounces first with the skin side down, then on the flesh side for just 1 minute, keeping them slightly translucent. Add salt and freshly ground black pepper.

... Add 1 tablespoon of butter to the braised endives and stir well. Taste and check the seasoning with salt and freshly ground black pepper.

... Then incorporate the reserved orange segments.

... Lay the cod fillets in a dish (or on individual plates) and distribute the stewed endives and oranges and the reserved endive leaves around them.

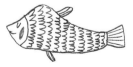

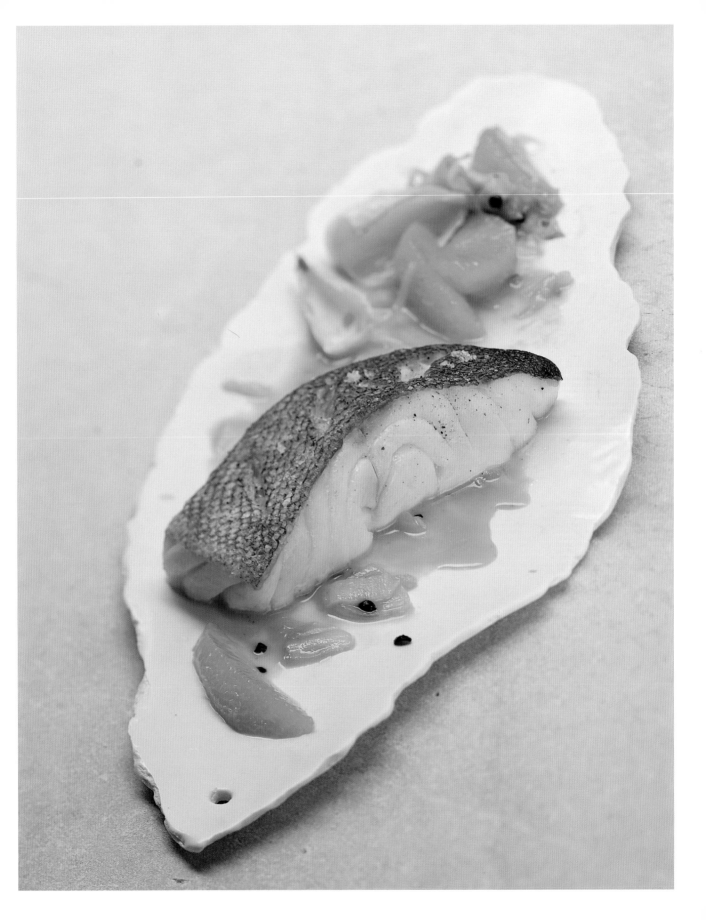

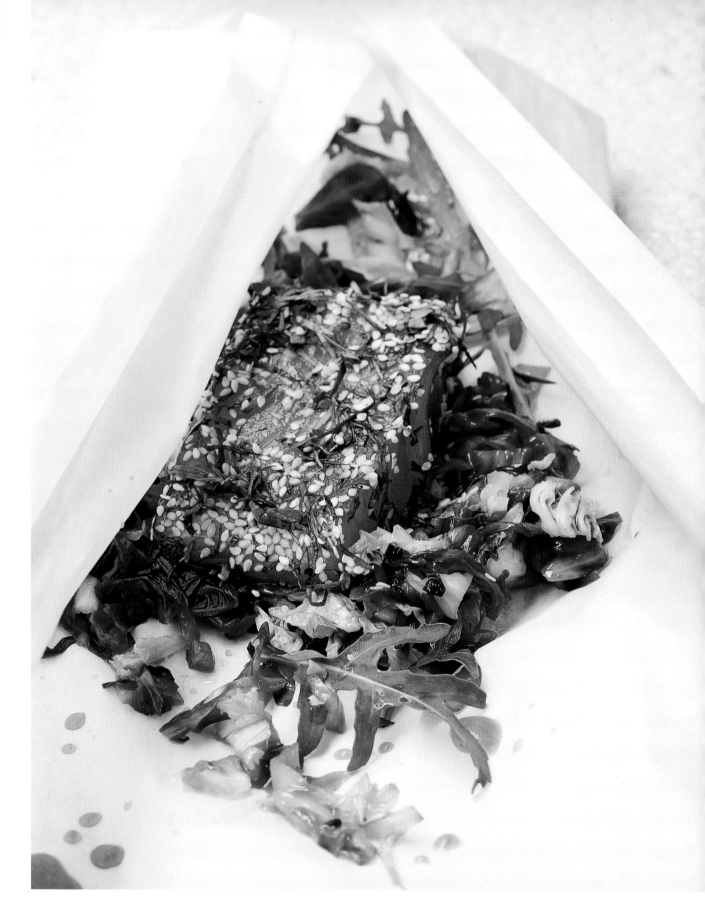

Pollock Parcels with Chinese Cabbage and Radicchio

… Serves 4

… Remove the skin from 4 pollock steaks weighing 4 ounces each. Put them in a dish and drizzle with 2 tablespoons of soy sauce. Leave to marinate for 15 minutes.

… In the meantime, wash 1 head of Chinese cabbage and 1 head of radicchio. Remove the outer leaves and chop the rest. Peel and crush 1 garlic clove.

… Heat a sauté pan with 2 tablespoons of olive oil, put in the greens and garlic, add salt, stir, cover the sauté pan, and sweat for 5 minutes.

… Pour in 3 tablespoons of wine vinegar and cook for an additional 10 minutes. Remove the sauté pan from the heat.

… Rinse and dry 4 sprigs of parsley and 4 sprigs of cilantro, pick off the leaves, and chop them. Mix with 2 teaspoons of sesame seeds and 1 teaspoon of mignonette pepper (see page 30).

… When the pollock steaks are sufficiently marinated, roll them in the parsley mixture, coating well on both sides.

… Preheat the oven to 325°F.

… Cut 4 sheets of parchment paper into 16-inch squares. Place a quarter of the sautéed greens on each one, then lay 1 pollock steak on top.

… Fold the right then the left side of the sheet of paper over the fish, half overlapping them. Then fold each sheet back underneath.

… Put the parcels on a baking dish and bake in the oven for 10 to 12 minutes. Serve in the parcels.

AD— This simple folding method allows you to open the parcel slightly to check when the fish is done. Prick it with a knife—it should be hot all the way through. PN— The flesh of pollock is very lean. It is sweet and has very few bones, which is always an advantage when cooking for children!

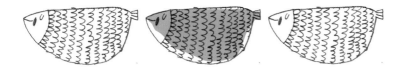

Steamed Whiting with Seaweed and Sautéed Greens

AD— *You can prepare the pea sauce and vegetables first, and keep them cool in containers covered with plastic wrap.*

PN— *Whiting is a lean fish. Cooking the vegetables quickly preserves all their vitamins. This is a particularly light dish.*

… Serves 4

Prepare the pea sauce

… Shell 1¼ pounds of fresh pea pods, sort out the smallest, and set them aside. De-string the pods and slice roughly.

… Heat a flameproof casserole dish with 1 tablespoon of olive oil, add the pods and the larger peas, a pinch of salt, and a pinch of superfine sugar, and sweat for 2 minutes, stirring. Add hot water to cover and bring to a boil quickly. Lower the heat and simmer gently for 4 minutes.

… Prepare a basin with water and ice cubes. Blend the sauce well, adjust the seasoning, pour into a salad bowl, and place in the ice cubes to cool quickly.

Prepare the vegetables

… Cut the tips of 8 small green asparagus spears into 3-inch lengths and then cut each one lengthwise into four. Rinse 1 small zucchini and slice into thin rounds. Wash and dry a handful of baby spinach leaves and 1 romaine lettuce heart; cut its leaves in half lengthwise. Wash a handful of French beans and cut into ½-inch pieces.

Prepare the whiting

… Remove the bones from 4 fillets of whiting each weighing 4 ounces.

… Rinse a handful of seaweed and cut into small strips. Heat water in a couscoussier or steamer.

Cook and finish your dish

… Heat a large skillet with 2 tablespoons of olive oil and cook and salt the reserved very small peas, asparagus tips, zucchini rounds, French beans, and 4 ounces of small shelled fava beans for approximately 3 minutes. Then add the baby spinach and romaine leaves. Stir, take the skillet off the heat, and transfer them into a serving dish. Reheat the pea sauce in the skillet and drizzle over the vegetables.

… Lay the whiting fillets in the upper basket of the steamer, sprinkle with sea salt, and put the seaweed on top. Cook for just 1 or 2 minutes. Place on top of the vegetables and serve right away.

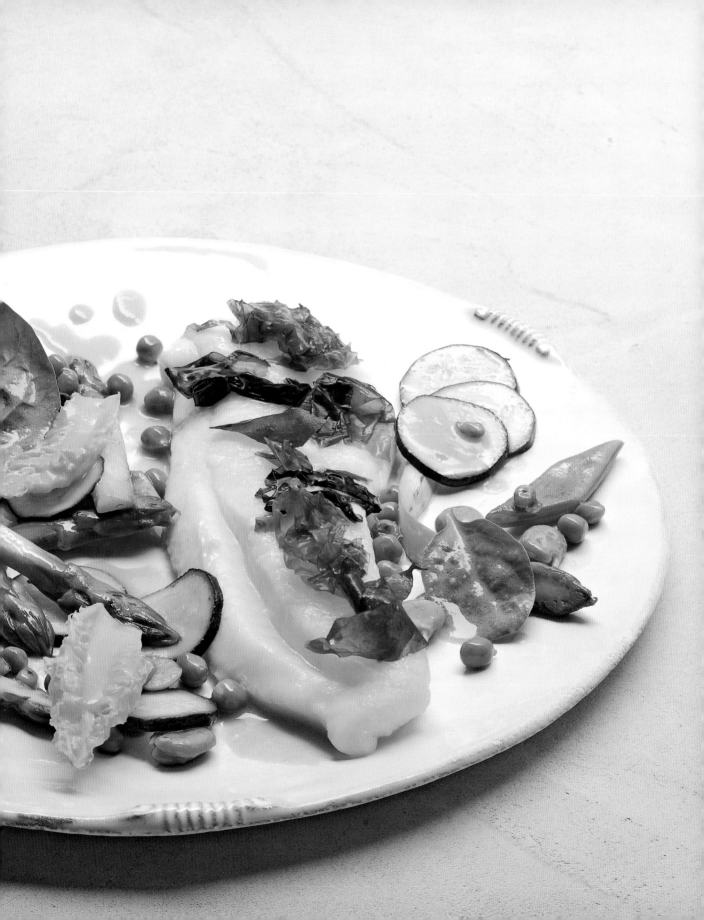

Salt Cod in Almond Pastry and Cannellini Beans with Garlic Confit

AD— It isn't easy to get rid of all the salt from salt cod, but if you do it this way, the salt sinks to the bottom of the basin and you can be sure that it will not end up too salty, which is often the case with other methods. When fresh cannellini beans are not in season, use dried white beans and soak them the day before.

PN— Salt cod is low in fat but rich in protein. With the slow carbohydrates, fiber, and minerals from the beans and almonds, this (light) dish is a excellent example of a balanced meal.

… Serves 4

Desalt the cod

… Put 1 pound of salt cod in a sieve, then place it in a basin filled with water. Leave to soak for 24 hours, changing the water at least four times.

Prepare the cannellini beans

… Put 7 ounces of fresh hulled cannellini beans, 1 crushed garlic clove, and 1 sprig of thyme (2 required in total for the recipe) in a saucepan.

… Cover well with water and cook gently for about 40 minutes, until the beans are soft. Add salt only at the end of cooking.

Cook the salt cod and the almond pastry

… In the meantime, chop ½ cup of unblanched almonds. Chop the leaves from 1 sprig of rosemary and 1 sprig of thyme. Mix all these ingredients together in a small bowl.

… Cut the skin of 1 salt-preserved lemon (page 15) into very small dice (brunoise).

… Drain the salt cod, wipe it dry, and cut into 4 equal pieces.

… Heat a skillet with a splash of olive oil, quickly brown the salt cod steaks on each side, drain, and transfer to a plate.

… Pour the contents of the bowl into the skillet and cook, stirring, until the almonds are lightly colored. Add ¾ tablespoons of butter and the preserved lemon brunoise and stir well.

To finish your dish

… Drain the beans, return them to their saucepan over very low heat, and add 4 cloves of garlic confit (page 12).

… Then return the salt cod steaks to the hot frying pan and, with a spoon, pile the almond, herb, and lemon mixture on top.

… Lift each one with a spatula and place them in the serving dish or on individual plates. Arrange the beans beside them and add freshly ground black pepper.

John Dory with Cooked and Raw Fennel

… Serves 4

… Get your fishmonger to fillet and remove the skin from 2 John Dory weighing 1 pound, and ask him to separate the fillets into their three parts.

… Peel and wash 4 fennel bulbs. Cut 2 of them in half and set the others aside.

… Peel and wash 4 spring onions.

… Heat a flameproof casserole dish with 2 tablespoons of olive oil. Place the half fennel bulbs face down in the casserole dish and add the spring onions. Add salt, cover the casserole dish with a lid, and brown for 3 minutes.

… Pour in 1¾ cups of chicken stock (page 10), sprinkle in 10 saffron threads, put the lid back on, and cook gently (simmering) for 15 minutes.

… In the meantime, slice the other 2 fennel bulbs into fine shavings with a mandoline and put in a salad bowl.

… Wash, dry, and take the leaves from 4 sprigs of dill and 4 sprigs of basil. Cut 1 tablespoon of pitted black olives into rounds, add all these to the salad bowl, and mix with the raw fennel. Season with 2 tablespoons of olive oil and the juice of half a lemon.

… When the fennel bulbs are cooked (check if they are done with a knife), lay the fillets in the casserole dish and cook for just 1 minute, basting them constantly with the stock from the casserole dish.

… Arrange the half fennel bulbs and fillets in a serving dish with a spring onion on top. Drizzle with the liquid from the casserole dish. Distribute 4 segments of tomato confit (page 16) on top and serve immediately with the bowl of raw fennel separately.

AD— The olives take care of salt for the raw fennel salad, so don't add any more, especially as the dill and basil enhance the flavors.
PN— A good idea! We eat too much salt. John Dory is a very lean fish, so it doesn't give us any good omega-3s. But given that fennel is bursting with antioxidants of all kinds, as well as vitamins and minerals, this doesn't much matter. If John Dory can't be found, turbot will also work for this recipe.

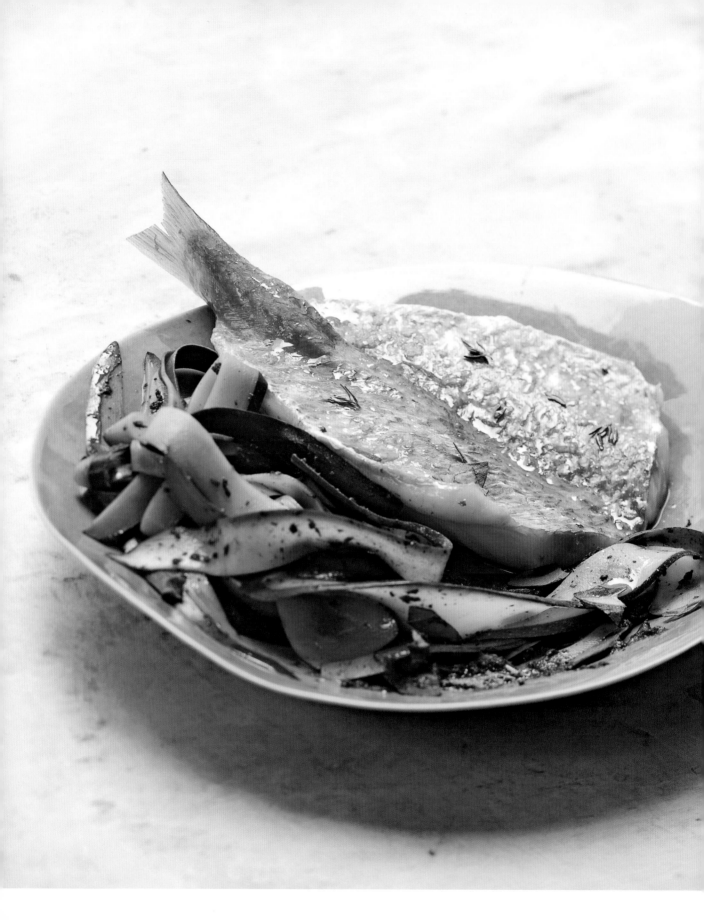

Fillets of Red Mullet, Zucchini, and Tapenade

... Serves 4

... Get your fishmonger to fillet 4 red mullet weighting about 8 ounces, and ask him to leave them attached at the tail. Check that there are no bones left in and keep cold.

... Wash and dry 6 medium zucchini. Cut them in half lengthwise, then slice each half into long strips with a mandoline, discarding the seeds from the middle.

... Wash and dry 3 sprigs of basil, take off the leaves, and crush them.

... Heat a drop of olive oil in a nonstick skillet and sauté the zucchini strips for just 1 minute. Add salt and freshly ground black pepper, then add the basil and 2 tablespoons of tapenade (page 40), mixing very gently.

... Heat the broiler.

... Salt and pepper the inside of the mullet fillets, then lay them on a baking sheet.

... Break up a small sprig of thyme on top.

... Slide the baking sheet under the broiler for just 1 or 2 minutes.

... Peel 1 garlic clove and rub 4 plates with it. Arrange the zucchini on the plates and place 1 mullet on top of each.

... Give a generous twist of freshly ground black pepper and serve immediately.

AD— Fishmongers and cooks have special pliers for removing fish bones. If you don't have these, ordinary tweezers will do, provided you clean them well.

PN— Don't use too much olive oil for sautéing the zucchini in the skillet or they will be too fatty, and this dish will lose its remarkable lightness (while being plentiful and satisfying).

Grilled Sardines with Chermoula

AD— There's no point in adding thyme or any other aromatic herb when grilling sardines. They are flavorful enough by themselves and it would only detract from the result. They can also be grilled on a plancha or griddle or under the broiler.

PN— Sardines are full of omega-3 oils, which are good for the heart and nervous system! This inexpensive fish makes a useful contribution to a healthy balanced diet. Eat it as often as you can . . . and if the smell from broiling it is too powerful, just open the windows!

… Serves 4

Prepare the sardines

… Scale and gut 16 very fresh sardines (or get your fishmonger to do it for you).

… Rinse well under running water and dry carefully with a clean dish towel. Keep in a cold place.

Make the chermoula condiment

… Peel 2 garlic cloves. Wash, dry, and take the leaves from 3 sprigs of cilantro and 3 sprigs of mint.

… Put the garlic cloves, a pinch of salt, and 2 pinches of Piment d'Espelette or hot paprika in a mortar.

… Crush the mixture to form a puree. Add 1 teaspoon of cumin and the cilantro and mint leaves.

… Continue to crush firmly and, when the mixture forms a paste, add the juice of 1 lemon then, gradually, 5 tablespoons of olive oil.

… Transfer the chermoula to a small saucepan.

… Heat gently, stirring, without allowing it to boil, until it begins to release its aroma. Allow to cool.

Grill the sardines and serve

… Salt the sardines lightly on each side.

… Grill on a hot charcoal grill for 2 minutes on each side.

… Add freshly ground black pepper. Arrange the fish on a serving dish with lemon wedges and serve the chermoula condiment separately.

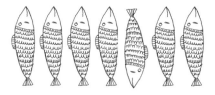

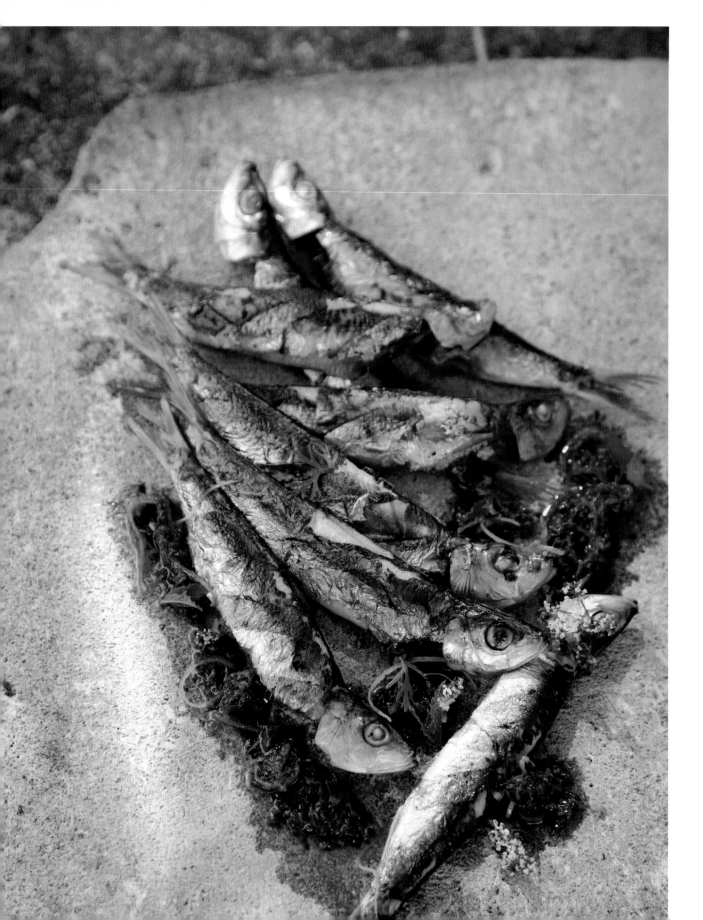

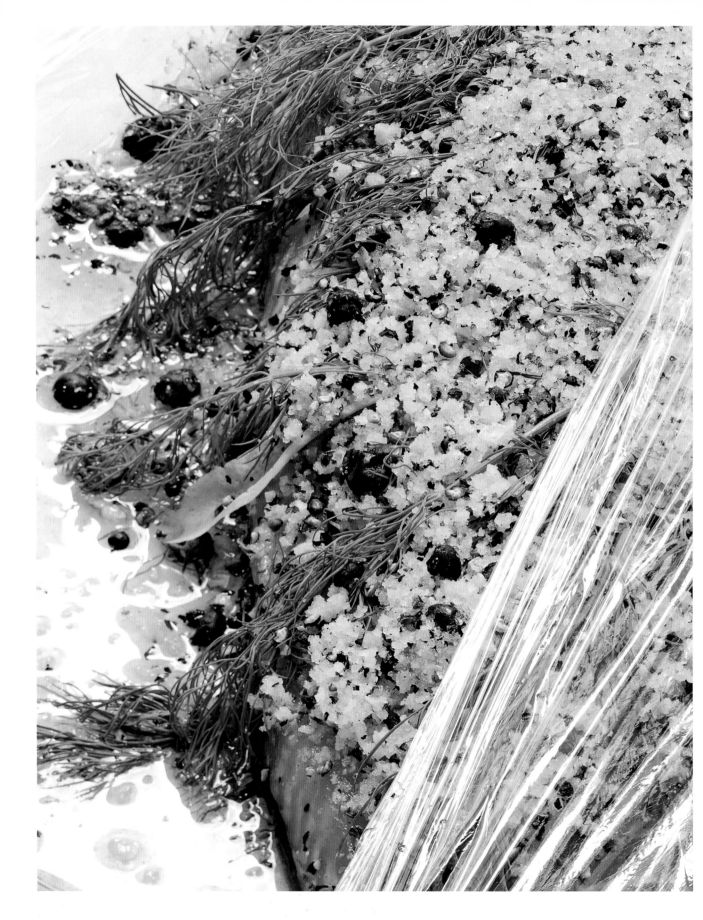

Salmon Gravalax, New Potatoes, and Arugula

… Serves 4

<u>24 hours before, prepare the salmon gravalax</u>

… Combine ½ cup of coarse gray sea salt, ½ cup of fine salt, ½ cup of superfine sugar, 3 tablespoons of mignonette pepper (see page 30), and 1½ tablespoons of crushed juniper berries in a bowl.

… Detach the leaves from a bunch of dill, pare the zest from 1 lemon (3 required in total for the recipe), and add them. Mix well.

… Put half of this marinade on a baking sheet or dish, then place 1 fillet of Scottish salmon weighing 1½ pounds on top, with its skin and bones.

… Cover with the rest of the marinade and leave in a cold place for 24 hours.

<u>On the day</u>

… Rinse the salmon fillet quickly under running water. Remove any bones with tweezers, then cut it at an angle into thin slices. Set them aside.

… Rub 2 pounds of new potatoes with coarse salt mixed with 1 cup of water to remove the skins.

… Cook them in salted boiling water for 15 minutes (check when they are done with a knife).

… In the meantime, wash and dry 4 handfuls of arugula and season with the juice of 1 lemon, a splash of olive oil, and a little sea salt.

… Also chop 1 bunch of chives.

… Drain the potatoes, cut in half immediately, and put in a dish. Drizzle with 5 tablespoons of olive oil and the juice of 1 lemon. Add the chopped chives and plenty of freshly ground black pepper. Mix well.

… Pile the arugula and salmon slices on top and serve immediately.

AD— The marinade enriches this finely flavored fish. And it's very quick to prepare, perfect for when you have friends round for dinner.
PN— The marinade does not spoil the superb nutritional qualities of the salmon (lots of omega-3s and good-quality proteins). With carbohydrates from the potatoes and fiber and vitamins from the arugula, this is a well-balanced dish.

Bonito Tartare with Herb Salad

AD— Bonito, also known as
skipjack tuna, belongs to the
tuna family. Its flesh is red like
red tuna—an endangered species
due to overfishing.
PN— There is a lot of omega-3s
in bonito, and a stack of vitamins,
antioxidants, and minerals in the
tomato confit and herb salad.
It's all good!

… Serves 4

… Cut half a cucumber into very small dice (brunoise), salt it, and leave to drain in a colander.

… Peel and mince or grate 1 red onion.

… Remove the skin and fat from 12 ounces of bonito and cut this into small dice too. Salt lightly.

… Chop 8 segments of tomato confit (page 16).

… Combine it all in a bowl. Season with 3 tablespoons of olive oil, salt, and freshly ground black pepper and 2 or 3 drops of Tabasco.

… Refrigerate this tartare.

… Toast 4 thin slices of whole-wheat or multigrain bread under the broiler. Break it up into small croutons and put in a salad bowl.

… Rinse and carefully dry 3 sprigs of basil, 3 sprigs of mint, and 6 sprigs of flat-leaf parsley and add their leaves to the salad bowl.

… Drizzle with a splash of olive oil and toss well.

… Divide the tartare among 4 serving plates, and arrange the herb salad with croutons decoratively on top. Serve immediately.

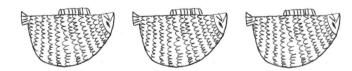

White-Flesh Tuna Steaks with Pepper and Tomato Condiment

… Serves 4

… Get your fishmonger to cut four 4-ounce steaks of white tuna about ¾ inch thick.

… Take them out of the fridge 1 hour before cooking.

… Peel and chop 2 shallots. Put in a saucepan and cover with red wine vinegar. Cook very gently until completely reduced (about 10 minutes).

… In the meantime, chop 2 tablespoons of capers and 2 tablespoons of black olives. Add them to the shallots when the vinegar has fully evaporated.

… Also add 6 tablespoons of chopped cooked tomatoes (page 21) and 1 tablespoon of olive oil.

… Salt the tuna steaks, then pepper copiously with mignonette pepper (see page 30).

… Heat a nonstick skillet with a splash of olive oil and cook them for just 30 seconds on each side.

… Lay them on plates or a serving dish. Pour the tomato condiment in a bowl or sauce boat and serve separately.

AD— Tuna needs to be cooked very rare; otherwise it becomes dry. You can make the flavors more interesting by coarsley grinding different peppercorns (black, white, or pink) over the steak. A watercress salad, fried tomatoes (page 156), and baked potatoes (pages 222 and 225) go very well with this tuna.

PN— This is an oily fish, much praised by nutritionists for its high levels of omega-3s, the champion among fatty acids, and also its vitamin A. White-flesh tuna is also called albacore; it is caught in the Bay of Biscay and the Atlantic.

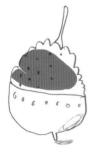

Fillets of Sole with Tomatoes and Mushrooms

AD— You can make this dish with other fillets of flat fish, such as turbot or flounder. A practical solution when entertaining is to make it in advance and put it in the oven at the last minute.

PN— Sole is a very lean fish, and its preparation here does not affect its low-fat status. Tomatoes, mushrooms, and spinach make this a super cocktail of vitamins, antioxidants, and minerals, which I think is really great!

… Serves 4

… Get your fishmonger to fillet two 1-pound soles. Then cut each fillet into three pieces.

… Take the base off 12 ounces of white mushrooms; wash and dry the caps. Cut them each into 3 slices.

… Wash and dry 6 handfuls of baby spinach leaves. Peel 2 garlic cloves, stick one on a fork, and crush the other one.

… Peel 4 pearl onions and cut into rings.

… Preheat the oven to 350°F.

… Heat a skillet with a splash of olive oil, pop in the spinach handful by handful, and stir with the fork with the garlic stuck on it until it has all wilted. Add salt and freshly ground black pepper. Transfer to a dish.

… Wipe your skillet, add a splash of olive oil, and sauté the mushroom slices and the onion rings with the crushed garlic clove over high heat for 3 minutes. Add salt and pepper.

… In a large ovenproof dish, make layers of 5 tablespoons of chopped cooked tomatoes (page 21), spinach, mushrooms, onions, and fillets of sole. Put in the oven for 10 minutes.

… Add a twist of freshly ground black pepper when you take it out of the oven and serve in the dish.

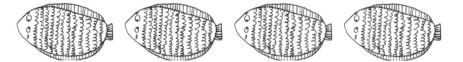

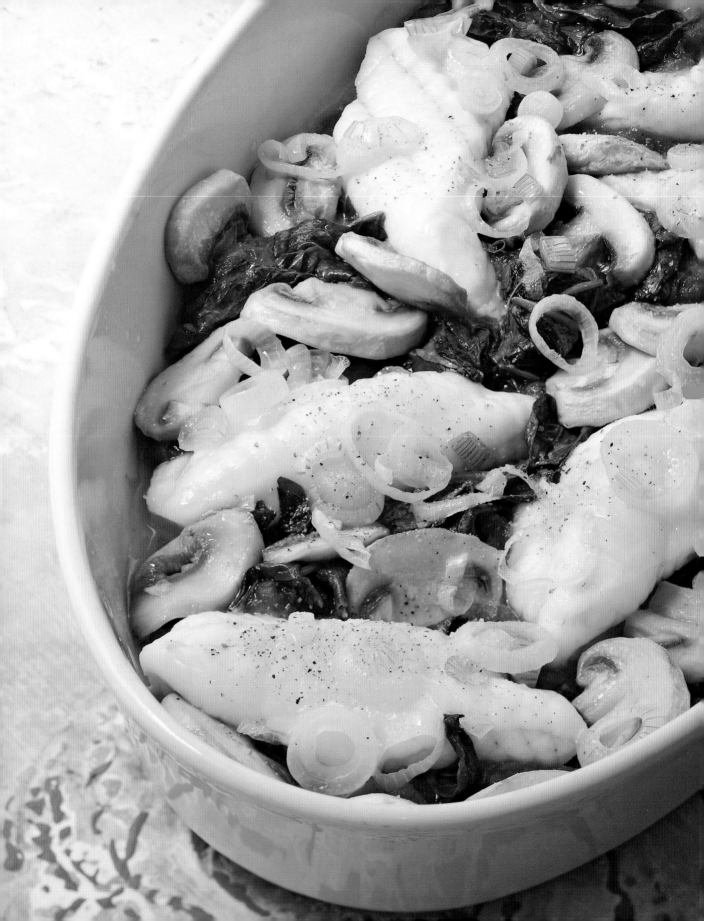

Finely Sliced Marinated Gray Mullet with Curried Vegetable Tartare

AD— *Sharpen your knife well before slicing the mullet fillet. Or ask your fishmonger to cut it into very thin carpaccio-style slices.*

PN— *The mullet is distinctive for its rich vitamin B$_6$ content, fairly rare in a fish. It is regarded as an "oily" fish because it contains health-giving omega-3s. Though not as rich, snapper can be substituted for the gray mullet.*

… Serves 4

Prepare the mullet

… Slice a 10-ounce fillet of gray mullet into very thin slices and lay them side by side in a dish.

… Grate the zest of 1 unwaxed lemon. Finely mince 2 scallions.

… Squeeze the juice of the unwaxed lemon into a small bowl, add 4 tablespoons of olive oil, 2 pinches of sea salt, 2 pinches of Piment d'Espelette or hot paprika, the grated lemon zest, and minced scallions.

… Spread this marinade over the slices of fish and leave in a cold place for 20 minutes.

Prepare the vegetable tartare

… In the meantime, peel and wash 1 carrot, 1 small fennel bulb, half a cucumber, 3 spears of green asparagus, and 10 radishes.

… Cut the half cucumber in two and scoop out the seeds. Cut the asparagus tips into 3- to 4-inch lengths. Cut all the other vegetables into small chunks.

… Peel and finely chop half a garlic clove. Wash 2 sprigs of basil, 1 sprig of parsley, and 1 sprig of cilantro and chop the leaves.

… Blitz the chunks of vegetables in a blender in short bursts so that they are not too fine and do not release their liquid.

… In a salad bowl, combine ½ cup Greek-style yogurt, the chopped garlic, 2 pinches of Indian curry powder, the chopped herbs, the juice of half a lime, and 2 tablespoons of olive oil and mix well with a whisk.

… Incorporate the chopped vegetables, stir delicately, and adjust the seasoning salt.

… Spoon the vegetable tartare into 4 individual bowls, then pile the mullet slices on top. Serve cold.

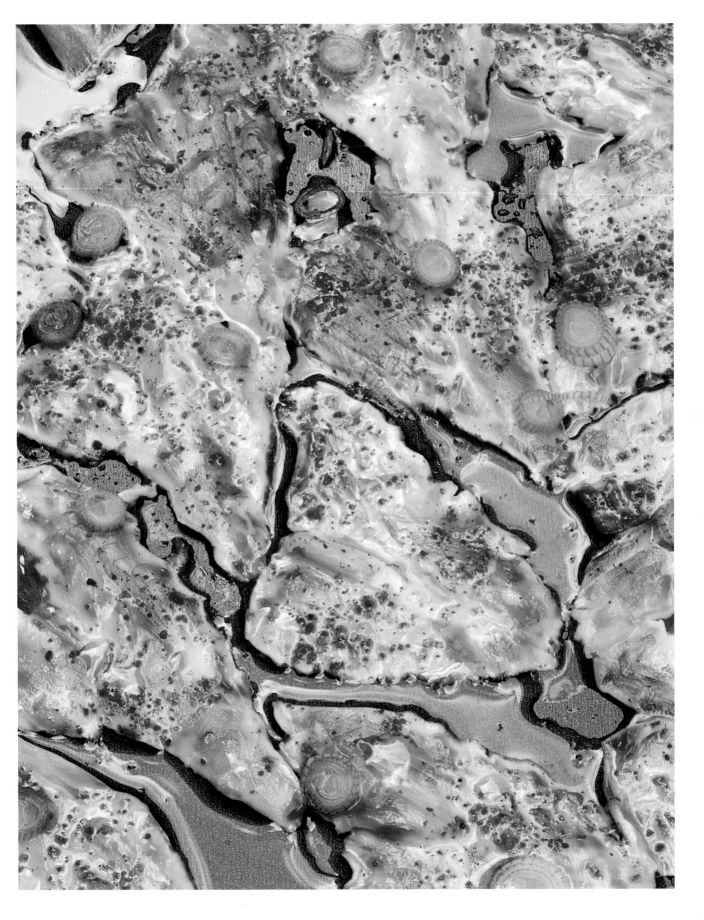

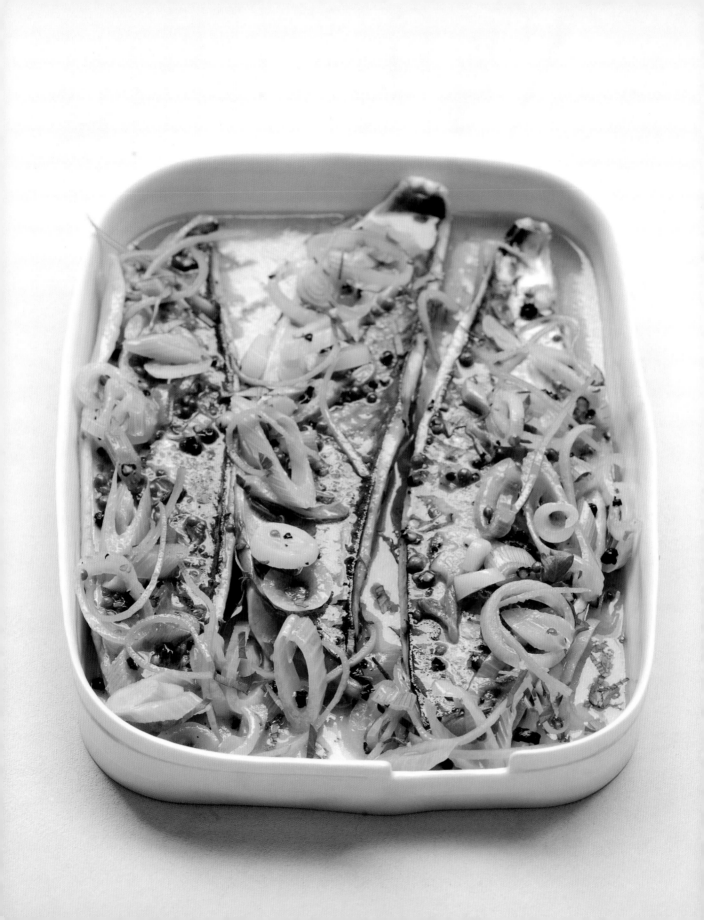

Mackerel Marinated in Orange

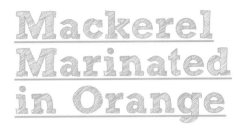

… Serves 4

… Gut two 1-pound mackerels, fillet them, and remove all the bones (or get your fishmonger to do it for you). Lay them on a dish.

… Rinse 2 unwaxed oranges and pare the zest from one of them. Cut it into small slivers (julienne), then immerse them in boiling water. Drain and refresh immediately. Repeat this twice in order to remove any bitterness from the zest.

… Squeeze the juice from both oranges and set aside.

… Peel, wash, and thinly slice 4 pearl onions and 4 small fennel bulbs.

… Crush 1 teaspoon of coriander seeds.

… Heat a flameproof casserole dish with a splash of olive oil and roll the onions and fennel bulbs in it for 1 minute.

… Salt lightly, then add the crushed coriander seeds and 1 teaspoon of mignonette pepper (see page 30).

… Pour in the juice from the oranges, stir, and cook for 5 minutes.

… Pour the contents of the casserole dish over the mackerel fillets. Cover immediately and seal with plastic wrap to keep in the heat.

… Leave the mackerel to cool in their cooking liquid for 1 hour at room temperature.

… Then chop 12 cilantro leaves. Sprinkle them over the mackerel. Serve in the dish.

AD— It is the heat from the orange juice that cooks the mackerel fillets. This way they stay nice and firm. If you get the fishmonger to fillet the fish, check carefully that there are no bones left in.

PN— Mackerel is an "oily" fish, full of good unsaturated fats (the majority of them omega-3s) but also vitamin A and minerals. The orange juice provides vitamin C, and it's nicer than the usual white wine!

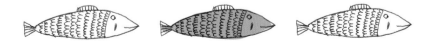

Whole Poached Sea Bass with Herb Cream

... Serves 4

... Get your fishmonger to trim, gut, and scale 1 sea bass weighing approximately 3 pounds.

... Heat 3 quarts of water in a flameproof casserole dish. Add the pared zest and slices of 1 lemon (3½ required in total for the recipe), 1 tablespoon of peppercorns, 1 tablespoon of coriander seeds, 1 handful of dried fennel stalks, and 1½ cups of white wine.

... When the water boils, immerse the bass in it. Lower the heat and simmer just under a boil for approximately 6 minutes.

... Turn off the heat and allow the fish to rest for 10 minutes.

... While the bass is cooking, prepare the herb cream. Rinse and dry the leaves of 6 sprigs of parsley and 4 sprigs of dill, then chop them finely.

... In a bowl or sauce boat, dilute 3 tablespoons of crème fraîche with the juice of half a lemon. Add the chopped herbs, some salt, and freshly ground black pepper and mix well.

... Take the bass out of its cooking liquid with a skimmer. Arrange it on the serving dish and add 2 lemons cut into wedges. Serve the sauce separately.

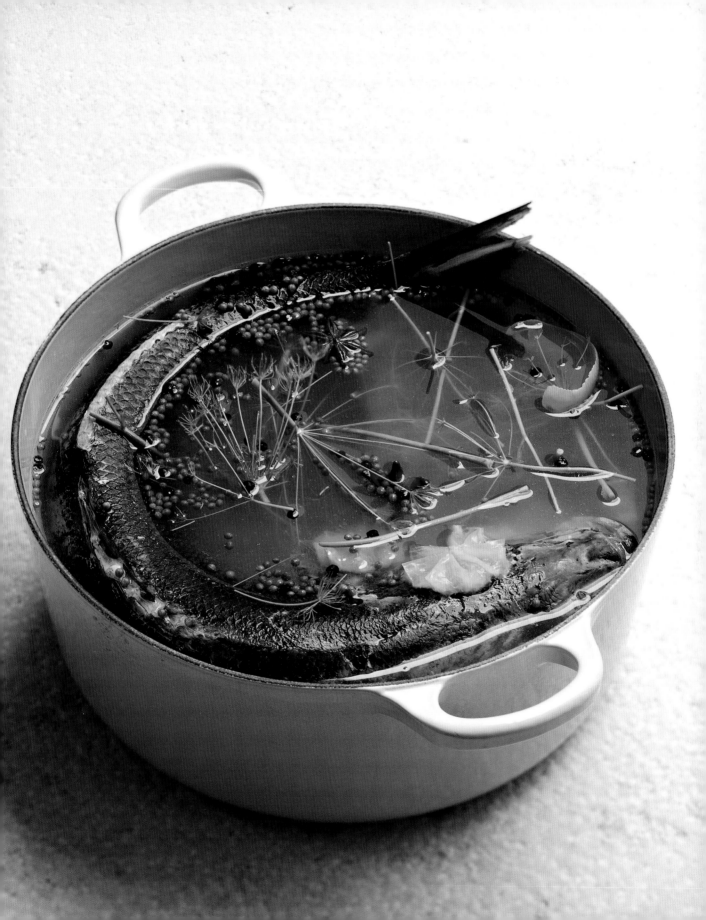

Grilled Salmon with Sesame Polenta Fingers

AD— It's a good idea to prepare the polenta the day before. It will keep for at least 24 hours in the refrigerator without any problem. PN— Sesame oil is rich in unsaturated fatty acids, which add to those of the salmon. For a balanced menu, don't forget a starter of vegetables and a dessert of fruits. There's no need for any cheese or other dairy product, as the polenta provides calcium.

… Serves 4

Prepare the salmon

… Remove the bones from a 1-pound fillet of salmon. Mix together 2½ tablespoons of coarse salt and 1½ tablespoons of superfine sugar and spread a layer of it on a dish. Lay the fillet of salmon on top and pour the rest of the salt-sugar mixture on top. Refrigerate and leave to marinate for 1 hour, turning the fillet over.

Prepare the polenta

… In the meantime, in a dry skillet, brown 2 tablespoons of sesame seeds and drain on paper towels.

… In a saucepan, heat 6 cups of lowfat milk with 3 tablespoons of sesame oil. When it boils, sprinkle in 10 ounces of polenta/cornmeal, beating vigorously. Cook for 6 minutes, stirring constantly. Add the sesame seeds and mix well.

… Pour the polenta into a dish between 2 sheets of wax paper. Flatten to a uniform thickness. Then put the dish in a cold place.

To finish your dish

… Heat a charcoal grill or broiler.

… Take out the salmon fillet, rinse under running water, and cut into 4 equal-sized pieces. Dry them well, then brush with a little olive oil on all sides.

… Cut the polenta into 12 rectangles. Heat a skillet with a good splash of olive oil and brown the polenta fingers on all sides. Drain on paper towels and keep warm.

… Lay the salmon steaks on the grill and cook for 1 or 2 minutes on each side.

… Put them in the serving dish or on individual plates and sprinkle with a few grains of sea salt. Arrange the polenta fingers all around them.

… Cut 2 lemons into wedges and add them. Add a generous twist of freshly ground black pepper and serve.

With Wilfrid, the chef at La Bastide de Moustiers

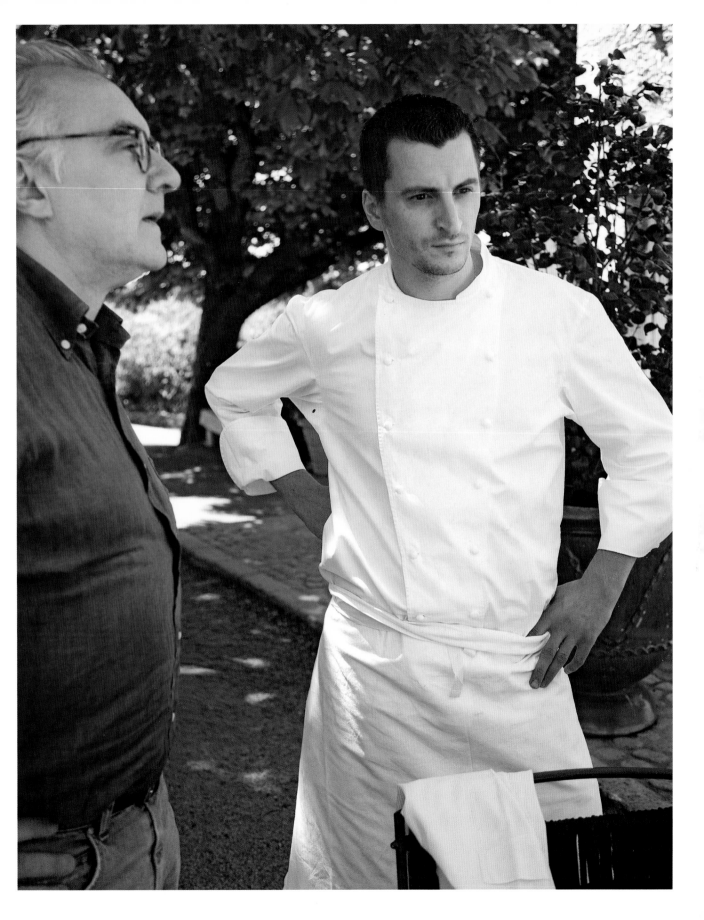

Tartare of Pink Trout and Condiments

AD— Salmon trout or sea trout, as its name suggests, is from the same family as salmon. It swims back up the coastal rivers of western France in the autumn, but it is also bred in fish farms. It has very fine flesh.

PN— A close relative to salmon, pink trout has the same nutritional qualities. It provides unsaturated fatty acids, including the famous omega-3s. Salmon can be used in place of the pink trout in this recipe.

… Serves 4

… Remove the skin and bones from a 1-pound fillet of pink trout (salmon trout).

… Cut into cubes of about ¼ inch.

… Put them in a dish, cover with plastic wrap, and refrigerate.

… Blanch 2 tomatoes and cut into quarters. Remove the seeds and chop the flesh into very small dice (brunoise).

… Cut 6 to 8 pickled gherkins into thin rounds.

… Trim and chop 4 scallions.

… Chop the leaves of a very small bunch of tarragon.

… Mix all the above in a bowl and refrigerate.

… Season the trout tartare with sea salt, Piment d'Espelette or hot paprika, and a splash of olive oil and divide it among individual plates.

… Drizzle with a few drops of balsamic vinegar.

… Arrange the condiment all around and serve nice and cold.

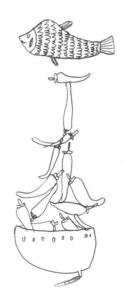

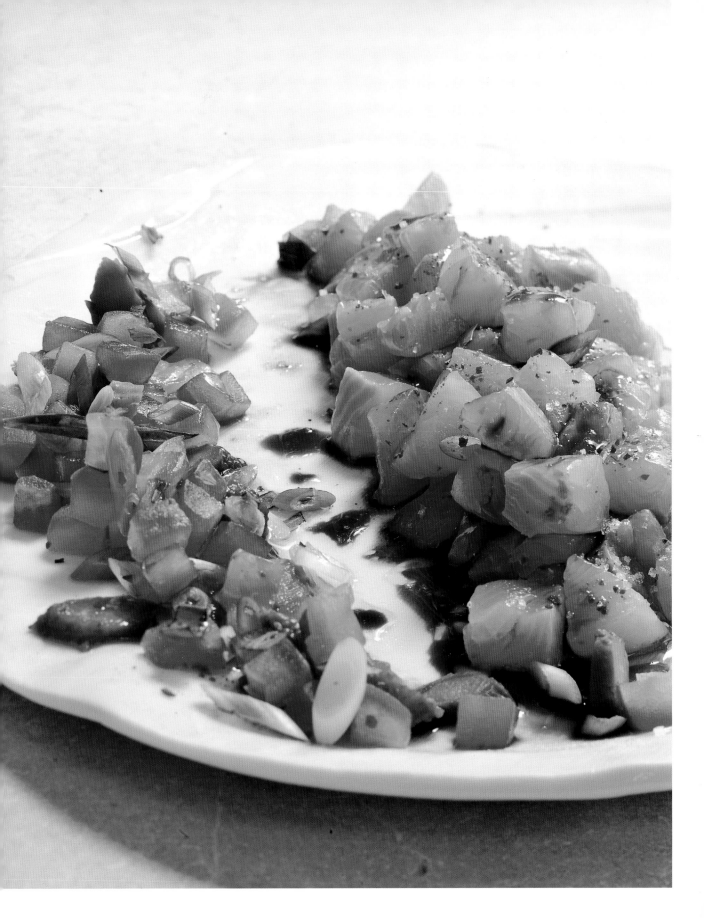

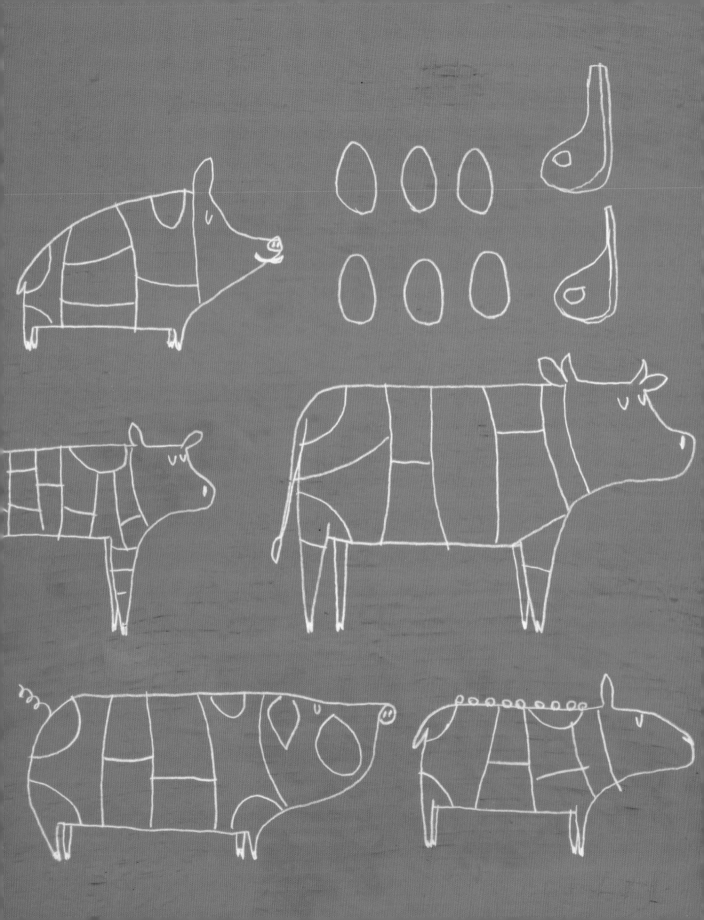

AD— Eggs, poultry, lamb, beef, pork, veal, and game. I am passionate about all these ingredients and with every new season they spark my imagination, steeped in my childhood experiences in the Landes.

PN— Don't overdo it, though! Because, apart from poultry and game, they contain too much saturated fat, which is not the best thing for your health. All these recipes keep the portions of meat quite small, and there are always some healthy vegetables to go with them.

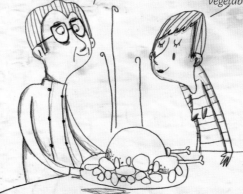

Land

Oeufs en Cocotte with Morels

AD— *If you find it difficult to get hold of fresh morels, use dried ones and rehydrate them in several changes of water. You can also use other mushrooms for this recipe.*
PN— *The proteins in eggs are the best balanced in terms of amino acids. They are used as a benchmark in nutritional codes.*

... Serves 4

... Remove the base from 5 ounces of fresh morels, then wash the caps in several changes of warm water until all traces of sand have been removed. Dry in a salad spinner. Cut any large ones in half.

... Peel and mince or grate 1 pearl onion.

... Heat a drop of olive oil in a flameproof casserole dish. Roll the morels and minced onion in it, add salt, and sweat for 3 minutes. Pour in 1 cup of chicken stock (page 10) and cook for about 20 minutes, until the morels are soft.

... Preheat the oven to 350°F.

... While the morels are cooking, stem and rinse and dry 2 handfuls of baby spinach leaves.

... Oil 4 ramekins with a brush, and rub with 1 peeled garlic clove.

... Add the baby spinach leaves to the casserole dish of morels, mix, then distribute the mixture among the ramekins, spreading it around the edges and leaving any excess liquid in the casserole dish. Take 4 eggs and break into the middle of each ramekin.

... Place the ramekins in a high-sided roasting pan, pour hot water a third of the way up and bake in the oven for 10 minutes, until the egg white is set.

... In the meantime, boil the remaining liquid from the morels in the casserole dish, add 1 tablespoon of crème fraîche, stir well until it melts, and pour this creamy liquid into the ramekins as soon as they come out of the oven. Add a twist of freshly ground black pepper and serve immediately.

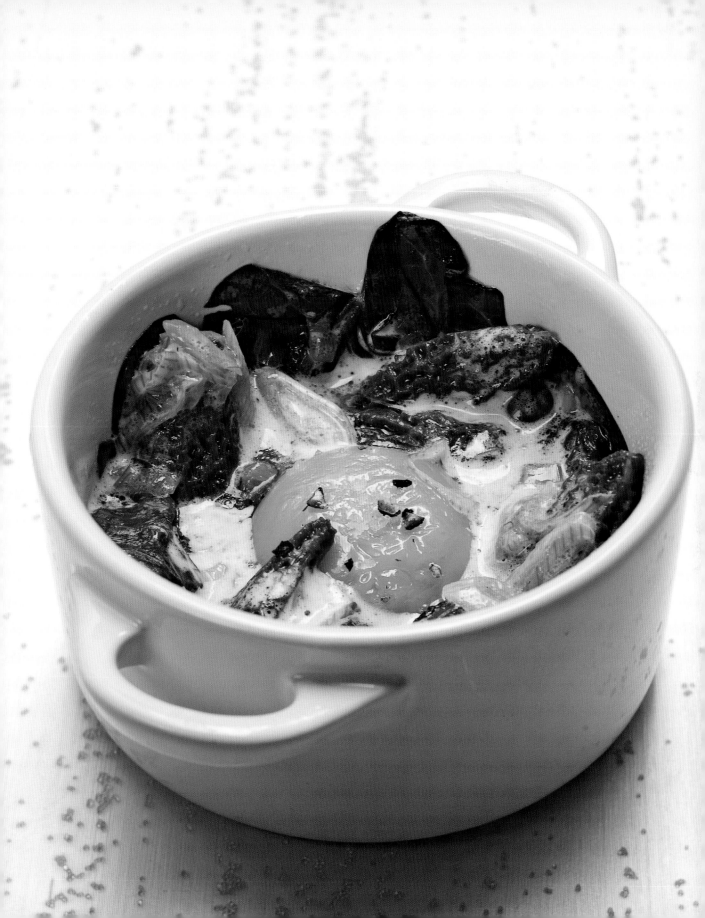

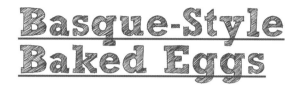

Basque-Style Baked Eggs

AD— Serve these Basque-style eggs with nice fresh slices of whole-wheat or multigrain bread. If you don't have a flameproof serving dish, use a skillet fit for serving at the table.

PN— If you cannot get Spanish Serrano ham, use an Italian cured ham, and trim the fat before cutting it. Peppers, onions, and tomatoes— plenty of antioxidants here!

… Serves 4

… Peel 2 white onions, and peel 1 red bell pepper, 1 green bell pepper, and 1 yellow bell pepper with a vegetable peeler and remove the seeds and membranes. Cut all these vegetables into thin slivers.

… Cut 4 tomatoes into quarters, remove their seeds, and cut their flesh similarly.

… Peel and chop 2 garlic cloves.

… Heat a splash of olive oil in a flameproof casserole dish and sweat the onions and peppers for 5 minutes, with the lid on.

… Add the tomatoes and garlic and cook gently with the lid off, until the liquid from the vegetables has evaporated.

… In the meantime, cut 4 ounces of Spanish Serrano ham into slivers and chop the leaves from a small bunch of basil.

… Add them when the vegetables are cooked and stir well. Taste and adjust the seasoning with salt and Piment d'Espelette or hot paprika.

… Spread the vegetables in a layer about 1½ inches deep in a large flameproof serving dish.

… Make 8 little hollows in the vegetable layer. Take 8 very fresh eggs and break one into each hollow. Cook gently until the white is set but the yolk is still runny.

… Sprinkle over a few grains of sea salt and serve.

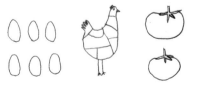

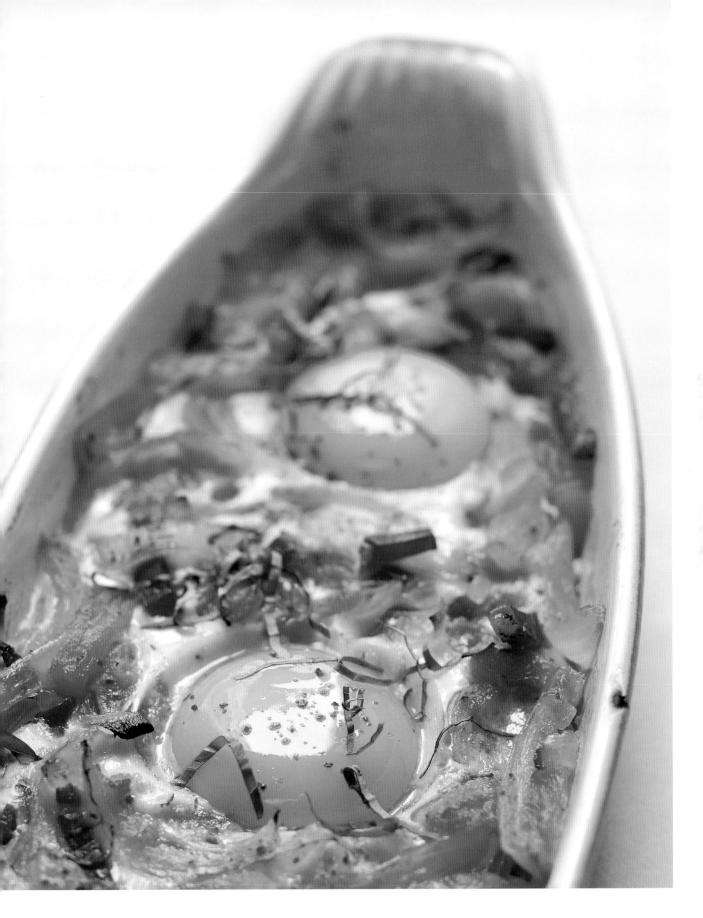

Cold Omelette Crespeou

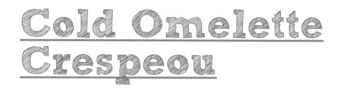

AD— *Crespeou is a Provençal cake of thin omelettes that look like crêpes, hence its name. If you like, season with a little balsamic vinegar. Serve with an herb salad (page 153).*

PN— *There's nothing to stop you from making one of these omelettes by itself! The herb one is bursting with vitamins, the crushed tomato one is full of antioxidants, and the tapenade one contains good healthy unsaturated fatty acids.*

… Serves 6

… This dish is prepared in advance.

Prepare the herb omelettes

… Finely chop 2 sprigs of thyme, 2 sprigs of savory, 20 chives, and the leaves of 2 sprigs of marjoram, 2 sprigs of tarragon, 5 sprigs of parsley, and 5 sprigs of basil.

… Combine them in a bowl, break 4 eggs (12 required in total for the recipe) on top, beat, and season with salt and freshly ground black pepper.

Prepare the tomato omelettes

… Pour 4 ounces of chopped cooked tomatoes (page 21) into another bowl.

… Break 4 eggs on top, mix together, and season.

Prepare the tapenade omelettes

… Beat 4 more eggs with 2 ounces of tapenade (page 40) into a third bowl and check the seasoning.

Cook the crespeou

… Heat a splash of olive oil in a small skillet (8 inches in diameter).

… Pour in a small ladleful of the egg and tomato mixture to make a very thin omelette. Once cooked, lay it on a dish.

… Then cook a small tapenade omelette in the same way, followed by an herb omelette, placing each omelette on top of the previous one.

… Continue in this way until all the egg mixture is used up.

… Cover the crespeou with a sheet of wax paper. Place a weight on top and refrigerate until you are ready to serve.

… Serve as is or cut into sections and arrange them on plates.

… Either way, season with a little sea salt and freshly ground black pepper.

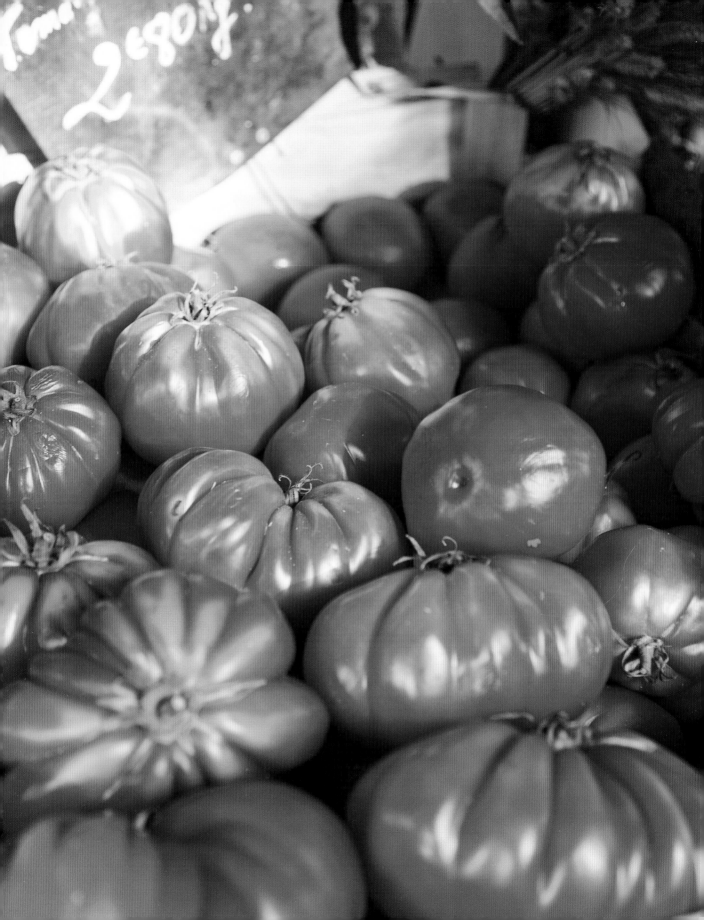

Poached Foie Gras with Turnips

AD— *This dish works best if you use turnips of different varieties. And if you ever come across yellow turnips called Boule d'Or snap them up, as their flesh is extraordinarily fine.*

PN— *The turnip's nutritional value is not stunning. But it does contain sulphur compounds that are among those elements believed to protect against certain cancers. As for foie gras, like the duck from which it comes, it contains good unsaturated fatty acids.*

… Serves 4

… Peel 2 bunches of turnips with their tops. Set aside the smallest 3, keeping ¼ inch of their tops on.

… Cut all the others into quarters, then cut each quarter into thin ⅟₁₆-inch slices.

… Heat 2 tablespoons of olive oil in a flameproof casserole dish. Add the turnip slices, salt them, and sweat for 2 minutes, stirring. Add 1 teaspoon of honey and allow to caramelize. Pour in 3 tablespoons of wine vinegar and stir well to deglaze. Cook until the vinegar has reduced by half.

… Then add 2 cups of chicken stock (page 10) and season with 3 pinches of quatre-épices (a four-spice mix featuring white pepper, ground ginger, nutmeg, and cloves) and salt. Cook for an additional 10 minutes, keeping the turnips fairly firm.

… In the meantime, cut the 3 reserved small turnips into thin slices with a mandoline.

… Using a knife that you have held under hot running water, cut 1 lobe of very fresh duck foie gras into cubes of around ¾ inch. Quickly remove the trimmings, nerves, and veins.

… Immerse the cubes of foie gras immediately in the stock and simmer just under a boil for 3 minutes.

… Take out the cubes of foie gras and turnips with a slotted spoon. Strain the stock through a conical strainer and adjust the seasoning.

… Arrange the foie gras and turnips in a serving dish or on individual plates. Sprinkle a little mignonette pepper (see page 30) onto the cubes of foie gras.

… Pour the stock into the plates and add a dash of balsamic vinegar.

… Top with the slices of raw turnip and serve immediately.

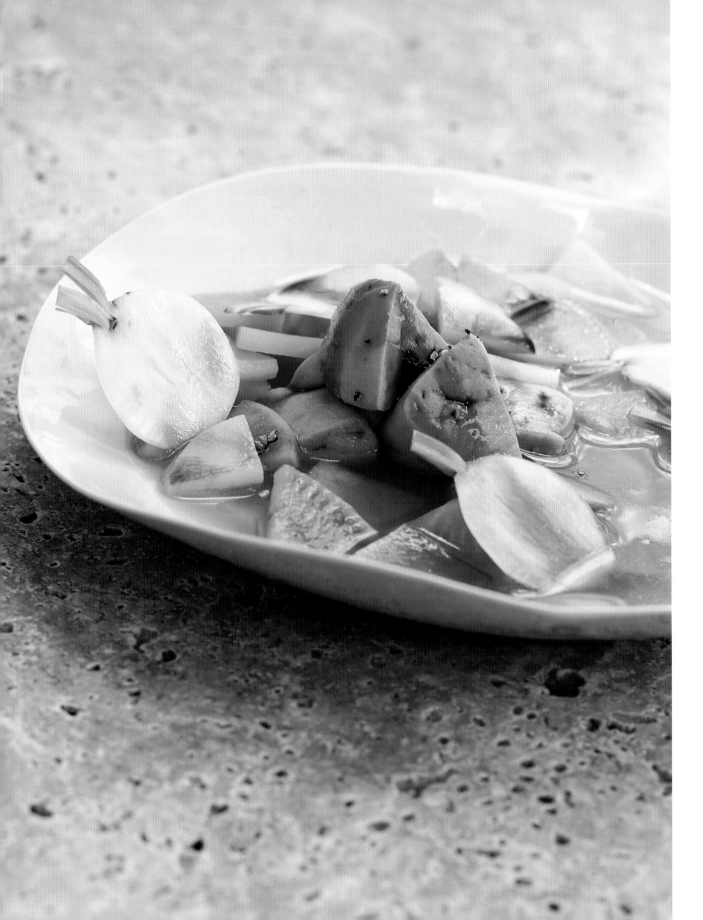

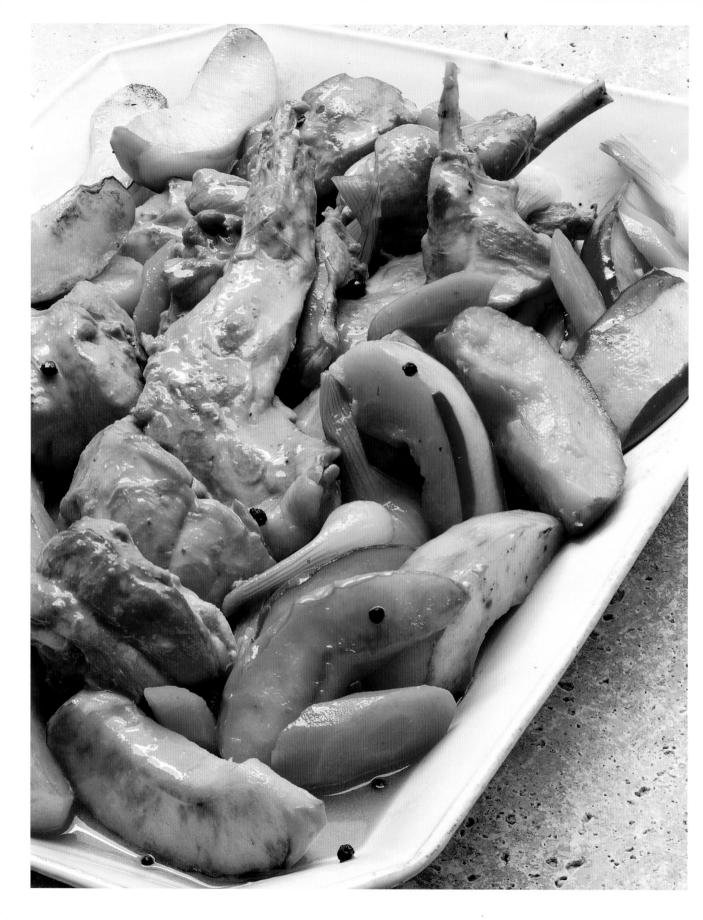

Sautéed Rabbit with Apples

… Serves 4 to 6

… Get your butcher to cut 1 fresh farmed rabbit weighing about 3½ pounds into pieces.

… Wash and peel 4 green and 4 red apples, leaving on a few strips of skin. Cut into wedges, remove the core, sprinkle with the juice of 1 lemon, and put in a salad bowl. Don't throw the peel away—you will need it for the sauce.

… Peel a bunch of fresh spring onions with stalks, keeping 1½ inches of stalk. Wash and peel 2 carrots and cut into rounds at an angle. Crush 2 garlic cloves without peeling them.

… Salt all the rabbit pieces. Heat 1 tablespoon of olive oil in a flameproof casserole dish and brown them lightly, then transfer them to a dish.

… In their place put the carrots, onions, and garlic and sweat for 3 minutes, stirring.

… Pour in 3 tablespoons of cider vinegar, scrape well to deglaze the juices, and allow to reduce by half. Then pour in a 750 ml bottle of dry cider and bring to a boil. Skim carefully, then put the rabbit back in. Add the apple peel and 10 peppercorns.

… Cook over low heat for 40 minutes, checking occasionally.

… Preheat the oven to 425°F.

… Before the rabbit finishes cooking, salt the apple segments. Pour a dash of olive oil into a dish and line them up side-by-side, turning so that they are all coated with oil.

… Put in the oven and cook until the apples are soft (for approximately 12 minutes).

… When the rabbit is cooked, take it out of the casserole dish, along with the carrots and onions, and put them all in the serving dish.

… Crush the apple parings in the sauce to thicken it. Adjust the seasoning and add a dash of cider vinegar if you like.

… Strain this sauce through a conical strainer onto the rabbit. Arrange the apples all around and serve nice and hot.

AD— You can adapt this recipe by using a chicken or a guinea fowl. For the red apples, you have plenty of choice, depending on the season: McIntosh, Red Delicious, and Granny Smith apples are available all year round.

PN— This is a good way to eat apples, which have scientifically recognized health-giving properties, justifying the old saying that "an apple a day keeps the doctor away."

Guinea Fowl with Cabbage

AD— This recipe is equally suitable for pheasant during the season. The flesh of guinea fowl is not white, but brown like a game bird. Its wild nature means that it has always been unsuitable for intensive rearing.

PN— The guinea fowl is the leanest of poultry. This is a nicely low-fat and well-rounded dish, with vitamins, fiber, and minerals from the vegetables, plus the super-healthy constituents of cabbage. Nothing but goodness!

... Serves 4

... Cut 1 good-sized free-range guinea fowl into 8 pieces (or get your butcher to do it for you) and keep all the trimmings.

... Take the outer leaves off 1 green cabbage, remove the stem end, cut the cabbage into quarters, and wash well. Put in a saucepan of cold water and bring to a boil. Drain, then refresh. Squeeze to remove as much water as possible, then slice into thin strips.

... Peel, wash, and thinly slice 2 carrots, 1 onion, and 4 stalks of celery.

... Preheat the oven to 325°F.

... Salt the pieces of guinea fowl and heat 2 tablespoons of olive oil in a flameproof casserole dish. Brown the guinea fowl on all sides, and then take the pieces out.

... In their place, put the cabbage, carrots, onion, celery, and trimmings from the guinea fowl and sweat for 3 minutes, stirring from time to time. Then put the pieces of guinea fowl back, pour in 2 cups of chicken stock (page 10), add 5 black peppercorns and 5 juniper berries, and bring to a boil.

... Then cover the casserole dish with a lid and put in the oven for 20 minutes.

... In the meantime, peel and wash 8 small, waxy potatoes.

... After it has been cooking for 20 minutes, take out the casserole dish, remove the wings of the guinea fowl, and replace them with the potatoes. Cook in the oven for an additional 30 minutes.

... Taste and adjust the seasoning of the cooking stock, remove the trimmings, return the wings to the casserole dish, and serve straight from the casserole dish.

Chicken Breasts in Yogurt with Stir-Fried Vegetables

… Serves 4

The day before, prepare the chicken

… Take the leaves from 5 sprigs of cilantro, peel 2 inches of ginger, remove the seeds from 1 bird's-eye chile, and chop all these ingredients.

… In a bowl, mix ½ cup of plain yogurt, 3 tablespoons of fromage blanc, 3 tablespoons of light cream, the cilantro, the bird's eye chile, chopped ginger, ½ teaspoon of ground mace, and a pinch of Piment d'Espelette or hot paprika. Stir well.

… Sprinkle salt on 4 free-range chicken breasts (boneless but with the skin on) and coat them entirely with this marinade. Wrap each one in plastic wrap and refrigerate for 24 hours.

On the day

… Peel and wash 2 carrots, 1 bunch of green asparagus, 2 heads of Belgian endive, 8 shiitake mushrooms, 1 head of cauliflower, and 3½ ounces of bean sprouts.

… Thinly slice the carrots, asparagus, endives, and shiitake mushrooms with a mandoline. Separate the cauliflower florets.

… Preheat the oven to 425°F.

… Take the chicken breasts out of the plastic wrap. Wipe them and cook on a grill pan or griddle skin side down for about 5 minutes, until they are a nice golden color. Then put them on a baking sheet and into the oven for 3 minutes to finish cooking. Keep warm.

… Heat 1 tablespoon of olive oil in a wok. Over high heat, sauté the carrots, cauliflower, asparagus, endives, and shiitake mushrooms until lightly colored.

… Salt lightly and add the bean sprouts. Continue to stir for 2 minutes and deglaze the wok with 3 tablespoons of soy sauce.

… Cut the chicken breasts into slices lengthwise and lay them on a serving dish or individual plates. Arrange the stir-fried vegetables alongside. Give a generous twist of freshly ground black pepper and serve.

AD— If you don't have mace, substitute a little grated nutmeg. Mace is the outer membrane of the nutmeg and it has a finer flavor. If you can get hold of red endives, use these! They will add an extra splash of color to your pan of vegetables. PN— A nice pan of winter vegetables with very healthy chicken breasts! The yogurt and fromage blanc in the marinade don't give you enough calcium, so this meal calls for a dairy product or cheese.

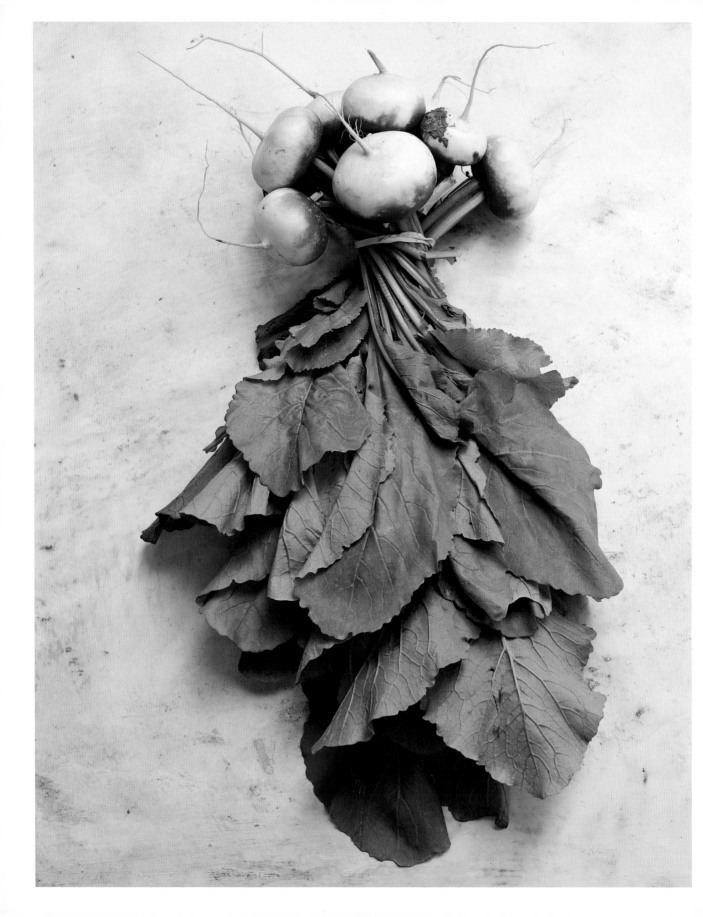

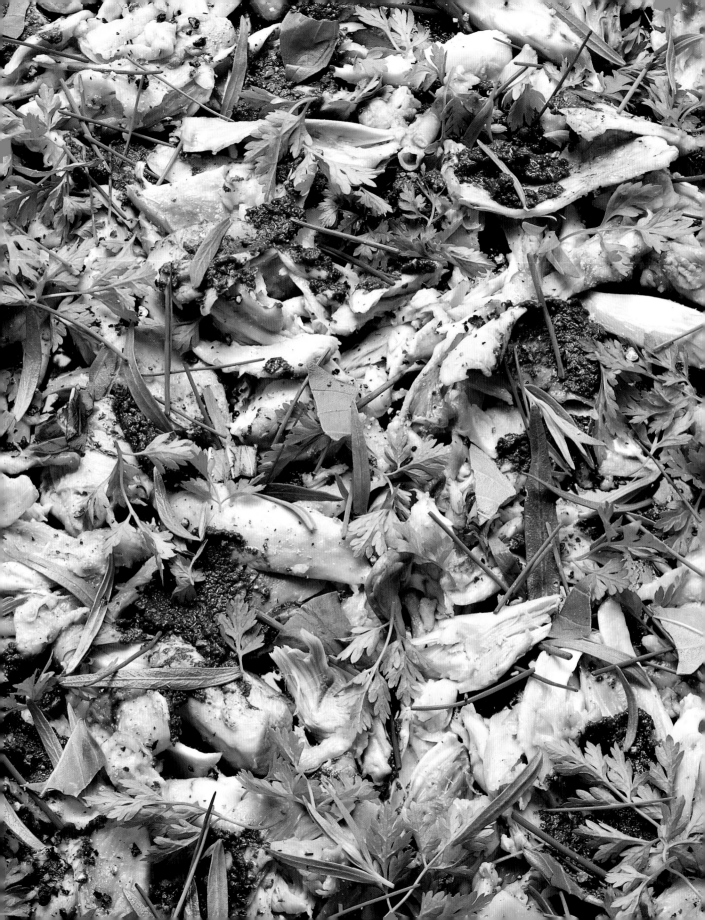

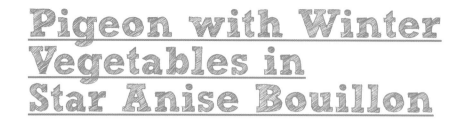

Pigeon with Winter Vegetables in Star Anise Bouillon

AD— Serve the rest of the bouillon in cups or keep and freeze for use in another dish. Skim frequently while cooking; it's tiresome, but you will end up with a nice clear bouillon.

PN— For small appetites, half a pigeon per person is enough, especially as there are plenty of vegetables. This bird is particularly low in fat and rich in protein and iron.

… Serves 4 to 8

… Get your butcher to prepare 4 pigeons weighing 1 pound, asking him to gut and singe them, take off the legs and separate the back of the breasts, open them out, and truss the wings.

… Peel and wash 4 small leeks, 8 carrots with tops, half a head of celery, 2 fennel bulbs, 1 bunch of turnips with tops, and half a green cabbage.

… Keep the tops and the tenderest trimmings.

… Put these vegetables in a large flameproof casserole dish along with the legs and carcasses of the pigeons and cover with 2 quarts of chicken stock (page 10). Add a pinch of coarse salt and 3 star anise and bring to a boil.

… Cook for 1 hour, skimming regularly.

… Off the heat, immerse the pigeon breasts in the broth for 4 minutes.

… With a slotted spoon, take out the vegetables and pigeon breasts.

… Strain the broth through a fine sieve and adjust its seasoning.

… Cut the vegetables into sections, arrange in a deep serving dish (preheated) and pour in 2 ladles of the broth. Add the pigeon breasts and legs and season with sea salt and freshly ground black pepper.

… Grate a small piece of horseradish on top and add all the reserved trimmings and the leaves from 2 sprigs of dill and 2 sprigs of chervil. Serve nice and hot.

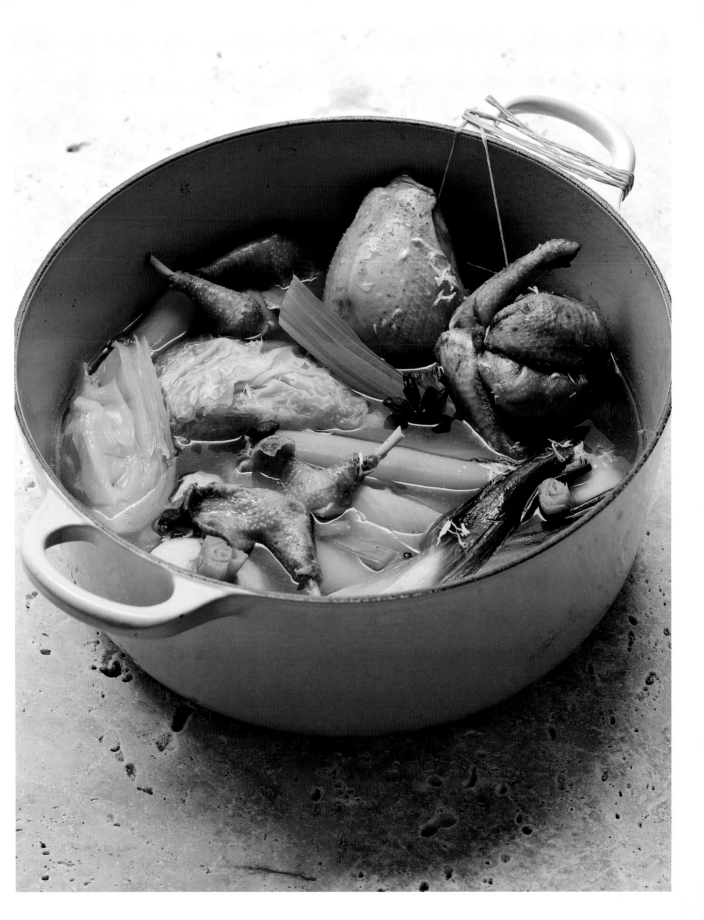

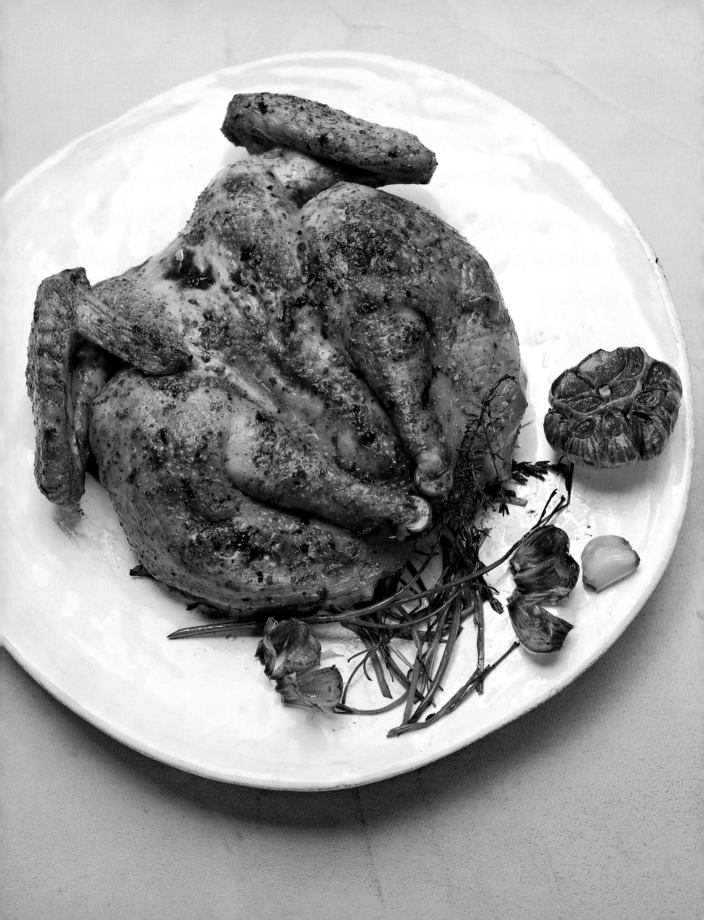

Herby Roast Chicken

… Serves 4 to 6

… Get your butcher to butterfly 1 good free-range chicken (severing the ends of the feet and wings, splitting the back lengthwise, and flattening it out). Ask him also to crush the neck.

… Preheat the oven to 400°F.

… Wash and dry a small bunch of parsley, a small bunch of chervil, and a very small bunch of tarragon. Chop the leaves and put them in a bowl. Don't throw away the stems.

… Cut the tops off 2 heads of garlic, then take 2 garlic cloves from them, chop these and add them to the bowl along with a pinch of freshly ground black pepper and 4 ounces of strained fromage blanc. Season with salt and mix well.

… Push this herb mixture under the skin of the chicken through the opening in the neck. Push with your fingers until the flesh of the breast and legs is well covered. Then salt inside the bird.

… In a baking pan, spread out 4 sprigs of thyme, 4 sprigs of rosemary, and the reserved herb stems. Lay the chicken on this aromatic bed and distribute around it the giblets and garlic heads, with the cut side down.

… Brush with 2 tablespoons of olive oil and roast in the oven for 20 minutes.

… Then lower the oven to 350°F and take out the garlic heads.

… Cook for an additional 20 to 30 minutes (depending on the size of your chicken), basting fairly regularly.

… When the chicken is cooked, transfer it to a dish, cover with aluminium foil, and allow to rest for 10 minutes.

… In the meantime, pour ½ cup of water onto the baking sheet and scrape up all the juices. Cut up the chicken and arrange the pieces on a serving dish.

… Drizzle the cooking juices over the chicken or serve separately.

AD— Always choose a good-quality free-range chicken so you can be sure that it has seen the sun and ended its life in semifreedom. All others, even "farm fresh" chickens, spend their entire lives in rearing sheds.
PN— An herb salad (page 153) goes particularly well with this chicken and gives you loads of vitamins and minerals as well.

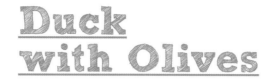

Duck with Olives

AD— Olives pretty much take care of any salt needed for the sauce. So it's vital to taste before adjusting your seasoning. You should of course always taste; otherwise how can you tell if the seasoning is right? PN— The duck is a fairly high-fat bird, but these are good unsaturated fatty acids, helping you maintain a healthy vascular system. The composition of duck fat is in fact quite similar to that of olive oil. The olives in this dish provide a generous stack of these healthy fatty acids as well.

… Serves 4

… Salt the inside and outside of 1 Muscovy duckling ready to cook.

… Preheat your oven to 350°F.

… Peel, wash, and thinly slice 2 carrots, 2 stalks of celery, 1 onion, and 1 fennel bulb.

… Heat a tablespoon of olive oil in a flameproof casserole dish. Brown the duck on all sides over medium heat. When it is nice and golden, drain.

… Discard the fat from the casserole dish.

… Put in all the vegetables with 1 sprig of thyme and 3 garlic cloves, squashed. Salt lightly.

… Place the duck on top and put the casserole dish in the oven for 30 to 50 minutes, depending on the size of the duck.

… Open the casserole dish, take out the bird and place it on a dish, cover with aluminium foil, and allow to rest for 10 minutes.

… Also take out the sprig of thyme and the skins of the garlic cloves.

… Add 4 ounces of pitted black olives to the casserole dish, and 2 tablespoons of ruby Port. Stir and scrape the bottom of the casserole dish with a wooden spatula.

… Add 1 cup of chicken stock (page 10). Mix again and reduce the liquid until it has a nice, slightly syrupy consistency.

… Taste and adjust the seasoning with salt and add freshly ground black pepper.

… Add a splash of wine vinegar.

… Carve the breasts and legs of the duck, arrange them in a dish, and pour the olive sauce all around. Serve immediately.

Christophe Saintagne

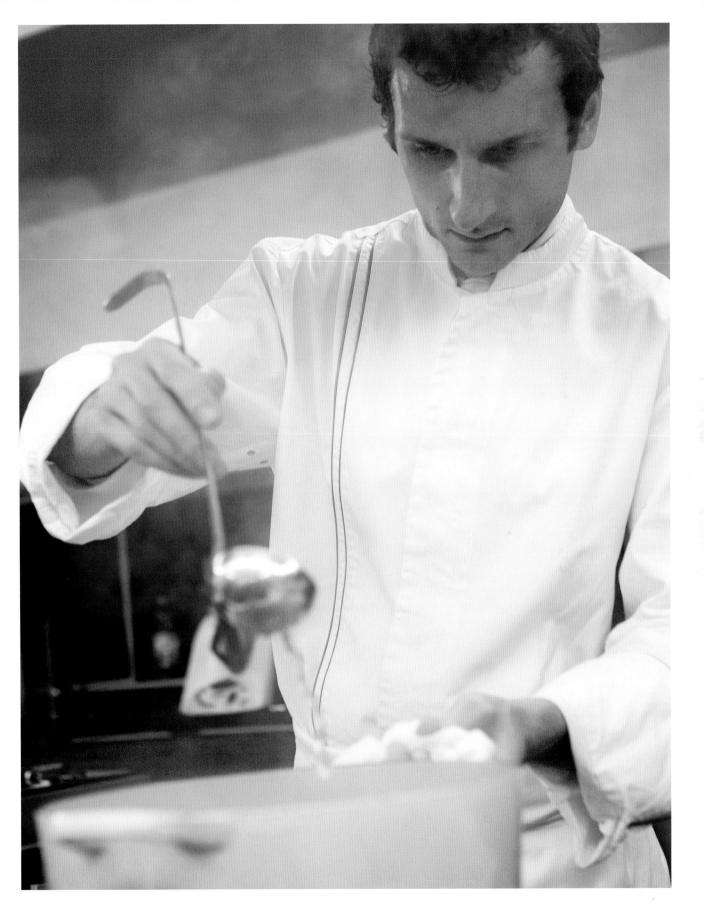

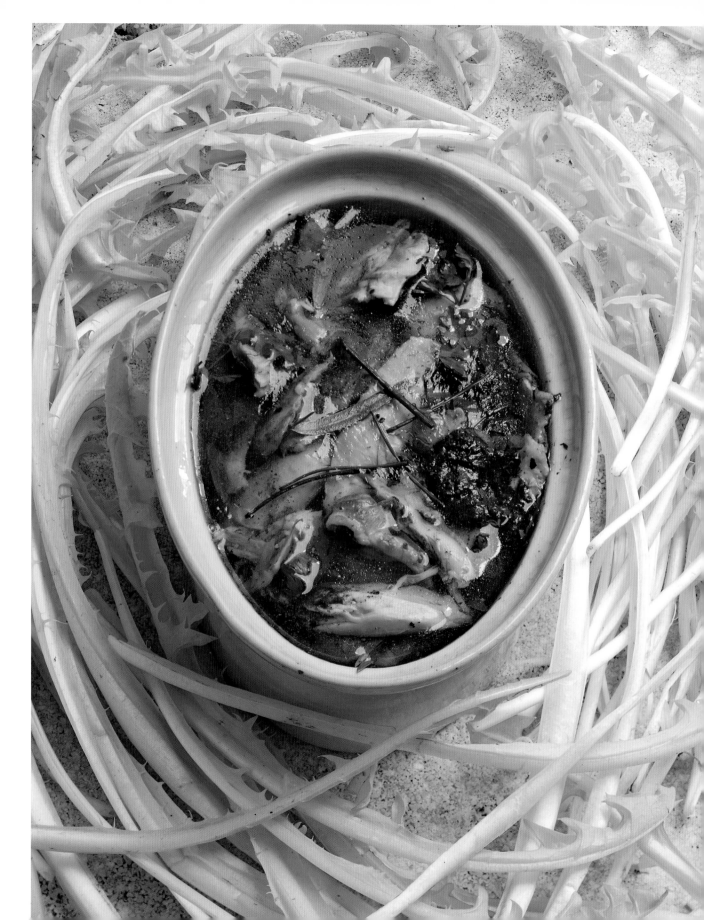

Young Rabbit en Gelée with Black Olive Puree

... Serves 6 to 8

<u>Prepare this dish the day before</u>

... Get your butcher to cut up 1 good-sized farmed rabbit with a knife.

... Peel and wash 2 onions, 2 carrots and 1 fennel bulb, and cut them into cubes of about ½ inch. Crush 5 garlic cloves (in their skins).

... Preheat your oven to 350°F.

... Heat a splash of olive oil in a flameproof casserole dish, and brown the pieces of rabbit until they are golden.

... Add the onions, carrots, fennel bulb, and garlic, salt lightly, and cook over medium heat for 5 minutes, stirring. Pour in 2 cups of white wine, stir again, and allow to reduce by half.

... Then add 1 quart of chicken stock (page 10), bring to a boil, and skim carefully.

... Add 5 small sprigs of thyme and 5 small sprigs of rosemary. Cover the casserole dish and put in the oven for 2½ hours.

... Take out the casserole dish and remove all the rabbit pieces.

... Strain the liquid through a sieve lined with a dish towel. Refrigerate for at least 12 hours. Then remove any fat that has solidified on the surface.

... Ladle into a saucepan, leaving any impurities that may remain at the bottom, and heat (without boiling).

... Soak 10 sheets of gelatin, then squeeze dry with your fingers and mix into the stock.

... While the stock is resting, debone the rabbit, carefully removing all the small bones, and shred the meat. Put in a large bowl.

... Wash and dry 3 sprigs of flat-leaf parsley, 3 sprigs of chervil, 3 sprigs of basil, and 1 sprig of tarragon and add the leaves to the bowl.

... Also add 3 tablespoons of tapenade (page 40). Mix gently and adjust the seasoning.

... Transfer the contents of the bowl to a terrine dish, then pour in the gelée. Cover with plastic wrap and refrigerate until the gelée is set firm.

AD— If you cut the rabbit with a knife, you can avoid the dangerous splinters of bone (difficult to get rid of later), whereas when cut with a cleaver it tends to leave lots. And if you prepare this terrine the day before, you are certain to have a perfect jelly.

PN— Serve this terrine with pickled gherkins, pickled onions, and a nice herb salad (page 153) or dandelion salad. Rabbit meat is lean; its fat is peripheral and will melt during cooking and can be removed when you allow the stock to rest.

Corn-Fed Chicken and Couscous with Citrus

AD— The free-range chicken of the Landes has long held the French Red Label for its guaranteed quality. It is fed with corn from the Landes region, which is what gives its flesh its yellow color.
PN— To balance the meal, serve a vegetable starter or a big salad of lamb's lettuce with cheese. Finish your meal with some fruit.

… Serves 6

Prepare the citrus zest

… Pare 5 zests from 4 oranges, 1 lemon, 1 lime, and 1 grapefruit, all unwaxed. Cut them into slivers (⅛ inch). Put these in a saucepan, cover with cold water, and bring to a boil. Drain, refresh with cold water, and repeat twice. Then cook gently for 2 hours with 2 tablespoons of superfine sugar and the juice of 2 oranges, the lime, and half of the grapefruit.

Prepare the citrus fruit and vegetables

… Peel and remove the inner membranes of the lemon, the other 2 oranges, and the other half grapefruit and separate into segments. Cut the bulbs of a bunch of fresh spring onions with stalks in two and cut the stalks into ½-inch pieces (set aside). Cut 1 fennel bulb into small cubes.

Cook the chicken

… Preheat the oven to 350°F. Chop a pinch of coriander seeds and crush 2 cardamom pods.

… Cut 1 large Landes or other corn-fed free-range chicken into pieces and salt. Brown in a flameproof casserole dish with 2 tablespoons of olive oil. Take them out. In their place, sweat the onions and fennel bulb for 3 minutes. Add the citrus segments, 2 pinches of coarsely ground black mignonette pepper (see page 30), the coriander, cardamom, and chicken pieces. Deglaze with ½ cup of water, cover the casserole dish with a lid, and put in the oven.

… Take out the breast pieces after 16 minutes and cook the legs for an additional 20 minutes. Take out the cardamom, chicken legs, and onions. Crush what is left in the pot with a fork. Add half of the citrus zests and the onion greens. Check the seasoning, put back the chicken pieces and onions, and stir. Keep the casserole dish hot.

Prepare the couscous and finish the dish

… Pour 2 cups of couscous into a bowl, add the rest of the cooked zests, some salt, a pinch of Piment d'Espelette or hot paprika, and 5 tablespoons of olive oil. Mix with your hands.

… Bring 2 cups of water to a boil and pour it over the couscous. Cover the bowl with plastic wrap and leave to swell for 10 minutes. Chop the leaves from a small bunch of basil.

… Fluff the couscous with a fork and add the basil. Serve the chicken in its casserole dish with the couscous in a separate dish.

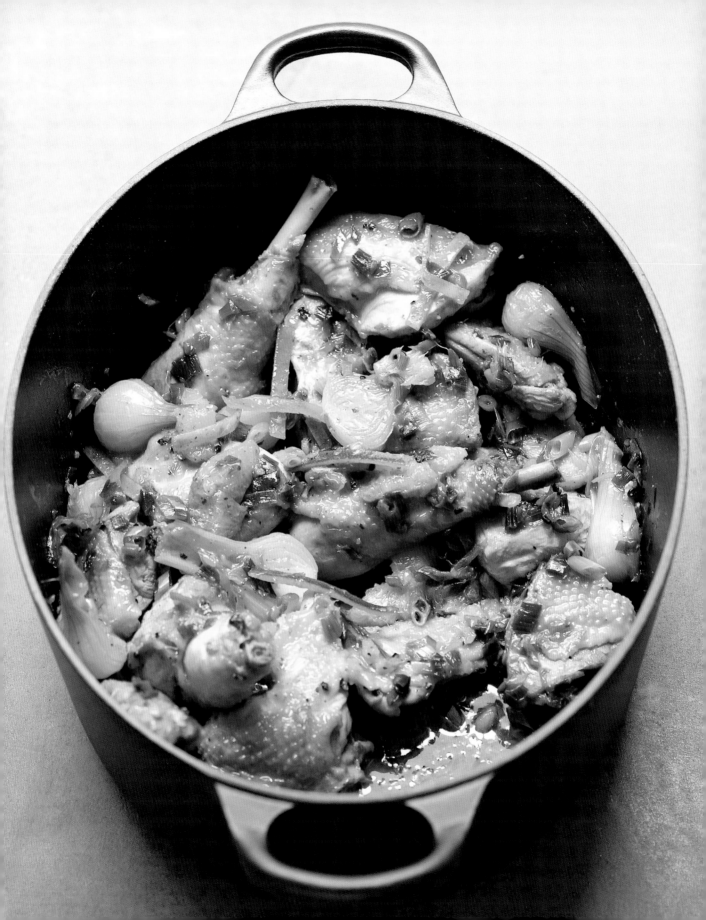

Rabbit Rillettes

AD— These rillettes improve if prepared the day before you eat them. Why not serve them as an aperitif with toasted whole-wheat or multigrain bread, or as a starter with a salad of lamb's lettuce or dandelion leaves.

PN— Onions are brimming with beneficial molecules, and goose or duck fat contain unsaturated fatty acids, so this is a healthy cocktail! Especially with a salad of lamb's lettuce, which is exceptionally concentrated nutritionally.

… Serves 4

… Cut half a farmed rabbit into pieces with a knife.

… Peel and thinly slice 5 onions.

… Heat a splash of olive oil in a flameproof casserole dish. Brown the rabbit pieces for 2 minutes.

… Add the onions, 3 whole garlic cloves, 2 sprigs of thyme, and 2 sprigs of rosemary.

… Pour in 2 cups of dry white wine, stir, salt, and cover the casserole dish. Cook gently for 1½ hours, stirring occasionally.

… Take out the rabbit pieces and shred the meat, carefully removing any bones, and put them in a large bowl.

… Strain the liquid through a conical strainer into a saucepan, reduce by three quarters, and add to the shredded meat.

… Take out the onions and garlic (remove the skins) and mix with the rabbit meat.

… Then incorporate 2 ounces of duck or goose fat and mix again.

… Taste and adjust the seasoning with 2 or 3 pinches of Piment d'Espelette or hot paprika.

… Pour the rillettes into a terrine dish, cover with plastic wrap, and keep refrigerated.

Peppercorned Duck Breasts in Bigarade Sauce

… Serves 4

Prepare the duck breasts

… Remove two thirds of the fat from 2 duck breasts, then make diagonal incisions in it with the tip of a knife, without piercing the flesh. Crush 2 tablespoons of mixed peppercorns and coat this side with them, pressing firmly to stick them on. Lightly salt the other side. Set these duck breasts aside.

Prepare the bigarade sauce

… Pour 1¾ cups of chicken stock (page 10) into a saucepan and reduce by three quarters.

… Squeeze the juice of 2 unwaxed oranges (keep the peel of one).

… Put 1 tablespoon of superfine sugar in a small saucepan with 1 tablespoon of water and cook until it forms a pale gold caramel. Add the orange juice and 1 tablespoon of white wine vinegar, stir well, and allow to reduce completely.

… Grate a quarter of the reserved orange zest into the saucepan, add the reduced chicken stock, stir well, and cook for an additional 5 minutes, until the sauce is nice and smooth. Season with freshly ground black pepper generously and add a splash of sherry vinegar. Keep hot.

Cook the duck breasts and finish your dish

… Put a skillet (or sauté pan) on the heat and when hot, lay the duck breasts in it skin side down. Cook for 3 to 5 minutes (depending on their thickness), then turn them over and cook for 3 minutes on the other side.

… Take them out and place on a rack or plate. Cover with aluminium foil and leave to rest for 5 minutes in a warm oven, with the door open.

… Cut the duck breasts into slices ¼ inch thick and arrange them on individual plates or in a serving dish.

… Coat with the bigarade sauce or serve this separately in a sauce boat.

AD— Resting the meat under aluminium foil allows it to relax after the stress of cooking, making it more tender and tasty. Adapt the cooking time to the way you like your duck breast, pink (better in my view) or more well done.

PN— Serve these duck breasts with a dish of vegetables and potatoes (for the carbohydrates). Duck is particularly rich in iron, which is a good thing, as it is often lacking in people's diets.

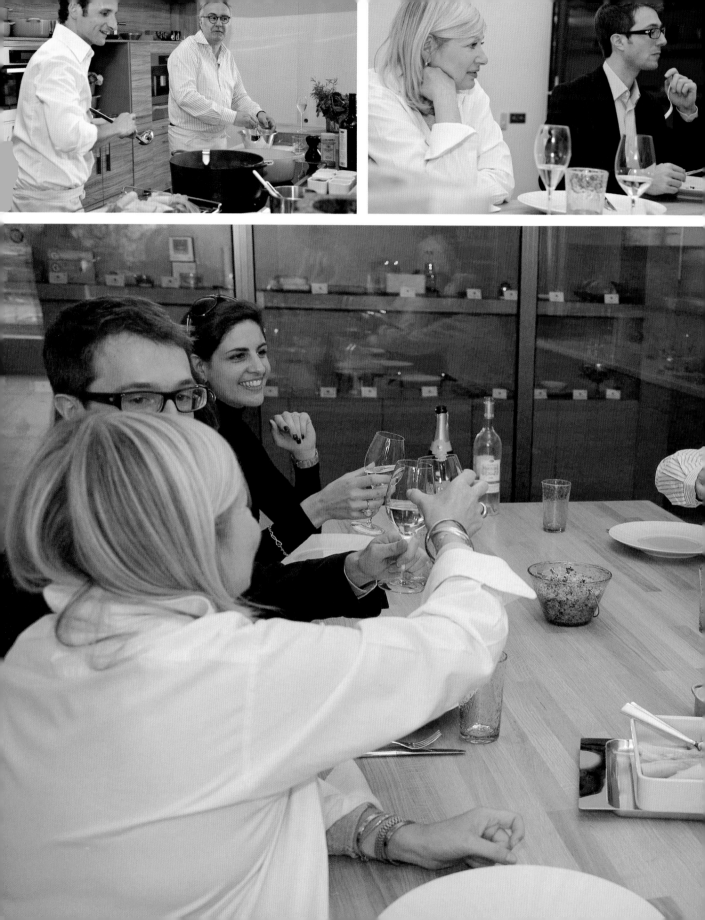

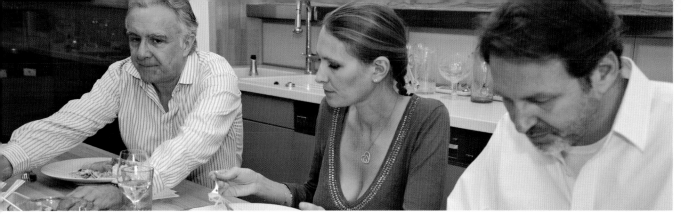

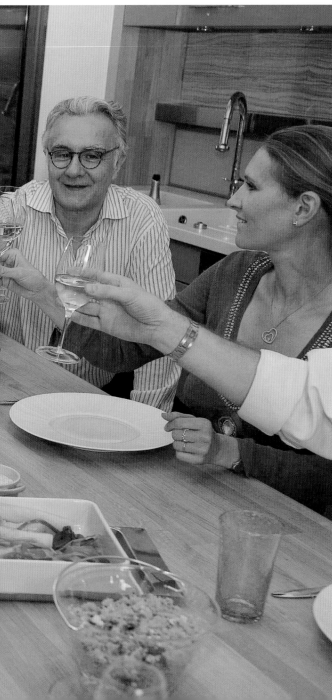

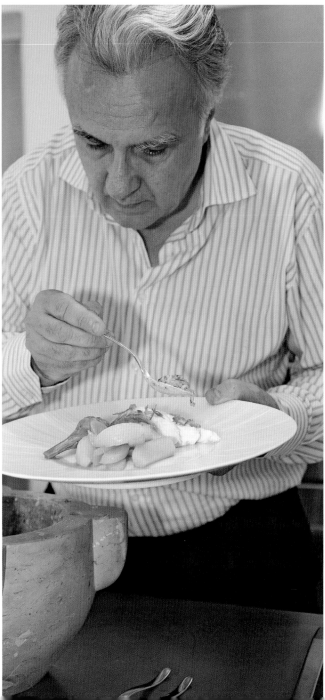

Rouelle of Pork with Oven-Roasted Vegetables

AD— Check when the vegetables are cooked with the tip of a knife. If some are cooked sooner than others, take them out and keep them warm. Rouelle is a French cut of pork from the leg, the part used for making ham. If you can't get this, buy 2 large pork loin chops (for 4) and remove the fat before cooking.

PN— You can cook pork pink without any worries. Farms have been Trichinella free for over twenty-five years. There is no longer any point in cooking for a long time and drying out the meat.

… Serves 4

… Remove the base of 4 heads of Belgian endive, wash, wipe dry, and cut in half lengthwise. Peel 4 carrots with tops, 4 turnips with tops, and 1 small black radish. Cut the radish into quarters. Peel half a celeriac and cut into wedges. Wash 4 apples, quarter them, and remove the core.

… Preheat the oven to 400°F.

… With the tip of a knife, make regular incisions in the rind of a 14-ounce rouelle (round) of pork. Then season with salt and mignonette pepper (see page 30).

… Put it in a large dish or in the broiler pan of the oven with a drop of olive oil, then put in the oven for 15 minutes.

… Add the vegetables, apples, and 2 garlic cloves, crushed. Add salt and continue to cook for an additional 15 minutes.

… Lower the oven temperature to 325°F, then add 1 small ladleful of chicken stock (page 10) and cook for an additional 15 minutes, basting frequently so that the meat stays nice and tender.

… Turn off the oven. Take the dish out, add 5 tablespoons of sherry vinegar, and deglaze the juices with a spatula.

… Cover the meat with aluminium foil and return the dish to the oven for 10 minutes, leaving the door half open.

… After its rest, cut the rouelle of pork into thick slices and place them in a serving dish or on individual plates. Add the vegetables and apples. Pour the cooking juices over them. Sprinkle with a few grains of sea salt and some freshly ground black pepper.

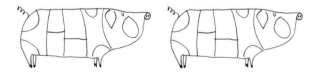

Pot-au-Feu

... Serves 8

<u>Prepare the meat and vegetables</u>

... Tie up a 1-pound chuck steak, 1-pound shoulder of beef, 1-pound shin, and 1 oxtail as for roasts, keeping a long length of string (or get your butcher to do this for you).

... Peel and wash 8 leeks. Cut the green part of the leeks and make it into a bouquet garni by tying it up with a sprig of thyme and a bay leaf. Set aside the white parts of the leek.

... Peel 3 yellow onions, take 2 cloves, and stick them into two of the onions.

<u>Cook the meat</u>

... Put all the meats in a stewpot. Cover well with water, then bring to a boil. Drain and rinse under running water.

... Empty and dry the stewpot. Put the meat back in, attaching the strings to one of the handles, cover well with water, add the bouquet garni and onions, then add 1 tablespoon of coarse salt.

... Bring to a boil and cook gently for 2 hours 15 minutes, skimming regularly.

<u>Cook the vegetables</u>

... Peel and wash 2 pounds of small turnips, 8 carrots, 1 head of celery, and 2 pounds of medium potatoes. Wash and cut 1 celeriac into 8 wedges.

... Add them to the stewpot with the reserved white leeks after 2 hours 15 minutes, then cook for an additional 45 minutes. Use a knife to check when the vegetables are cooked.

<u>To finish the pot-au-feu</u>

... Turn off the heat and wait for about 10 minutes. With a small ladle, remove the film of fat that has formed on the surface. Fish out the bouquet garni and throw it away.

... Take out the parcels of meat, put them in a large hot dish, and remove the strings. Cut into thick slices.

... Take out all the whole vegetables with a slotted spoon and arrange alongside the meat.

... Season the pot-au-feu with sea salt and mignonette pepper (see page 30). Then grate 1 inch of fresh horseradish on top.

... Serve in the dish, with the stock in bowls, a small dish of sea salt, and another of mignonette pepper, some pickled gherkins, and pickled onions.

AD— Strain any leftover stock put it in the fridge, and the next day take off the film of fat that has formed. Then freeze the stock: You can use it for sauces.
PN— Granted, this dish does take a long time to cook, but it's a really healthy winter dish!
You can make it in two stages: Prepare the meat the day before (and then the fat will separate from the stock in the cold), then reheat the meat gently the next day while you are cooking the vegetables.

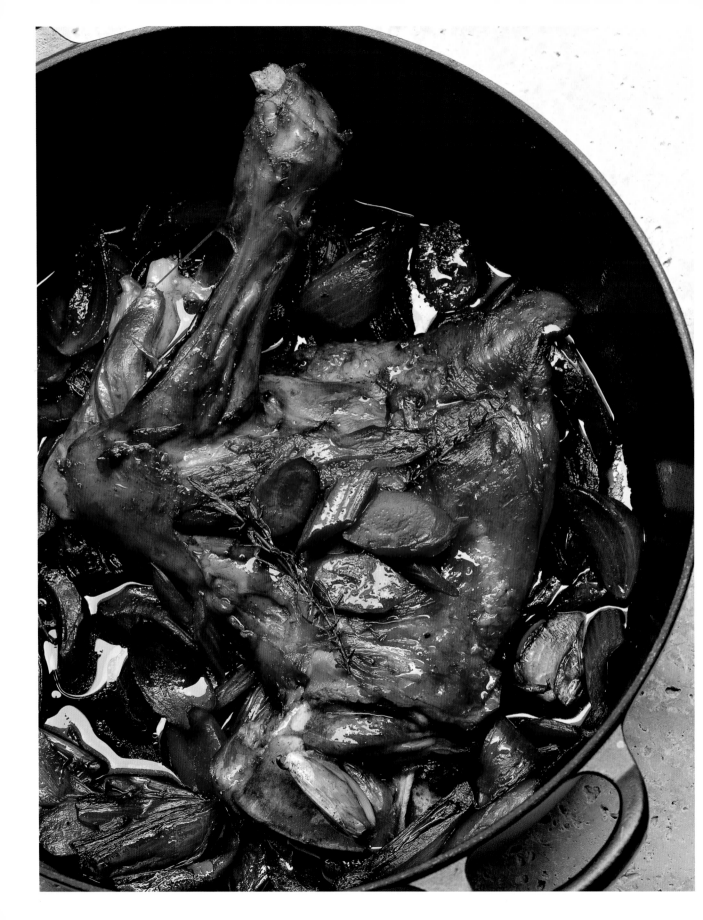

Slow-Cooked Lamb with Sage and Pearl Barley

… Serves 4 to 6

… Trim the fat from 1 shoulder of young lamb. Peel, wash, and thinly slice 4 carrots and 2 stalks of celery. Peel 4 red onions and cut into small wedges.

Cook the shoulder of lamb

… Preheat the oven to 300°F. Heat a flameproof casserole dish with a splash of olive oil and brown the shoulder on all sides. Take it out, throw away the cooking fat, wipe the casserole dish clean, and put it back on the heat with an additional splash of olive oil.

… Put in half the vegetables and sweat for 2 to 3 minutes, stirring. Add 3 squashed garlic cloves, 12 sage leaves, and 8 peppercorns, mix well, and return the shoulder of lamb to the casserole dish.

… Pour in 1¼ cups of red wine and reduce by half. Then add 1¼ cups of chicken stock (page 10), cover the casserole dish with a lid, and put in the oven for 2½ hours, basting the shoulder from time to time.

… Take out the casserole dish. Remove the shoulder, wrap it in aluminium foil, and keep warm. Keep the casserole dish on hand.

Prepare the pearl barley

… Shortly before the end of cooking the lamb, put ¾ cup of pearl barley to soak for 10 minutes.

… Heat another casserole dish with a splash of olive oil, put in the rest of the vegetables, and cook for 2 minutes, stirring. Drain the pearl barley and add to the vegetables. Stir, season with salt, and cook for 1 to 2 minutes.

… Take a ladleful of the cooking liquid from the lamb casserole dish and pour it into the barley casserole dish. Let it swell with the liquid and cook for 15 to 18 minutes, adding more of the liquid as and when it is absorbed.

… Peel 12 fresh almonds and add them at the end of cooking with a splash of olive oil. Stir and check the seasoning.

To finish your dish

… Cut the shoulder into large pieces and return them to their casserole dish. Add the contents of the other casserole dish and a generous twist of freshly ground black pepper and serve in the casserole dish.

AD— If you have cooking juices left over in the lamb casserole dish and it seems too much, put it back on the heat and reduce.

PN— In pearl barley all the husks have been removed. As a result it keeps its richness in carbohydrates but loses most of its vitamins and minerals. Fortunately, the vegetables make up for this.

Calf's Liver with Parsley and Shaved Jerusalem Artichokes

AD— A frisée lettuce goes very well with this dish. Make sure that your butcher cuts the calf's liver into very uniform slices and that they are well trimmed, with any veins removed.

PN— Calf's liver is very rich in iron and vitamins, especially vitamin A. It is quite high in cholesterol, but that is no reason to do without, unless you have serious problems in that regard.

… Serves 4

… Get your butcher to cut 4 slices of calf's liver weighing 4 ounces and about ½ inch thick.

… Peel 1 pound of Jerusalem artichokes, wash them, and slice thinly with a knife. Peel 2 garlic cloves; crush 1 of them and chop the other. Rinse and dry 10 sprigs of flat-leaf parsley and chop the leaves.

… Heat 1 tablespoon of olive oil in a nonstick skillet, and sauté the slices of Jerusalem artichoke with the crushed garlic clove over high heat for 5 minutes. Add salt.

… Lower the heat, add 1 tablespoon of butter, and continue to cook for 10 to 15 minutes, until the Jerusalem artichokes are golden on the outside and soft inside.

… In the meantime, salt the slices of calf's liver. Heat a splash of olive oil in a skillet, add the liver, and cook for about 1½ minutes on each side if you like your liver rare, 2½ minutes if you prefer it medium.

… Put them in the serving dish.

… Put the chopped parsley and chopped garlic into the skillet. Stir for 20 seconds, then add 2 tablespoons of wine vinegar. Stir once more and pour this liquid over the slices of calf's liver.

… Add a generous twist of freshly ground black pepper. Arrange the Jerusalem artichokes around the meat, or serve them separately.

Sesame-Coated Steamed Beef Patties with Coconut Condiment

... Serves 4

Make the patties

... Peel 4 white onions and 1 small green bell pepper and cut into the finest possible slivers. Heat a splash of olive oil in a sauté pan and soften the onions for 1 minute. Add the pepper, stir, season with salt, and cook until quite soft.

... Chop the leaves from a bunch of marjoram and a bunch of flat-leaf parsley. In a bowl, mix 1 pound of lean ground beef, 4 eggs, and the parsley and marjoram. Add the cooked onions and peppers, stir, and season to taste.

... Put 1½ cups white sesame seeds on a plate. Take 1 tablespoon of the meat mixture and roll it between the palms of your hands, forming a ball about 1 inch in diameter. Then roll it in the sesame seeds. Prepare the other patties similarly and keep in the fridge until you are ready to cook them.

Prepare the coconut condiment

... In a bowl, combine 1½ cups of desiccated coconut and ½ cup of lowfat milk. Stir and leave to swell.

... Take the leaves from a very small bunch of mint and a very small bunch of cilantro. Crush 5 shelled walnuts. Combine in the bowl of a blender and add the coconut soaked in milk, 3 pinches of Piment d'Espelette or hot paprika, and 4 pinches of curry powder. Blend until the mixture is nice and smooth. Warm in a saucepan and add 3 tablespoons of olive oil, stirring vigorously. Add the juice of half a lemon (2 required in total for the recipe), season to taste, and keep warm.

To finish your dish

... Rinse and dry 4 handfuls of baby spinach leaves. Season with the juice of 1 lemon, salt, and freshly ground black pepper.

... Put the patties into 4 small bamboo baskets. Place them over a pan of boiling water and steam for 5 minutes. Then divide the baby spinach leaves among the baskets. Serve in the baskets, with the coconut condiment in a separate dish.

AD— If you don't have bamboo steamer baskets, cook the patties in a steamer or even in a sieve over a pan of boiling water (but don't put too much water in the pan, as the patties should not soak in it!).

PN— Another way of eating ground beef! Serve these patties with a dish of vegetables or an herb salad (page 153). It's true that coconut is rich in saturated fatty acids, but this doesn't matter once in a while—you don't eat it every day.

Ham Hock with Red Lentils

AD— *Keep any leftover cooking stock (freeze if necessary); you can use it instead of chicken stock.*
PN— *Pork and ham are excellent! The meat of the pig is richest in vitamin B₁ and you are strongly advised to eat it at least once a week to ensure that you get enough. Furthermore, it's not really fatty, especially the meat from the front leg.*

… Serves 4

… Put 1 half-salted ham hock in a basin of water and leave to de-salt for 2 hours, in several changes of water.

… Transfer to a flameproof casserole dish, not too large, cover with water, and bring to a boil. Skim until the stock is clear, then add 1 bay leaf.

… In the meantime, peel and wash 3 carrots, 3 stalks of celery, and 4 small young spring onions with stalks. Slice them thinly, set aside, and add the trimmings (the carrot and celery ends, the onion stalks) to the casserole dish with the ham.

… Simmer gently, just below a boil, for 2 hours.

… Then take out the vegetable trimmings. Rinse 1 cup of red lentils and add to the casserole dish.

… Cook for an additional 10 minutes or so, until the lentils are soft.

… In the meantime, in a sauté pan with a drop of olive oil, sweat the sliced vegetables with a pinch of salt for 4 minutes, with a lid on the pan.

… Chop the leaves of 3 sprigs of parsley and 1 sprig of tarragon.

… Take out the ham hock and keep it warm on a serving dish.

… Drain the lentils in a sieve over a bowl and add them to the sauté pan of vegetables.

… Add ¾ cup of the cooking stock, 2 tablespoons of Dijon mustard, the chopped herbs, and stir well.

… Add a twist of freshly ground black pepper and arrange the lentils around the ham. Serve immediately.

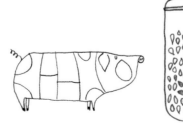

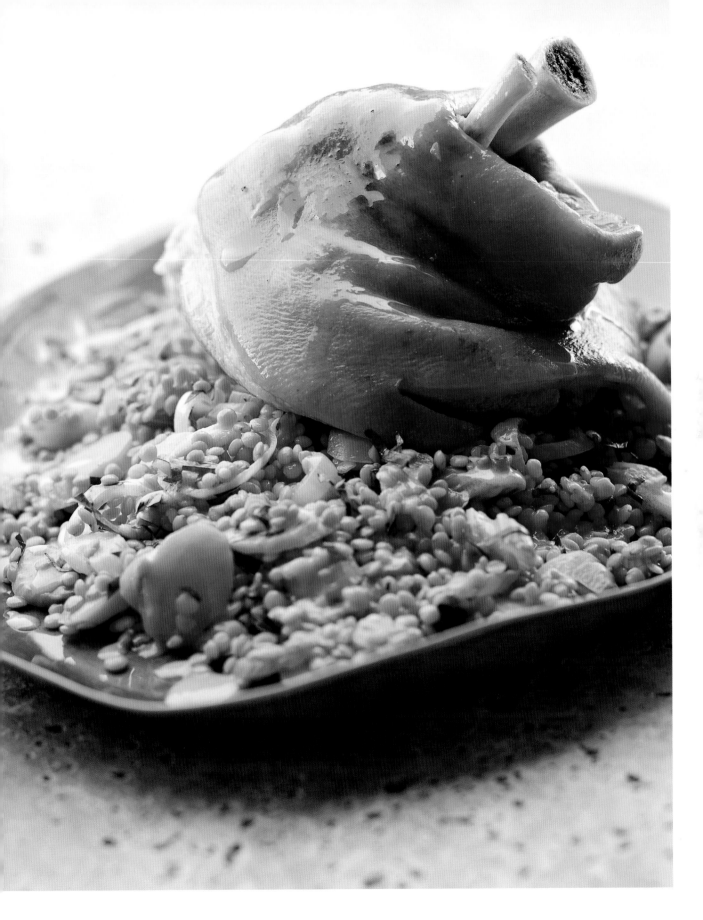

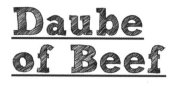

Daube of Beef

AD— *If the sauce is too thin, put the casserole dish back on the heat and reduce it. If it is too thick, add the necessary amount of chicken stock. You can use the leftovers of this daube to make dishes such as whole-wheat pasta casseroles (page 84).*

PN— *Oxtail is a fairly fatty meat, but it gives the daube an incomparably mellow texture. Do trim off the fat all the same. Serve a dish of pasta (for the carbohydrates) with this daube, and perhaps a starter of vegetables, as it does not contain enough.*

... Serves 4

Two days in advance

... Get your butcher to trim the fat off half an oxtail, 1 pound of beef shin and 1 pound of chuck and cut into 1-inch cubes.

... Peel and wash 4 carrots and 3 stalks of celery, and cut at an angle into rounds. Peel 2 white onions and 2 garlic cloves; cut the onions into small wedges and crush the garlic cloves.

... Cut 1 unwaxed orange into slices.

... Combine all these ingredients in a bowl. Add 15 peppercorns and 2 sprigs of thyme.

... Pour in a bottle of red wine and leave to marinate in the fridge for 48 hours.

On the day

... Preheat the oven to 300°F.

... Drain the meat. Strain the marinade directly into a saucepan, but keep the solids.

... Boil the wine of the marinade for 2 minutes and skim.

... Heat a splash of olive oil in a cast-iron casserole dish and brown the cubes of meat on all sides. Then take them out with a slotted spoon and put the solids from the marinade in their place, without the oranges. Stir for 2 minutes, sprinkle with 3 tablespoons of flour, and stir again.

... Return the pieces of beef and slices of orange to the casserole dish. Pour in the wine, then 4 to 6 cups of chicken stock (page 10) to just cover the meat.

... Salt lightly and boil, skimming well. Then cover the casserole dish with a lid and put in the oven for 3 hours.

... Serve the daube in its casserole dish or in a deep serving dish.

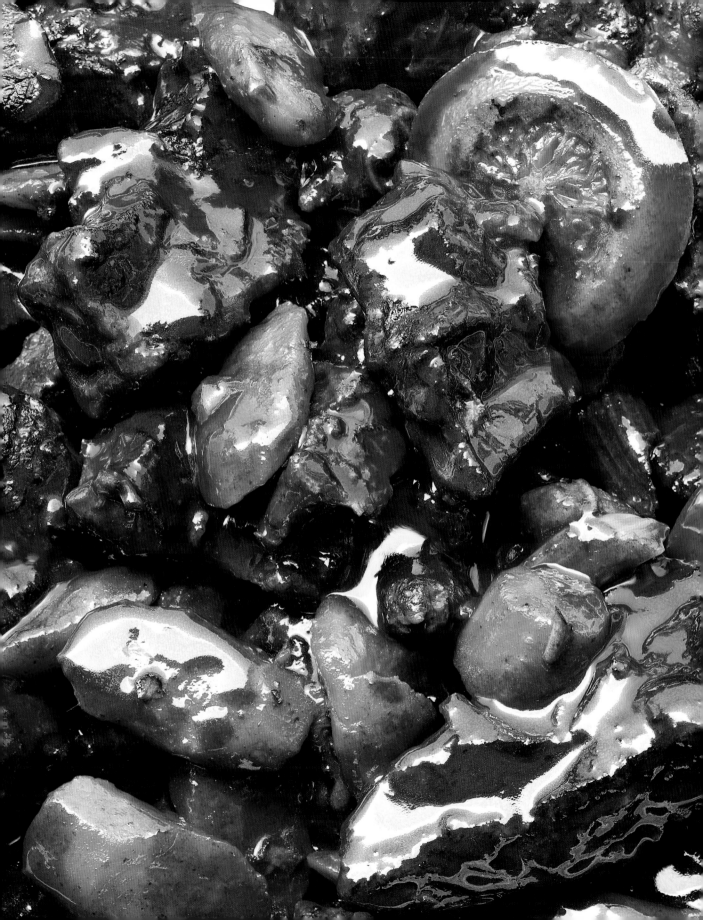

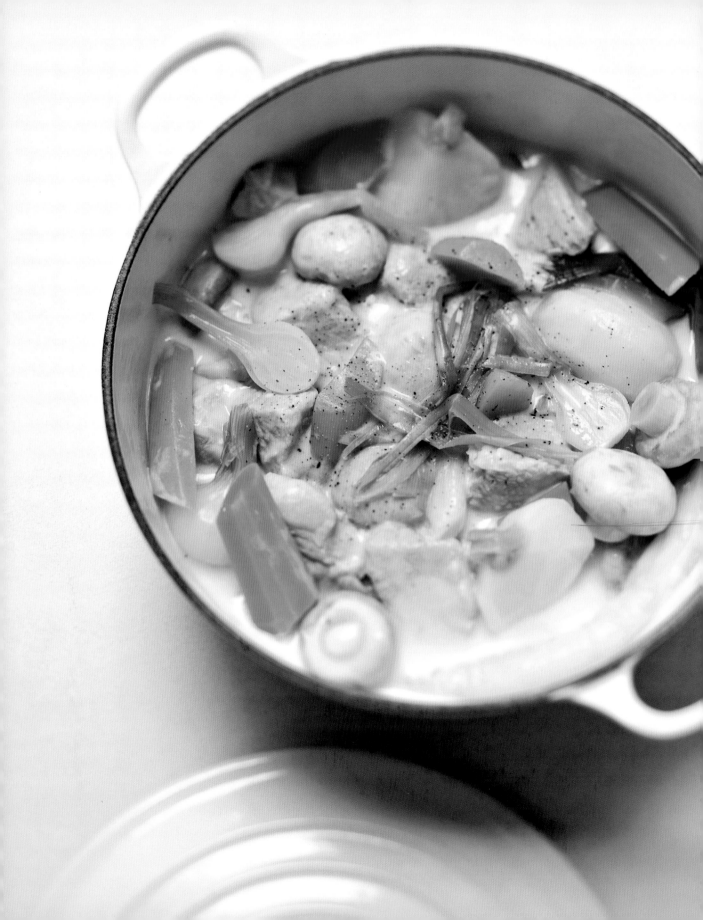

Blanquette of Veal with Spring Vegetables

… Serves 4

… Get your butcher to cut 4 ounces of knuckle, 4 ounces of chuck, 4 ounces of flank, and 4 ounces of shoulder of veal into approximately 1⅓-inch chunks.

<u>Prepare the blanquette</u>

… Peel and wash 4 baby leeks, 4 stalks of celery, 1 bunch of carrots with tops, and 1 bunch of young spring onions. Cut the leeks in half and the celery and carrots into sections. Leave 2 inches of stalk on the onions and cut them in half.

… Put the pieces of veal in a flameproof casserole dish and just cover with cold water. Boil for 3 minutes, then drain, discard the water, and wipe the casserole dish with paper towels.

… Rinse the pieces of veal under running water, return them to the casserole dish, and cover with 2 quarts of cold water. Bring to a boil and skim until the stock is clear.

… Add all the prepared vegetables and 5 black peppercorns. Add some coarse salt, cover, and simmer gently for 1 hour, skimming regularly.

… In the meantime, clean 7 ounces of white mushrooms and cut into quarters. Add to the casserole dish after it has been cooking for 1 hour and cook for an additional 10 minutes.

… Then take out the pieces of veal and vegetables with a slotted spoon and keep them warm in a dish.

<u>Prepare the sauce</u>

… Strain the cooking stock through a fine sieve. Clean the casserole dish.

… In it, melt 1½ tablespoons of butter and mix with 3 tablespoons of all-purpose flour. Cook this roux for 1 minute, then pour in 1 cup of the cooking stock.

… Bring to a boil and add ½ cup Greek yogurt. Beat well and season the sauce with the juice of half a lemon. Taste and correct the seasoning with salt and freshly ground black pepper.

… Return the meat and vegetables to the casserole dish. Serve nice and hot straight from the casserole dish.

AD— Freeze any leftover veal stock. It will be useful in a number of recipes. Veal is at its best quality in the spring, but you can find it all year round. In other seasons make this blanquette with whatever vegetables are in season.

PN— A blanquette sauce without egg yolk! This will be welcome for for anyone who has to avoid eggs because they are high in cholesterol or due to allergy.

Lamb Meatballs with Couscous-Style Vegetables

AD— To check when the lamb meatballs are done, stick a knife into one. If it comes out hot, they are cooked. The lamb sweetbreads can be replaced with brain, depending on what is available.

PN— Protein from the meat (but not too much); slow carbohydrates from the chickpeas; fiber, vitamins, and minerals in these and in the vegetables; and little fat: What better balanced dish could you dream of?

The couscous in the recipe title refers to the method of cooking the vegetables.

… Serves 4

The day before

… Soak ¾ cup of dried chickpeas.

On the day, cook the chickpeas

… Peel 1 small onion and 1 carrot (5 required in total for the recipe), then cut into pieces.

… Drain the chickpeas and put in a saucepan with the vegetables and 1 bay leaf. Cover well with water and cook for 1½ hours. Add salt only at the end of cooking.

Prepare the lamb meatballs

… Grind 12 ounces of trimmed lamb (shoulder or leg) and 2 lamb sweetbreads. Put the ground meat into a bowl.

… Peel and chop 1 garlic clove (3 required in total for the recipe). Wash and dry the leaves of 3 sprigs of cilantro and 3 sprigs of parsley and chop them (keeping aside a few leaves for decoration). Add to the bowl and mix.

… Season the ground beef with 2 pinches of ground coriander, ¾ teaspoon of salt, and 2 pinches of Piment d'Espelette or hot paprika.

… Mix well by hand, then form into 4 balls. Set aside.

Cook and finish your dish

… Peel 4 red onions and cut into wedges. Peel and wash 4 stalks of celery, 4 carrots, and 2 fennel bulbs and cut into sections. Crush 2 garlic cloves.

… Heat 3 tablespoons of olive oil in a sauté pan. Put in all these vegetables, season with salt, add 3 pinches of ras al-hanout, stir, and cover the pan with a lid. Cook gently for about 10 minutes.

… Drain the chickpeas and pour three quarters of their cooking liquid into the sauté pan. Stir and cook for 5 minutes.

… Then add the lamb meatballs and the chickpeas, cover the sauté pan, and simmer gently for 10 minutes.

… Arrange the chickpeas, vegetables, and lamb meatballs in a dish.

… Strain the cooking liquid on top through a conical strainer. Sprinkle with the reserved parsley leaves and serve.

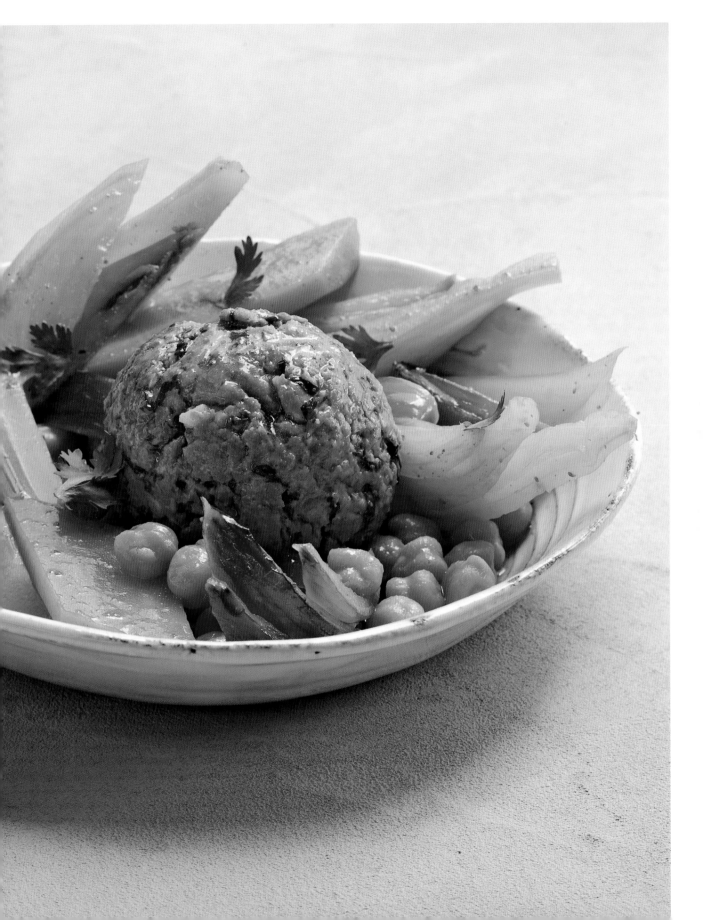

Grenadins of Veal with Spinach and Baked Tomatoes

AD— *If you cook veal too much, it becomes dry and stringy. Better to keep it pink. Choose a good-quality outdoor-reared rosé veal.*

PN— *There's quite a lot of iron in the spinach. The combination with veal is good because this meat contains little. Antioxidants in the tomatoes, and a little drop of calcium from the sheep's curd: It all adds up!*

Fromage blanc or cottage cheese may be used if fresh curd cannot be found.

... Serves 4

... Preheat the oven to 250°F. Blanch 4 nice big tomatoes and cut in half horizontally. Squeeze them between your fingers to remove the juice and seeds. Line them up on a baking sheet, drizzle with a good splash of olive oil, and sprinkle with 1 teaspoon of superfine sugar and salt. Add 3 crushed garlic cloves (6 required in total for the recipe), cover, and put in the oven for 1½ hours.

... Stem, wash, and dry 1¼ pounds of spinach and set aside.

... Take the sheet of tomatoes out of the oven and increase the temperature to 350°F. Take 8 tablespoons of sheep's curd and 8 segments of tomato confit (page 16) and spread one of each on the 8 tomato halves in the sheet. Then spread some fine shavings cut from 1½ ounces of hard sheep's cheese with a vegetable peeler. Return the sheet to the oven for a few minutes.

... Heat a sauté pan with a splash of olive oil. Peel 1 garlic clove and stick it onto a fork. Put the spinach into the sauté pan by the handful and cook quickly, stirring with the fork. Add salt and freshly ground black pepper.

... Heat a splash of olive oil in another sauté pan. Brown 4 grenadins (fillets cut from the loin) of veal, each weighing 4 ounces, on each side. Add 2 crushed garlic cloves and 1 sprig of thyme, then cook over medium heat for 3 to 4 minutes on each side (depending on their thickness). Place on a dish and keep in a warm place covered with aluminium foil.

... Return the sauté pan to the heat. Pour in 1 cup of chicken stock (page 10) and scrape well with a spatula to deglaze the juices. Bring to a boil and cook until the juices are slightly syrupy. Season to taste.

... Place the spinach, then the tomatoes in the center of the dish or on each individual plate and then top with 1 grenadin on each one.

... Pour the juices over, strained through a fine wire-mesh sieve, and serve immediately.

Vitello Tonnato Gremolata

… Serves 4

<u>Prepare the veal</u>

… Trim 1 pound of veal eye of round and salt it. Heat a flameproof casserole dish with a splash of olive oil, sear the meat lightly on all sides, then add 1 cup of chicken stock (page 10). Add 1 sprig of thyme and 1 bay leaf. Cook over very low heat for about 40 minutes. Then take out of the casserole dish and allow to cool. Keep it cold and set aside the cooking liquid.

<u>Prepare the gremolata</u>

… Preheat the oven to 175°F. Grate the zest of 1 unwaxed orange and spread it on a baking sheet covered with a sheet of silicone or parchment paper, sprinkle with the leaves of 1 sprig of thyme, and dry in the oven for 1 hour.

… Wash and peel a quarter of a green bell pepper and a quarter of a red bell pepper with a vegetable peeler, remove the seeds, then chop the flesh into very small dice (1/16 inch).

… Put them in a corner of the veal casserole dish for just 1 minute, then drain into a bowl. Pour 2 tablespoons of olive oil on top and marinate in the refrigerator.

<u>Prepare the tonnato sauce</u>

… Blend together the contents of a small can of tuna in oil, 3 anchovy fillets in oil, 2 egg yolks, ½ cup of sherry vinegar, 1 teaspoon of Dijon mustard, 1 tablespoon of olive oil, and 2 spoonfuls of the reserved veal cooking liquid.

… Pour into a bowl and refrigerate.

<u>To finish your dish</u>

… Before serving, cut the veal into thin slices (1/16 inch thick) and arrange in a circle on a serving dish or on individual plates, then salt lightly and add freshly ground black pepper.

… Pour the tonnato sauce on top and sprinkle with the dried orange zest. Drain the peppers of their marinade and distribute them around the meat. With a vegetable peeler, shave ¾ ounces of Parmesan and sprinkle the shavings over the peppers, then scatter 2 tablespoons of pitted black olives over them.

… Serve nice and cold.

AD— As this is a dish served cold, you can make it the day before (at least the veal and the dried orange zest). Flake the tuna and chop up the anchovies, which makes them easier to blend. PN— Accompany this vitello tonnato with a nice herb salad (page 153) and lightly toasted slices of whole-wheat or multigrain bread.

Veal Piccata with Sage and Steamed Carrots

AD— Choose milk-fed veal if you can get it—it is much better! Veal from calves that have been reared outdoors with their mother until ready for slaughter is still fairly rare, but is becoming more available.

PN— Veal is a particularly lean meat, and the carrots are cooked with practically no fat. This makes for a very low-fat dish that will not put a strain on your calorie allowance but will give you loads of carotenoids, which are good for the skin and all the cells.

… Serves 4

… Get your butcher to cut twelve 1¼-ounce piccata (scallops) of veal from the filet mignon.

… Wash and peel 3 orange carrots, 3 yellow carrots, and 3 purple carrots and cut them into rounds at an angle. Keep the trimmings (tops and tails). Peel and crush 1 garlic clove.

… Salt the carrot rounds. Heat a flameproof casserole dish with 1 tablespoon of olive oil and sweat them with the crushed garlic clove over low heat for 3 minutes. Squeeze the juice of 2 oranges and add it. Cover and cook for 8 minutes.

… In the meantime, chop the carrot trimmings, and wash and mince 2 spring onions. Combine in a bowl and add 2 tablespoons of mustard and 1 tablespoon of capers. Put this crunchy condiment aside.

… Take 12 small sage leaves and place one on each veal piccata, pressing down lightly so that it sticks to the meat.

… Get a skillet nice and hot with a splash of olive oil. Place the piccata sage side down, cook for 30 seconds, turn over, and cook for an additional 30 seconds on the other side. Then add them to the serving dish, or onto individual plates.

… Pour in ¼ cup of chicken stock (page 10), deglaze the pan, bring to a boil to reduce a little, then add the crunchy condiment. Stir well and pour over the dish (or plates).

… Arrange the carrots at the side, add a twist of freshly ground black pepper, and serve nice and hot.

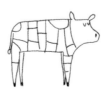

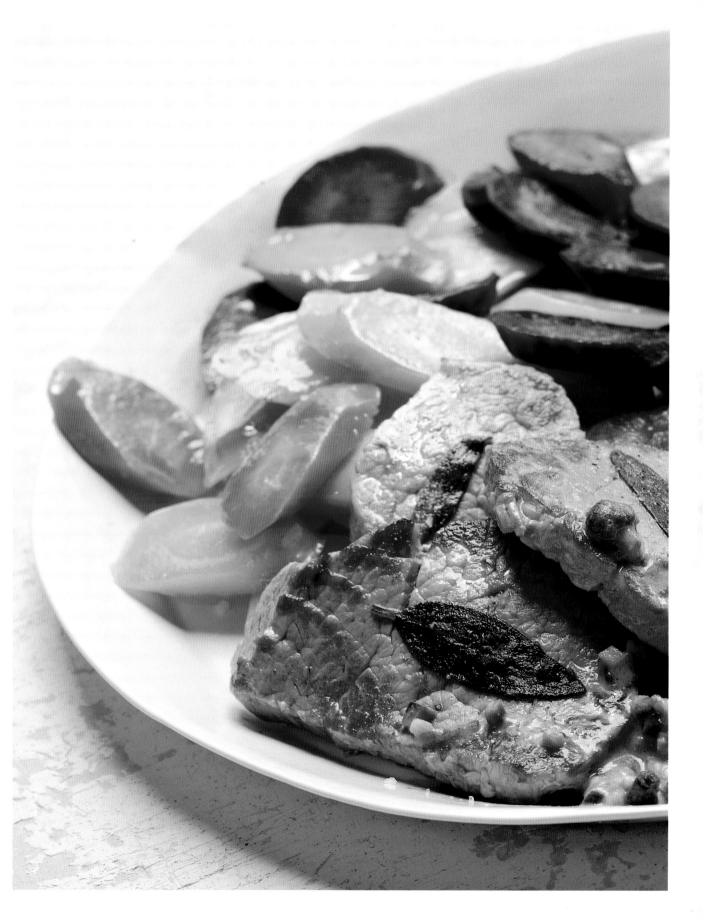

Shoulder of Wild Boar with Chestnuts

… Serves 4

The day before

… Cut 1 pound of boneless shoulder of wild boar into chunks (about 1½ ounces each) and put them in a large bowl.

… Wash and peel 2 white onions, 6 stalks of celery, and 2 carrots and cut into sections. Peel 3 garlic cloves (5 required in total for the recipe). Gradually add all these vegetables to the bowl and complete with 1 sprig of thyme, 1 bay leaf, 10 black peppercorns, and 6 juniper berries. Pour in a bottle of good red wine and leave overnight to marinate in the refrigerator.

On the day

… Preheat the oven to 325°F. Drain the wild boar, reserving the marinade solids and wine. Salt the pieces, sear on all sides in a flameproof casserole dish with 1 tablespoon of olive oil, then take them out.

… In their place, put the solids from the marinade, except for the peppercorns. Brown it, then put on the lid and cook gently for 5 minutes. Put the wild boar back in and sprinkle with 2 tablespoons of flour. Stir well and cook for 2 minutes.

… Deglaze with ½ cup of cognac. Then pour in the wine of the marinade, along with ½ to 1 cup of chicken stock (1 to 1½ cups of stock required in total for the recipe) (page 10) to just cover. Then add the peppercorns. Heat until this liquid is simmering and skim well. Then cover the casserole dish with a lid and put in the oven for 2 hours.

… About 30 minutes before the end of the cooking time, peel 7 ounces of white mushrooms and cut into quarters.

… Heat another flameproof casserole dish with 2 tablespoons of olive oil. Roast 10 ounces of vacuum-packed or frozen chestnuts, the mushrooms, and 2 crushed garlic cloves in it for 4 minutes. Pour in another ½ cup of chicken stock, cover, and simmer for 10 minutes.

… Take out the casserole dish containing the wild boar, lift out the pieces of meat, and put them in with the chestnuts. Correct the seasoning of the wild boar liquid with salt and freshly ground black pepper, then strain into the casserole dish through a conical strainer and serve directly from this pot.

Venison Noisettes with Sautéed Wild Mushrooms

… Serves 4

… Prepare 1 bowl of dried fruit condiment (page 47), replacing the saffron with 2 inches of grated ginger and the orange with the zest of 1 lime.

… Stem and wash 2 ounces of horn of plenty mushrooms and 7 ounces of chanterelles. Cut the biggest ones in half. Clean 7 ounces of porcini and slice them. Wash, dry, and chop the leaves of a bunch of parsley. Peel and chop 2 garlic cloves.

… In a hot skillet with 1 tablespoon of olive oil, sauté the mushrooms in batches for 2 minutes, adding salt. Drain in a sieve as you go.

… Melt 1 tablespoon of butter (1¾ tablespoons in total required for the recipe) in the same skillet, and add all the mushrooms. Cook over high heat for 5 minutes. Add freshly ground black pepper, then add the chopped parsley and chopped garlic, and sauté for just 1 minute.

… Crush 4 juniper berries. Mix with 2 pinches of mignonette pepper (see page 30) and salt, then use this to season twelve 1½-ounce noisettes of venison filet on each side.

… Heat a splash of olive oil in a skillet and cook them for 1½ minutes on each side.

… Add them to a warm serving dish. Deglaze the cooking juices with a splash of cognac, add ½ cup of chicken stock (page 10), and reduce to three-quarters. Then quickly add ¾ tablespoons of butter and stir well as it melts in order to thicken the sauce.

… Pour the sauce onto the venison noisettes. Distribute the mushrooms all around and serve the dried fruit condiment separately.

AD— This recipe can also be made with venison from the doe of the roe deer. Check that the venison hasn't been frozen prior to sale, which is often the case. PN— Venison is a lean meat, but rich in iron. And as this is a trace element often found wanting in people's diets, this is a welcome dish, especially as the mushrooms contain a little iron too.

———

Noisettes are small, round steaks taken from the filet known to be especially tender. If horn of plenty or black trumpet mushrooms cannot be found, increase the amount of chanterelles.

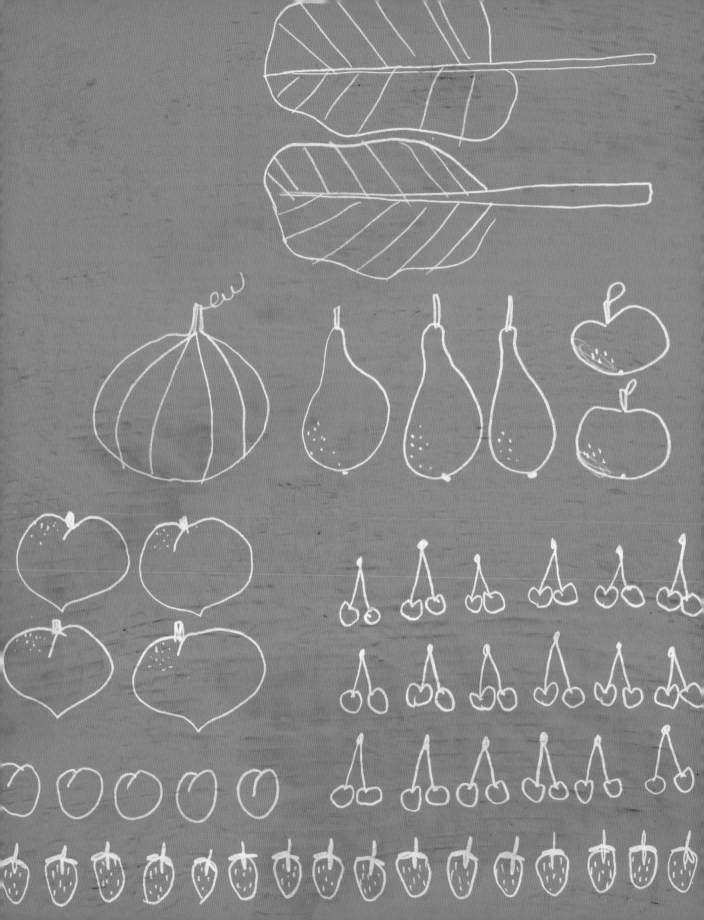

AD— I'm not too keen on very sugary desserts because sugar overloads the taste buds and destroys the flavors. All the following desserts are chef's dessert recipes, easy to make (well!) but sophisticated.

PN— It's not so much the sugar that adds the calories but the butter. In these desserts, we have used little sugar, but also small amounts of butter in the tart pastry. And above all plenty of fruit!

Desserts

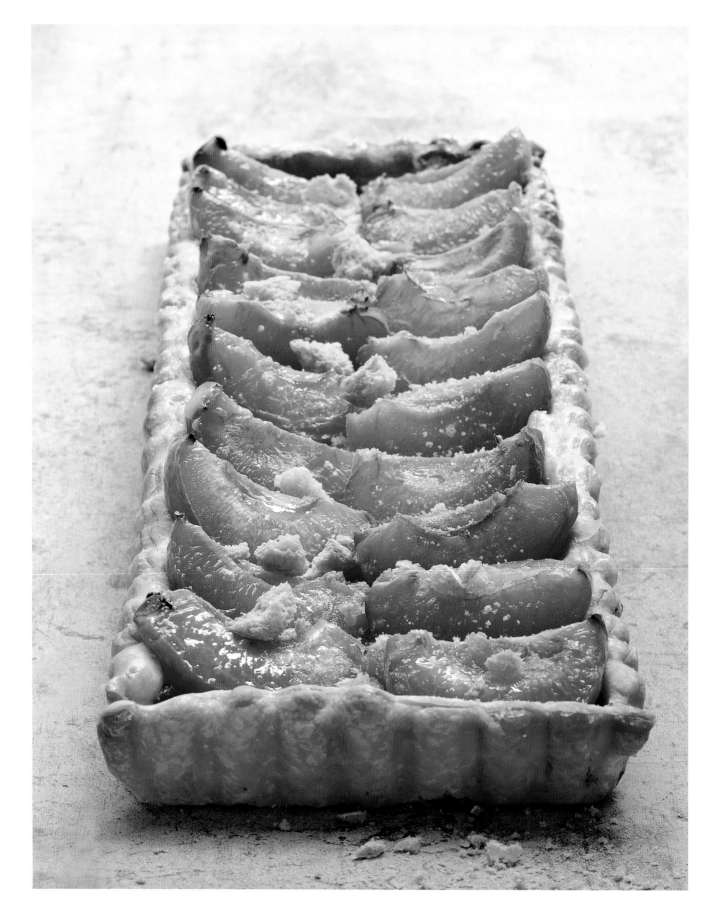

Apricot Tart

… Serves 4

The day before, prepare the rhubarb

… Trim 1½ pounds of rhubarb, cut into small sections, put them in a bowl, and sprinkle with 5 tablespoons of superfine sugar (10 required in total for the recipe). Cover the bowl with plastic wrap and refrigerate for 12 hours.

… Then drain the rhubarb in a colander and put it in a flameproof casserole dish. Cover with a lid and cook slowly until softened well.

On the day, prepare the tart

… Butter a flan dish 10 inches in diameter or a rectangular baking pan about 3½ by 12 inches. Sprinkle with 2 tablespoons of superfine sugar and keep in the refrigerator.

… Roll out 8 ounces good-quality butter puff pastry on a lightly floured worktop to about ⅛ inch thick, then place it in the pan. Press gently all over to fit it into the corners. Roll the rolling pin across to cut off any excess. Prick the bottom with a fork, then leave to rest in the refrigerator for about 20 minutes.

… In the meantime, prepare about 20 nice big apricots: Rinse and dry them, cut them in half, and remove the pits. Then cut each half-apricot in two.

… Preheat the oven to 415°F.

… Cut an 11-inch circle or a 3½-by-12-inch rectangle of parchment paper and lay it in the crust.

… Cover the bottom with a layer of ceramic baking beans or dried beans and bake in the oven for 20 minutes.

… Take out the baking beans and the paper, then allow the crust to cool. Spread the rhubarb evenly in the crust. Take 4 ladyfingers and crumble 3 on top, reserving 1. Arrange the apricot quarters on top. Sprinkle with the remaining 3 tablespoons of superfine sugar. Bake in the oven for an additional 20 to 25 minutes.

… Take out the tart and crumble the last ladyfinger on top. Serve warm.

AD— Choose apricots that are nice and ripe, if possible red Roussillon apricots, which are the best and the ones I prefer.
PN— The apricot is a fruit particularly rich in carotenoids, whose antioxidant virtues and beneficial effects on the skin are widely recognized. It is also rich in fiber, as is rhubarb.

Cherries in Their Juice

AD— *You can serve these cherries with a scoop of pistachio ice cream; the flavors go very well together. Melt the butter over very low heat—it must not be allowed to darken!*

PN— *Cherries are fairly rich in fiber, and part of their carbohydrates is sorbitol, a substance that promotes intestinal transit. They also contain plenty of minerals.*

... Serves 4

... Rinse 1¼ pounds of cherries and remove their stems and pits. Split a vanilla bean open lengthwise.

... Melt 1½ tablespoons of butter and 3 tablespoons of superfine sugar together in a skillet, add the cherries, and cook them for 2 minutes over high heat, stirring to coat them well.

... Cut the vanilla bean in half and scrape with the blade of a knife to detach the seeds and mix with the cherries.

... Pour in ¾ cup of red wine and cook for just 1 minute, stirring continuously and gently.

... Pour the cherries and their juice into a fruit dish and refrigerate until you are ready to serve.

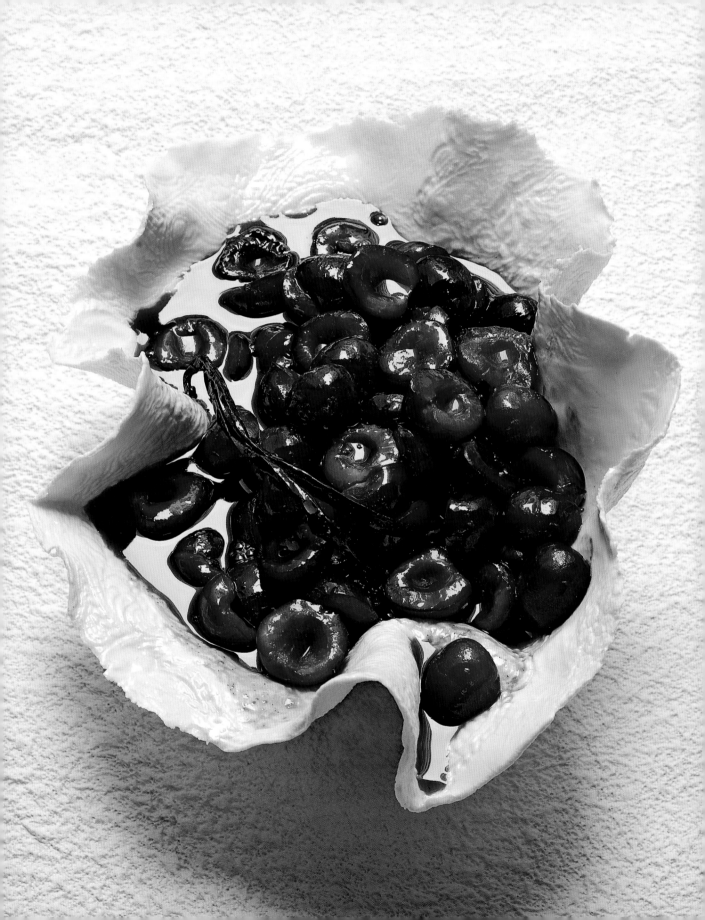

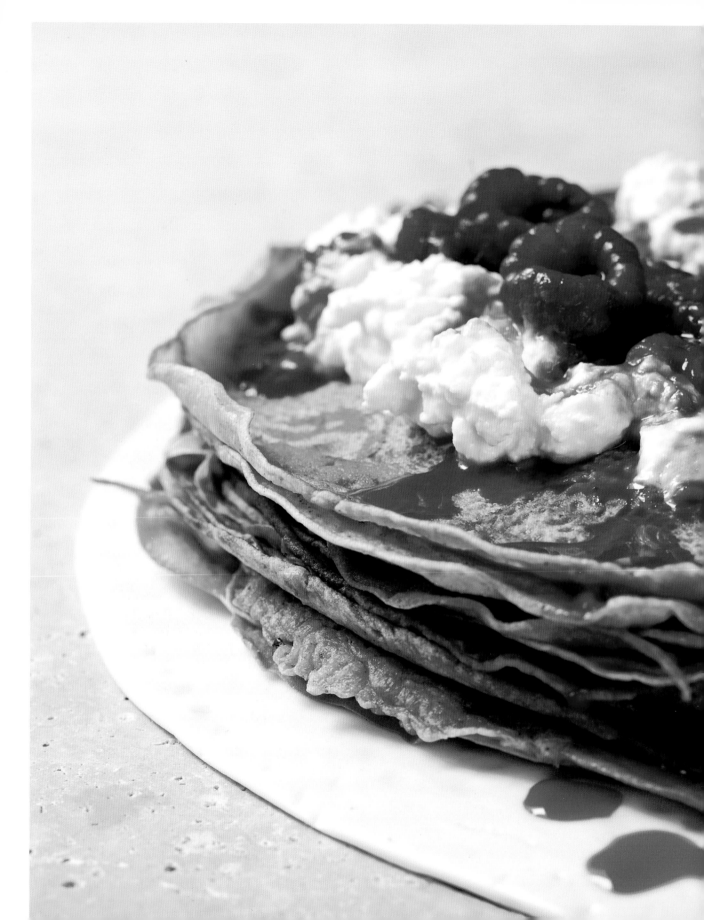

Chestnut Crêpes with Pan-Fried Raspberries and Brocciu

... Serves 4

Prepare the crêpe batter

... Combine 2 cups of chestnut flour, 1 cup of all-purpose flour, and 4 pinches of salt in a bowl and stir together. Make a well in the center and break 2 eggs into it. Mix well, then pour in ¾ cup of water and ¾ cup of milk, stirring continuously.

... When the batter is nice and smooth, cover the bowl with a cloth and leave to rest in a warm place for 1 hour.

Cook the crêpes

... Melt ¾ tablespoon of butter (1½ tablespoons required in total for the recipe) in the microwave and brush a skillet with it.

... Pour in a small ladleful of crêpe batter and spread it over the whole of the skillet. Cook until the edges of the crêpe begin to color, then toss or turn with a spatula and cook for about 1 minute on the other side.

... Lay the crêpe on a plate and keep warm. Cook the other crêpes similarly.

Prepare the pan-fried raspberries

... Melt ¾ tablespoon of butter with 1½ tablespoons of superfine sugar in a skillet, add 2 pints of raspberries (3 pints required in total for the recipe) and cook, shaking the pan, for 1 minute. Add 1 tablespoon of crème de framboise raspberry liqueur, stir delicately, and take the pan off the heat.

To finish your dessert

... Place a small quenelle of very fresh Brocciu and a spoonful of stir-fried raspberries in the center of each crêpe, fold them, and arrange on a serving dish.

... Sprinkle another pint of raspberries on top.

AD— Brocciu is a Corsican fresh cheese, made not from milk but from the whey of goat's or ewe's milk. It has a very distinctive texture and flavor. If you can't get hold of this, substitute Brousse de Brebis ewe's milk cheese or simply fromage blanc.

PN— The crêpes provide good slow carbohydrates, the raspberries provide pectin and antioxidants, and the Brocciu provides calcium. There is practically no fat or sugar in this recipe, making this a fabulously light dessert!

Pan-Fried Summer or Winter Fruits

AD— Whatever the season, vary the fruit according to your own inspiration. But always finish the dish with a fresh fruit that will give it a note of acidity.

PN— The vitamin C of the fruits doesn't have time to oxidize in the very short cooking time over a moderate heat. It's win, win!

… Serves 4

Pan-fried summer fruits

… Wash 2 apricots, 2 nectarines, and 2 handfuls of cherries, and peel 2 yellow or white peaches. Rinse and hull 1 pint of strawberries.

… Cut the apricots, nectarines, and peaches in half and remove their pits. Cut each half-fruit into wedges. Stem the cherries and remove their pits too.

… Heat a skillet with 1 tablespoon of olive oil, 1 tablespoon of honey, 1 split vanilla bean, and 1 sprig of thyme and cook gently until the honey is lightly caramelized. Add the fruits, stir them delicately to coat with this caramel, and cook for 2 to 3 minutes.

… Take out the thyme and vanilla. Pour the fruit into a serving dish or distribute into fruit bowls. Sprinkle 1 pint of raspberries on top. Serve warm.

Pan-fried winter fruits

… Peel 1 Granny Smith apple and 1 large pear. Cut in half, remove the cores, and cut into wedges.

… With a large knife, cut the skin from 1 small pineapple. Cut into slices, remove the fibrous center, then cut these slices into four.

… Peel 2 baby bananas, and cut them in half lengthwise.

… Heat a skillet with 1 tablespoon of olive oil, 1 tablespoon of honey, 1 split vanilla bean, and 1 sprig of thyme and cook gently until the honey is lightly caramelized. Add the fruits, stir them delicately to coat with this caramel, and cook for 3 to 4 minutes. Squeeze the juice of 1 orange, pour it into the skillet, stir quickly, and take off the heat.

… Peel 2 clementines and separate the segments.

… Take out the thyme and vanilla. Pour the fruit into a serving dish or distribute into fruit bowls. Sprinkle the clementines on top. Serve warm.

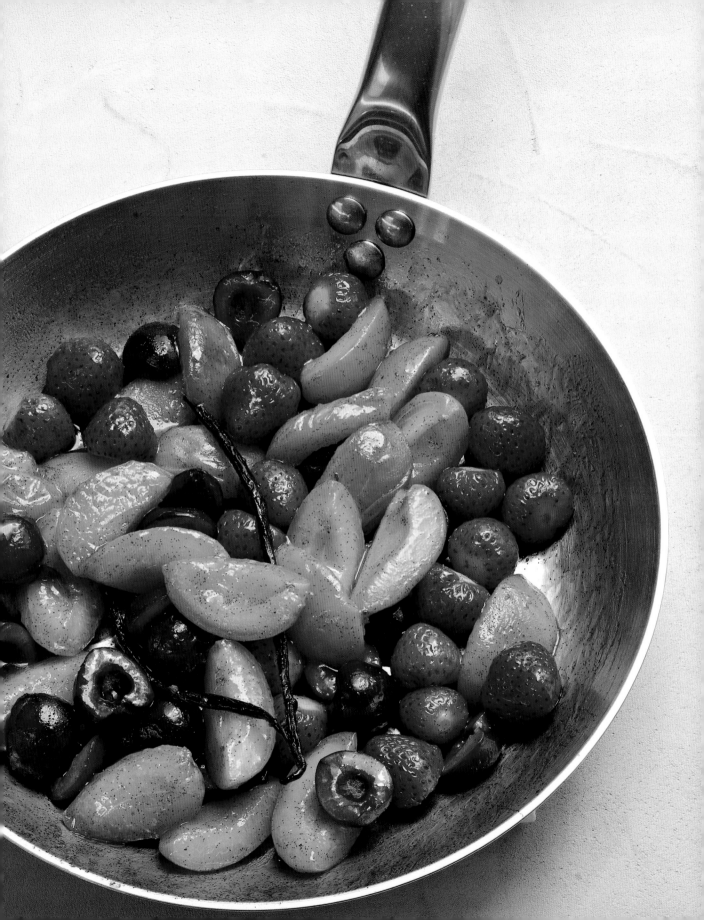

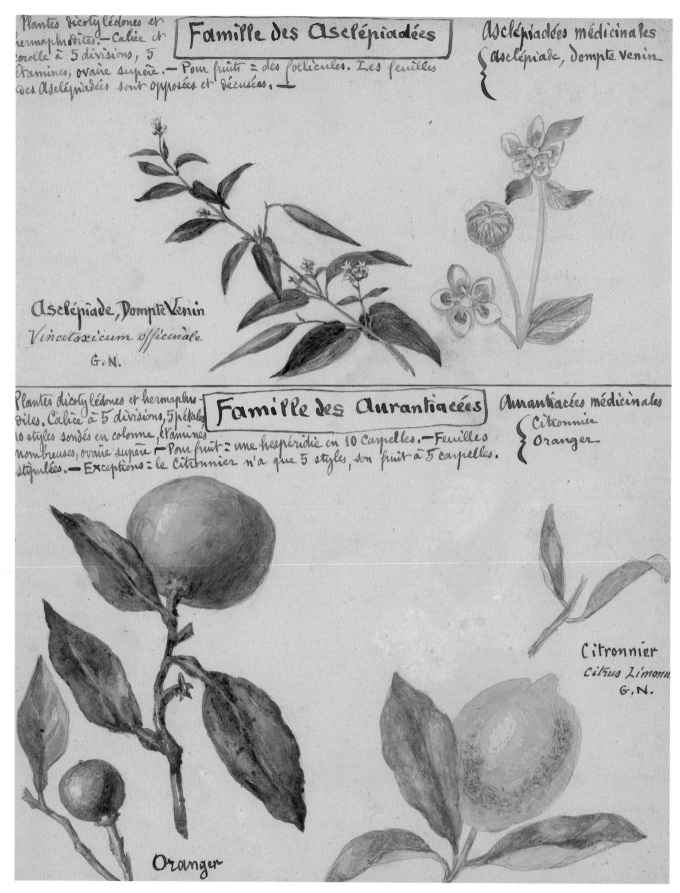

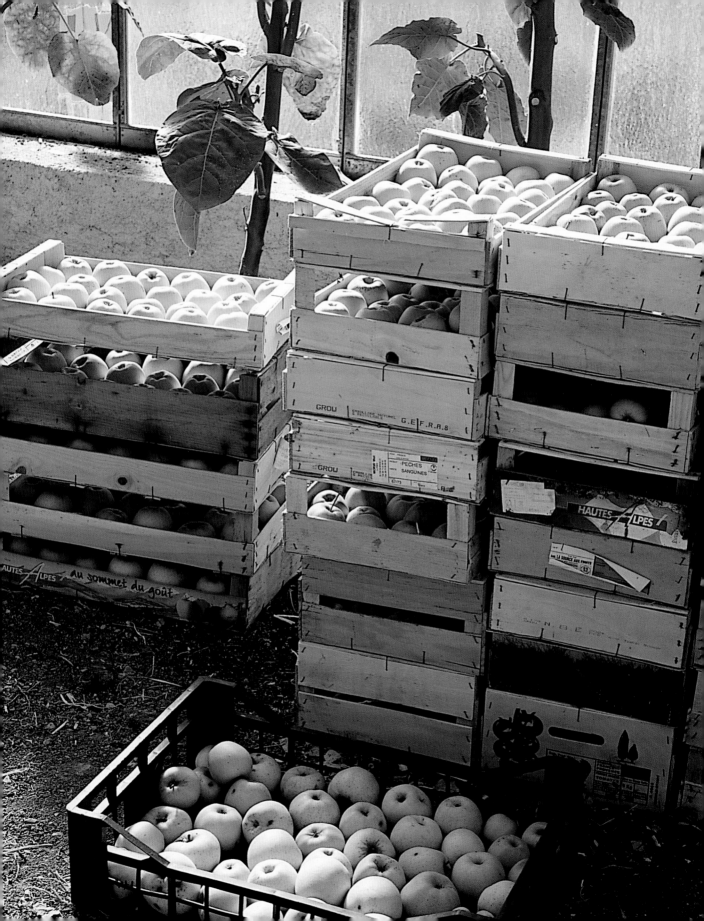

Poached Pears, Pear Sorbet, and Chocolate Sauce

AD— The pears should be fully immersed in the syrup or they won't cook properly. Choose your saucepan accordingly. And baste them with their syrup from time to time while they are cooking.

PN— The taste and nutritional virtues of chocolate are well known! So enjoy this dessert without guilt, because pleasure, as is less well known, is one of the components of a healthy balanced diet.

… Serves 4

… Make a pear sorbet (opposite).

… Wash 4 ripe Bartlett pears. Peel, leaving the stem on, and don't throw away the peel.

… In a saucepan, combine 3 cups of water, ½ cup of superfine sugar, the juice of half a lemon, 1 vanilla bean, opened and scraped, and the pear peel. Bring to a boil.

… Then immerse the pears upright in this syrup and cook for 15 minutes.

… Take the saucepan off the heat and leave the pears in it while they cool.

… Break 4½ ounces of 70% dark chocolate into pieces and melt in a bain-marie or in the microwave. Add 2 tablespoons of light cream and 2 to 3 spoonfuls of the pear cooking syrup and mix well.

… Put a scoop of pear sorbet in each dish. Top with a pear, pour chocolate sauce over, and serve immediately.

Fruit Sorbets

… Serves 4

Strawberry or raspberry sorbet

… Rinse 1 pound of strawberries, remove the stems, and halve them. If you prefer, use 1 pound of raspberries, but you must not wash them, just remove any stems.

… Put the strawberries or raspberries in the bowl of a food processor. Add the juice of half a lemon. Blend, incorporating ½ cup of superfine sugar. Pour into the sorbet maker and follow the manufacturer's instructions.

Peach or pear sorbet

… Peel 4 white peaches or 4 very ripe pears. Take out the peach pits or the pear cores. Cut the fruit into small chunks. Blend the peaches or pears with ¼ cup of superfine sugar, pour into the sorbet maker, and follow the manufacturer's instructions.

Orange or grapefruit sorbet

… Squeeze 8 oranges or 4 grapefruits, strain the juice, and mix with ½ cup of superfine sugar. For the grapefruit, add the quantity of sugar to suit your taste.

… Add the juice of half a lemon to the orange juice—don't add this to the grapefruit juice.

… In either one, you can if you like add 2 tablespoons of Cointreau or Grand Marnier. Pour into the sorbet maker and follow the manufacturer's instructions.

Prune sorbet

… Put 14 ounces of prunes in a saucepan and pour in 2½ cups water and ¼ cup of superfine sugar. Break up 1 stick of cinnamon, peel and grate 2 inches of ginger, and add them. Cook for about 20 minutes.

… Take out the cinnamon, blend well, then strain through a fine sieve to remove any bits of skin.

… Add the juice of 1 lemon. Leave to cool, then put in the sorbet maker and follow the manufacturer's instructions.

AD— Once made, keep all these sorbets in plastic containers in the freezer. The recipe for raspberry sorbet also works for other fruits such as blackcurrants and blackberries. Make the most of the fruit season and make these sorbets in larger quantities.

PN— All the vitamins of the fruits are preserved when you freeze them. These sorbets are as good for you as fresh fruits, but much more fun. The prune sorbet will work like a charm if you suffer from constipation!

Strawberry Granita

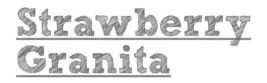

AD— Nothing could be simpler than making this granita! It keeps in the freezer without any problems and you can add it to any fruit salad for a touch of sophistication. In winter, make it with frozen strawberries.
PN— Strawberries are just as rich in vitamin C as citrus fruits. They are also rich in pectin, which is good for the digestive tract. And these qualities remain intact when kept in the freezer.

… Serves 4

… Rinse and hull ½ pound of ripe and fragrant strawberries.

… Set aside about 4 ounces of the smaller fruits.

… Cut the rest into chunks and blend with 3½ tablespoons of superfine sugar.

… Pour the resulting juice into a dish and put in the freezer for at least 4 hours.

… Stir from time to time with a fork until ice crystals form.

… Put 4 fruit dishes in the freezer to chill thoroughly.

… When serving, divide the reserved strawberries among these dishes and scrape the granita on top.

… Decorate with fresh mint leaves.

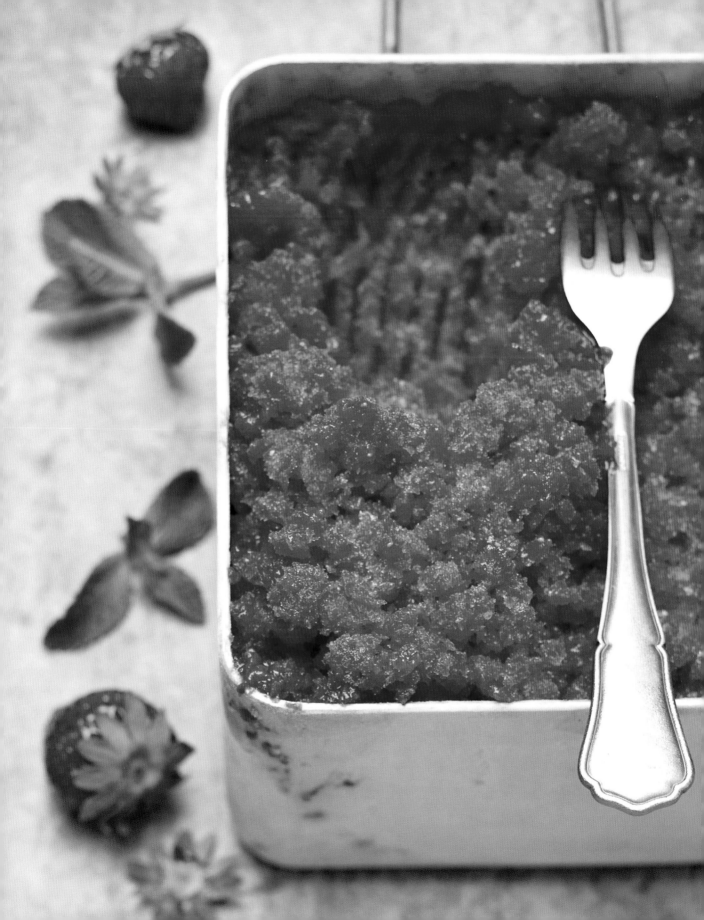

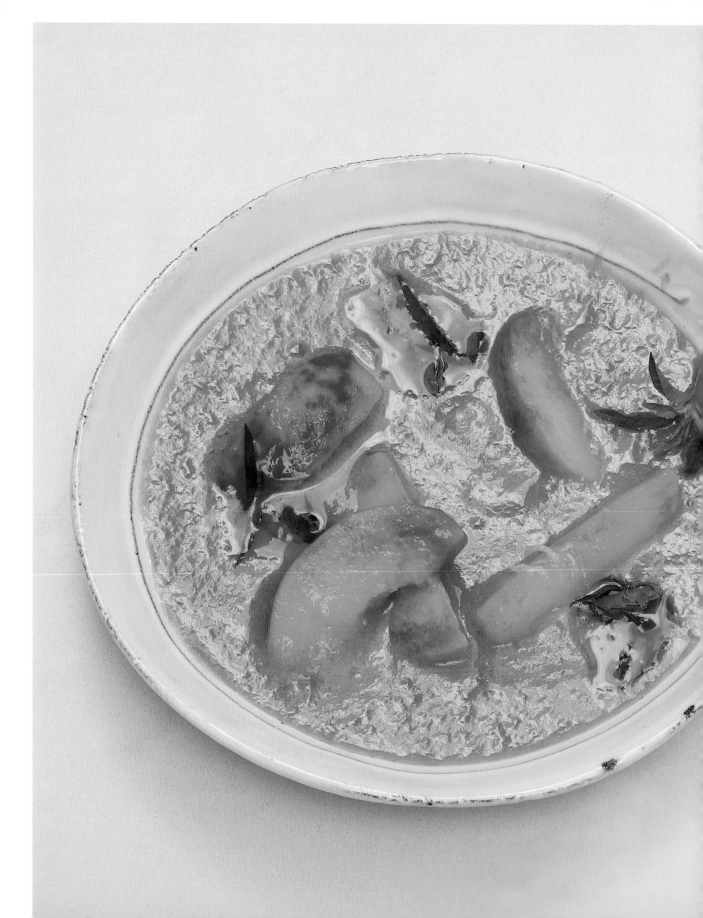

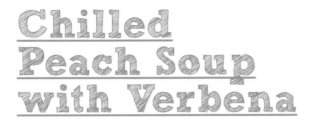

Chilled Peach Soup with Verbena

… Serves 4

Make the verbena jelly

… Pour 1¼ cups of water and 2 tablespoons of superfine sugar (6 tablespoons required in total for the recipe) into a saucepan and bring to a boil. Remove the pan from the heat, add 3 sprigs of verbena, and leave to infuse for 10 minutes.

… Soak 3 sheets of gelatin in a small bowl of water.

… When the verbena is infused, add the juice of 1 lemon (2 lemons required in total for the recipe). Stir and strain through a conical strainer. Drain the gelatin between your fingers and add it to the verbena infusion. Take the leaves from 1 sprig of the infused verbena, chop them up, and add them. (Reserve the remaining verbena.)

… Pour the mixture into a large bowl. Refrigerate for at least 2 hours.

Prepare the peaches

… Peel 6 large yellow peaches, cut them in half, and remove the pits. Then cut each one into 6 wedges. Set 12 of these aside on a plate in a cold place.

… Blend the others with ¼ cup of superfine sugar and the juice of 1 lemon. If the puree is too thick, thin with a little water. Keep cold until serving.

To serve your dessert

… Put 4 soup plates in the freezer to chill thoroughly.

… Take the plates out of the fridge and pour the chilled peach soup into each plate. Distribute the reserved peach wedges on top, then add spoonfuls of verbena jelly. Decorate with the leaves from another sprig of the infused verbena. Serve immediately.

AD— Use very ripe peaches! First because they are better, but also because they're easy to peel. But you can also immerse them in boiling water for 30 seconds to make the task easier.

PN— Yellow peaches are rich in carotenes but low in vitamin C. The lemon juice makes up for this. They also contain flavonoids, which strengthen the blood vessels. Verbena is known for its digestive properties; there's no need for a digestive herbal tea after this meal!

Apple Pie

AD— The pastry can also be made in an electric mixer: Put the butter in small pieces in the bowl and turn on slowly to soften it. Then add, in this order, the egg yolks, the superfine sugar, the ground almonds, and the flour sifted with the baking powder.
PN— This pastry is not high in fat, as it contains little butter. Apples, with their happy combination of fiber, magnesium, and vitamin C, do you nothing but good.

... Serves 4

... Make your sweet shortcrust pastry. Cut ½ cup (1 stick) of butter into small pieces and leave to soften. Then sift 1½ cups of fine pastry flour and 1¼ teaspoons baking powder onto your work surface or into a large bowl. Add 1 cup of finely ground almonds and ½ teaspoon of salt, then mix together with your fingers. Make a well in the middle. Drop in 2 egg yolks, the softened butter, and 7 tablespoons superfine sugar and combine well until the pastry forms a ball.

... Flatten the ball of pastry, wrap it in plastic wrap, and refrigerate for at least 30 minutes.

... In the meantime, peel 4 Granny Smith apples, cut them in half, and remove the core and pits. Then cut each half into slices ⅛ inch thick and place them in a dish.

... Squeeze the juice of 2 unwaxed lemons into a glass (don't throw away the peels), add 1 teaspoon of calvados, and pour it all over the apples and stir gently so that they soak it up (otherwise they will discolor). Leave to marinate for 1 hour.

... Preheat your oven to 410°F. Butter and flour a 9-inch pie dish. Take the pastry out of the fridge. Cut two thirds of it and roll out this piece into a 10-inch circle. Lay it in the bottom of the pie dish, pressing the edges down well.

... Then lay the apple slices, one by one, in a circle, beginning with the outside of the pie and working toward the middle. Grate a little zest from 1 or 2 of the lemon peels on top. Sprinkle it all with 3 tablespoons of superfine sugar.

... Then roll out the other piece of pastry into a circle 9 inches in diameter. Place it over the pie and pinch the two circles of pastry together around the edges to seal.

... Gently pierce the top of the pie with a fork to release the steam during cooking and bake in the oven for 45 minutes.

... Take the pie out of the oven. Sprinkle with confectioners' sugar and put it under the broiler for just 5 minutes to caramelize. Then allow the pie to rest in its dish for about 15 minutes and serve warm.

Chilled Melon Soup with Mint Ice Cubes

... Serves 4

Make the mint ice cubes

... Take the leaves from 2 bunches of mint.

... Fill a large bowl with water and ice cubes and place another bowl on top.

... Heat 2 cups of water in a saucepan. When it boils, immerse the mint leaves for 4 minutes. Drain with a slotted spoon.

... Blend them with a ladleful of cooking liquid until you have a smooth and even puree. Cool immediately in the bowl on top of the ice.

... Distribute this mint puree in ice-cube trays and freeze.

Make the melon soup

... Put 4 bowls or fruit dishes to chill in the freezer.

... Cut 3 large melons in half and remove the seeds and all the membranes.

... Cut the flesh from 2 of the melons, blend into a smooth soup, adding a little water if it's too thick. Put in the fridge.

... With a melon baller, scoop the flesh from the whole of the third melon. Reserve these balls in the fridge too.

... When you are ready to serve, distribute the melon soup among the chilled bowls or dishes. Drop the small melon balls on top, add a few mint ice cubes, and serve immediately.

AD— This melon soup is just as good served as a starter. The ice cubes can of course be made the day before, and why not double the quantities so you can use them in a fruit juice cocktail or another chilled fruit soup.

PN— A real health-giving dessert! Melon beats all the records in terms of antioxidant carotenoids, good for all the body's cells (and for tanning!). Mint is also rich in them. Their action is strengthened by that of vitamin C, which is also plentiful in both. And no sugar, which makes this a dessert you can eat without moderation!

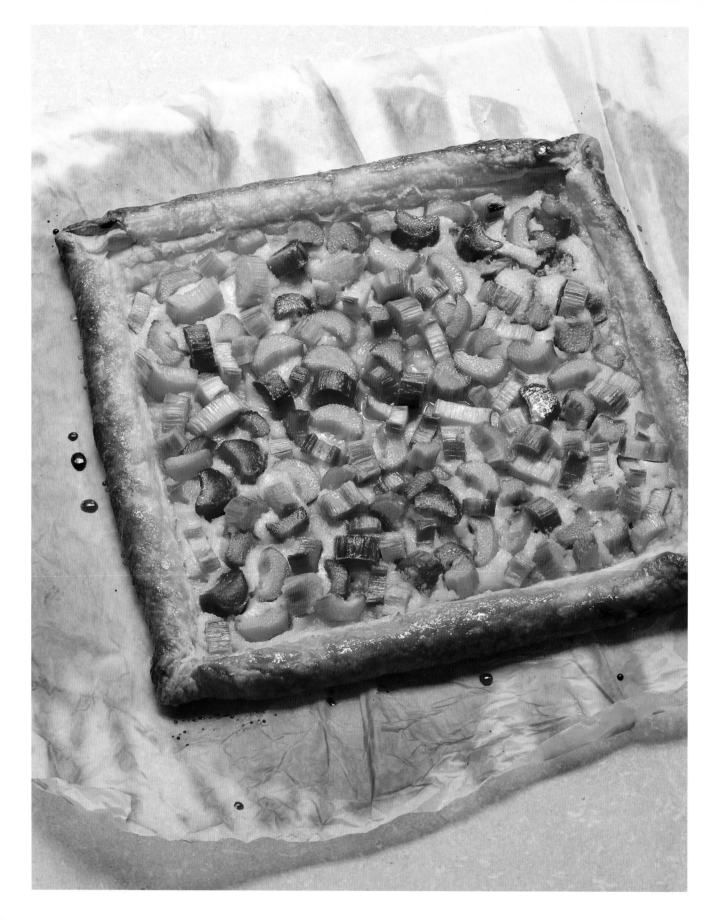

Rhubarb Tart

… Serves 4 to 6

… Peel 1 pound rhubarb stalks and cut into cubes. Put in a large bowl with 3½ tablespoons of superfine sugar (6½ tablespoons required in total for the recipe) and leave to drain for 1 hour.

… Roll out 8 ounces of all-butter puff pastry into a square. Then roll the edges in and pinch the pastry at each corner.

… Cover a baking sheet with a sheet of parchment paper and lay the pastry on top.

… Prick the bottom with a fork and leave to rest for 30 minutes in the fridge.

… Preheat the oven to 400°F.

… After its rest, lay another sheet of parchment paper over the pastry, spread baking beans on top, and bake in the oven for 20 minutes.

… Into a bowl, stirring constantly, pour ¼ cup of yogurt, ½ cup ground almonds, 1 egg, 2 teaspoons vanilla sugar, and 1 tablespoon superfine sugar.

… Peel and grate 1 inch of ginger, add, and mix well.

… Take the pastry out of the oven, leave it to cool, and, with a spoon, spread the almond cream on top. Smooth with the back of the spoon.

… Drain the rhubarb pieces and arrange them evenly on top.

… Sprinkle with the remaining 2 tablespoons superfine sugar and put the tart back in the oven at 350°F for 20 minutes. Serve warm or at room temperature.

AD— Like all fruits, rhubarb is full of water. So, you need to remove the excess water, otherwise the pastry will get too wet and will not cook.
PN— Always buy good quality puff pastry made with butter. Admittedly, this is not a low-fat pastry, but it is delicious and can be eaten in small quantities, which is the case with this tart. Don't forget that enjoying your food is part of a healthy balanced diet.

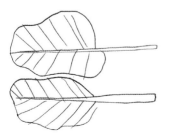

Lemon Caramel Custard

AD— This baked caramel custard tastes even better if you make it the day before. Experience shows that a long rest improves both flavor and consistency.

PN— With the protein from the eggs and milk this dessert is very nourishing. So, serve it as part of a light menu, without meat or fish. Needless to say, there's no need for cheese or any other dairy product, as the milk provides plenty of calcium.

... Serves 6 to 8

... Pour 1 quart of lowfat milk into a saucepan with 1 vanilla bean slit open and scraped, and heat.

... Mix 8 egg yolks, 4 whole eggs, and 7 tablespoons of superfine sugar (17 tablespoons required in total for the recipe) in a bowl.

... Beat until the mixture is nice and smooth, then gradually pour in the warm milk, beating as you go.

... Strain through a conical strainer.

... Preheat your oven to 350°F.

... Then make the caramel. Squeeze the juice of 2 lemons. Put the remaining 10 tablespoons of superfine sugar into a saucepan and melt gently until it turns golden. Quickly pour in the lemon juice, stirring well as you do so.

... Pour this hot caramel into small glass dishes, ramekins, or a baking dish.

... Pour the egg mixture on top.

... Put the glass dishes, ramekins, or baking dish into a deep baking pan, add water to come halfway up, and bake in the oven for 20 to 25 minutes.

... Take out the sheet. Allow the baked egg custard to cool, then keep it cold until you are ready to serve.

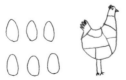

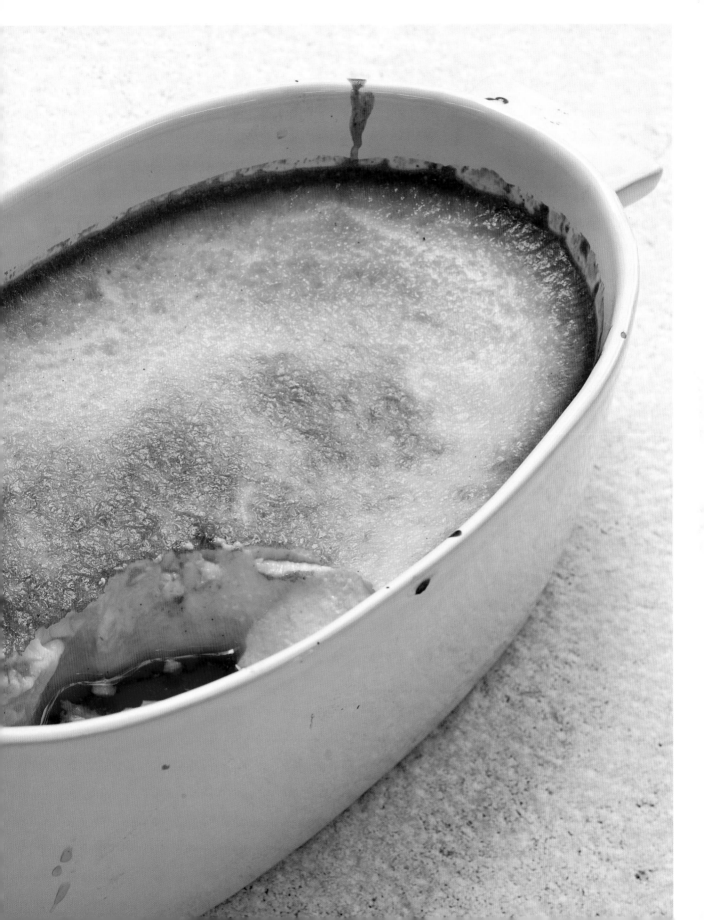

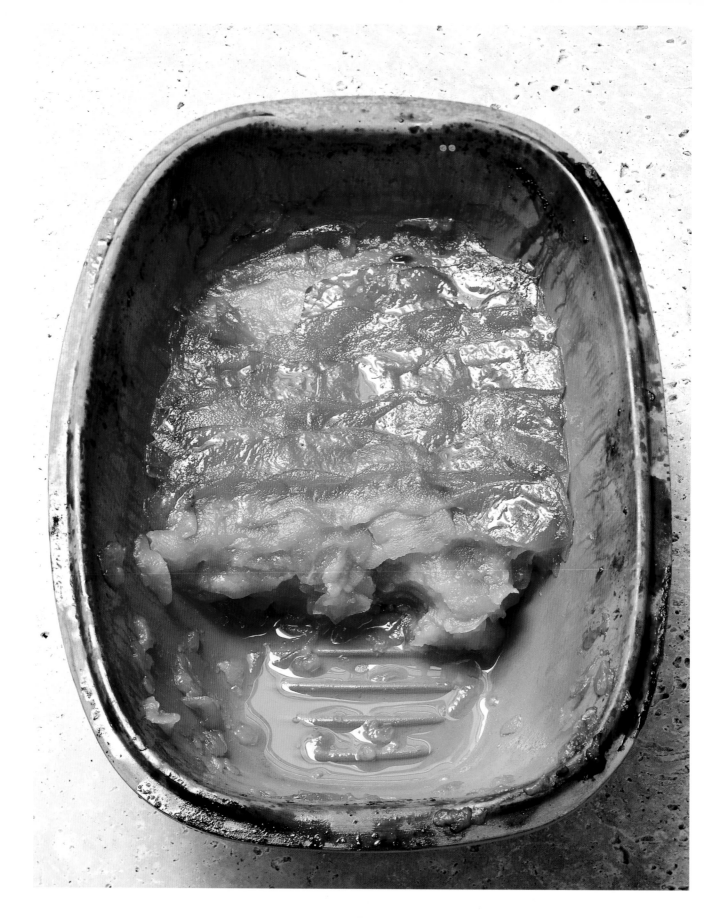

Apples and Pears Gently Stewed in a Römertopf

… Serves 8

<u>The day before</u>

… Put the Römertopf clay baker and its lid to soak in water.

<u>On the day</u>

… Preheat the oven to 400°F.

… Peel 8 large apples and 8 large pears. Quarter them and remove the cores. Then cut each quarter into thin slices.

… Measure ¾ cup of light brown sugar.

… Arrange the slices of fruit in the Römertopf in flat, even layers, alternating pears and apples and sprinkling each layer with a little light brown sugar. Fill the whole pot in this way to ¾ inch below the edge.

… Cover, taking care to wedge the lid tightly, and put the Römertopf in the oven for 2½ to 3 hours, until the fruit has turned a nice golden color.

… Serve warm or cold.

AD— It is essential to soak your Römertopf. The clay absorbs the water, which then turns into steam when cooking. This cooking method is particularly gentle, and preserves the full aromas of the fruit.

PN— The fruit reduces a great deal, so you eat more than if they were fresh, and this is good for your dietary balance and health. A little crème fraîche to accompany it will do no harm, especially if you serve the Römertopf warm. Or you could even serve it with a scoop of sorbet (page 337). There's really very little sugar in this dessert, so there's nothing to worry about!

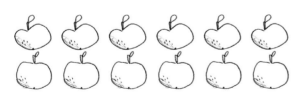

Pears in Red Wine

AD— This classic dessert will be even better if you make it the day before. After a night in the fridge, the pears will be even more impregnated with the flavors of the wine and spices. Why not serve it with a blackcurrant sorbet? PN— The pear is not so dazzling from a nutritional point of view. Apart from its plentiful fiber, it doesn't have a lot of vitamins and minerals. Red wine has the great merit of providing plenty of protective molecules that support the cardiovascular system. And ginger gives you energy!

… Serves 4

… Pour a bottle of good red wine into a saucepan, bring to a boil, and flambé.

… Wash 4 ripe Bartlett pears, then peel them, but leave the stems on. Cut them in half, remove the core, and squeeze the juice of 1 lemon over as soon as they are peeled. Put the peelings in the flambéed red wine.

… Pare the zest from 1 unwaxed orange, then remove the skin and outer membrane and cut into slices. Peel and thinly slice 1½ inches of ginger.

… Add ½ cup of superfine sugar to the flambéed red wine, add 1 vanilla bean slit open and scraped, the orange zest, the ginger, and a generous twist of freshly ground white pepper.

… Bring back to a boil, then lower the heat and immerse the half pears in this wonderfully fragrant wine.

… Cook gently, at a low simmer, for about 25 minutes. Take the saucepan off the heat and leave the fruit to rest in its cooking liquid.

… Then put them in a glass bowl. Strain the wine through a conical strainer and pour it over the pears.

… Keep the pears in the fridge until you are ready to serve them.

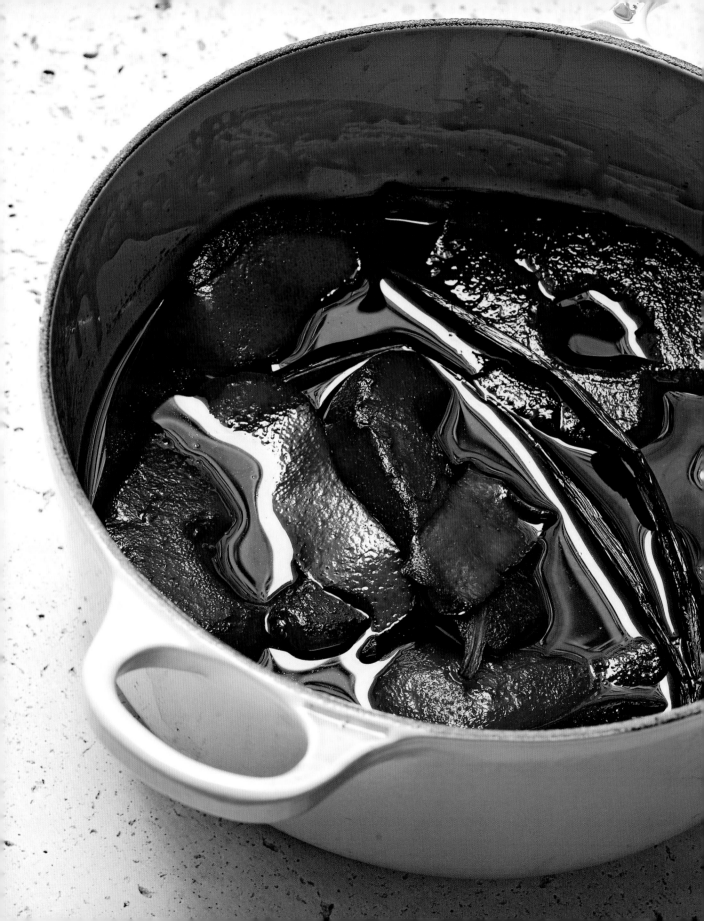

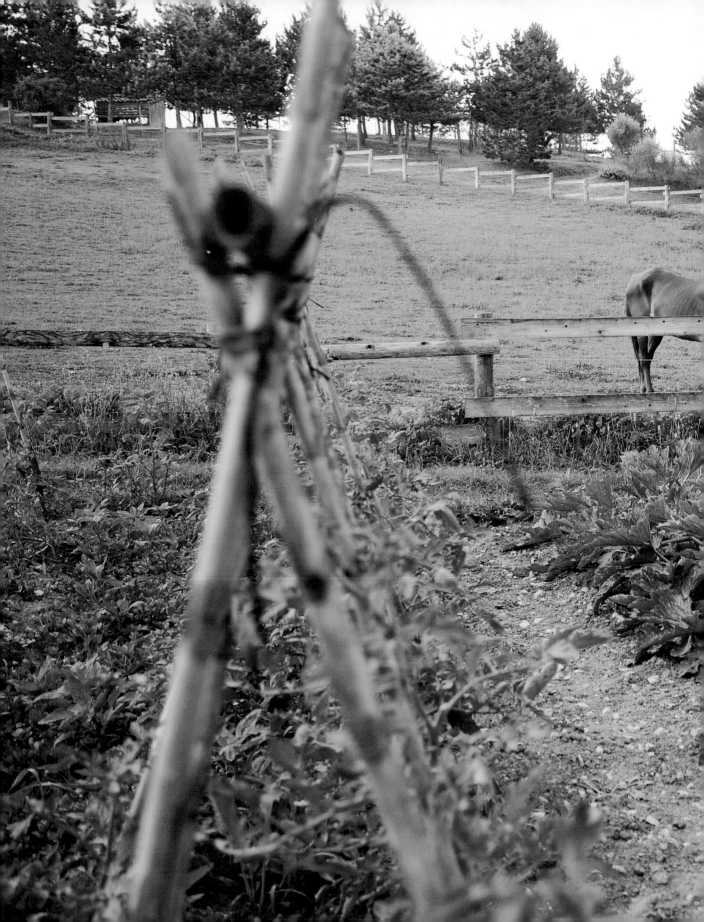

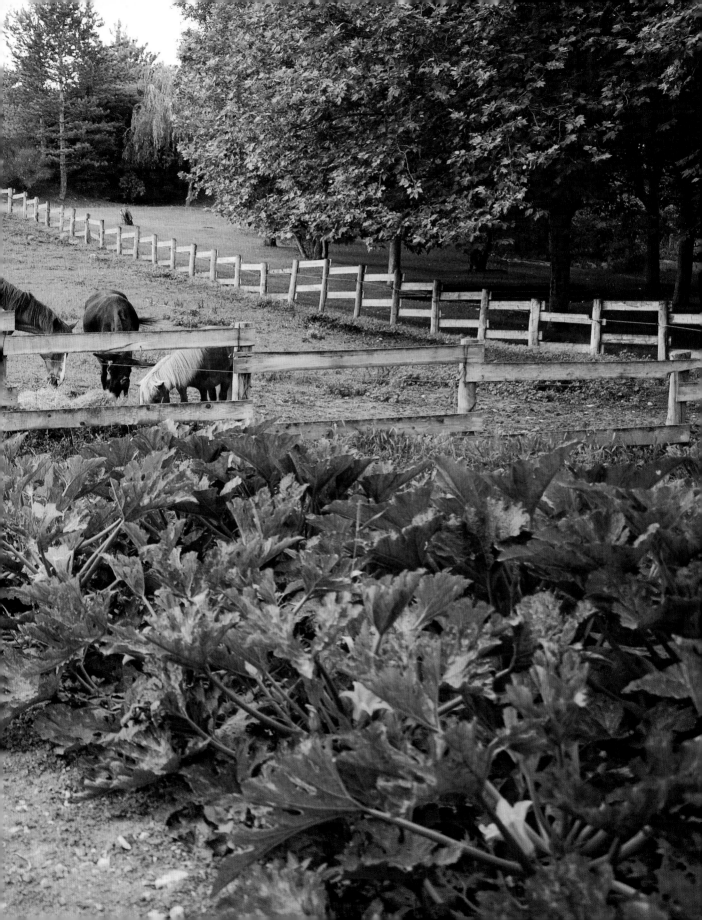

First published in the United States of America in 2011
by Rizzoli International Publications, Inc.
300 Park Avenue South
New York, NY 10010
www.rizzoliusa.com

Nature, simple, sain et bon © 2009 LEC Alain Ducasse Editions

Originally published in French in 2009
by LEC Alain Ducasse Editions
www.alain-ducasse.com

First published in English in 2011
by Hardie Grant Books
www.hardiegrant.co.uk

English translation by Gilla Evans

2012 2013 2014 / 10 9 8 7 6 5 4 3

Distributed in the U.S. trade by Random House, New York

Printed in China

ISBN-13: 978-0-8478-3840-0
Library of Congress Control Number: 2011935848

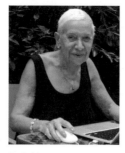
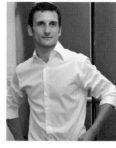

Paule Neyrat   Christophe Saintagne

CREDITS

PROPS

ASTIER DE VILLATTE
www.astierdevillatte.com

BERNADETTE ANDRIEU CRÉATIONS
www.atelier-ceramique.fr

GARGANTUA
www.gargantua.ch

CAROLINE GOMEZ, COLOR DESIGNER
www.carolinegomez.com

ISABELLE POUPINEL, CREATOR OF USEFUL ART
www.isabellepoupinel-atable.com

JARS CÉRAMISTES
www.jarsceramistes.com

LE CREUSET
www.lecreuset.fr

PILLIVUYT
www.pillivuyt.com

SENTOU GALERIE
www.sentou.fr

WASARA BY Shinichiro Ogata
www.virages.fr

FUNDS

AC MATIÈRE
www.acmatiere.fr

LES GRÈS DE COLOGNE
www.lesgresdecologne.com

MATIÈRES MARIUS AURENTI
www.mariusaurenti.com

DIRECTOR OF PUBLISHING
Emmanuel Jirou-Najou

EDITOR
Hortense Jablonski

ARTISTIC DIRECTION / CONCEPT
Pierre Tachon / Soins graphiques

ILLUSTRATIONS
Christine Roussey

PHOTOGRAPHERS
Françoise Nicol
Jean-Marie del Moral (page 335)

RECIPE STYLISTS
Virginie Michelin,
Gladys Palatin

EXECUTION AND MODEL
Anne Chaponnay & Key Graphic

COLOR CORRECTION
Isabelle Cappelli & Correctif

PRE-PRESS
MDP Group

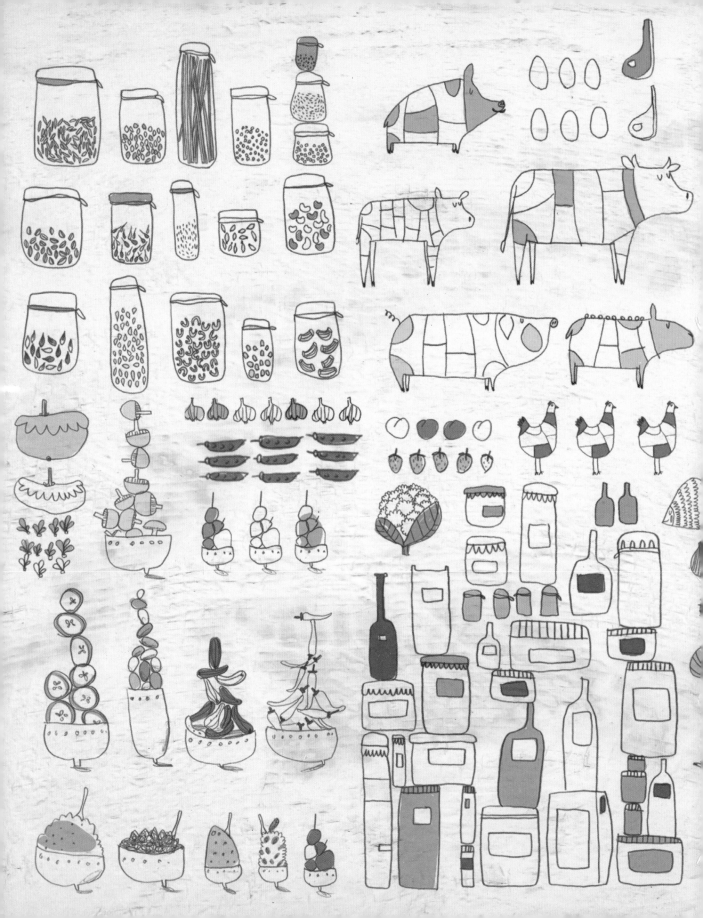